Neurology Self-Assessment

Neurology Self-Assessment: A Companion to Bradley's Neurology in Clinical Practice

JUSTIN T. JORDAN, MD
Assistant in Neurology, Massachusetts General Hospital;
Instructor in Neurology, Harvard Medical School,
Boston, MA

DAVID R. MAYANS, MD
Neurology Consultants of Kansas;
Clinical Assistant Professor, University of Kansas School of
Medicine, Wichita, KS

MICHAEL J. SOILEAU, MD
Director, Plummer Movement Disorder Center, Baylor Scott
& White Health, Temple, TX;
Clinical Assistant Professor and Assistant Program Director,
Neurology Residency, Texas A&M Health Science Center,
Temple, TX

Foreword by

JOHN C. MAZZIOTTA, MD, PHD
Vice Chancellor, UCLA Health Sciences;
Dean, David Geffen School of Medicine;
CEO, UCLA Health,
University of California, Los Angeles, CA

For additional online content visit ExpertConsult.com

ELSEVIER
Edinburgh London New York Oxford Philadelphia St Louis Sydney Toronto 2017

ELSEVIER

ISBN: 978-0-323-37709-6
eISBN: 978-0-323-39221-1

Senior Content Strategist: Lotta Kryhl
Senior Content Development Specialist: Ailsa Laing
Project Manager: Louisa Talbott
Designer: Miles Hitchen
Marketing Manager: Michele Milano

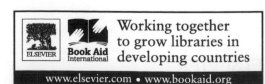

Contents

Contents

To my father, who inspired my career, and my family for their endless support.

JTJ

I want to thank Laura and Gabriella for their patience with me while writing this book. I would like to thank my mentors, particularly Nikhil Balakrishnan, for his encouragement through this process. Finally, I want to thank JJ for giving me the opportunity to be part of this exceptional book.

DRM

I wish to thank my wife Janiece and son Mason for supporting me throughout my career and for their love each day. I'd also like to thank the many mentors and colleagues along the way who have molded me into the physician I am today and for igniting excitement for the field of neurology.

MJS

Foreword

It is difficult to write self-assessment texts. They need to be comprehensive in scope and practical in usage. *Neurology Self-Assessment* by Drs. Jordan, Mayans, and Soileau accomplishes these goals admirably and is the perfect companion for *Bradley's Neurology in Clinical Practice*, Seventh Edition.

Physicians, in general, and neurologists, in particular, are always motivated to test their knowledge. A multiple-choice question is an opportunity to see how deep one's knowledge is. When I was preparing for my board examination in Psychiatry and Neurology, I obtained a recent edition of one of the most comprehensive texts in the field at that time. I went through the book, page-by-page, table-by-table, and figure-by-figure and made mental multiple-choice questions out of its content. This was a laborious but rewarding task. After that exercise, I felt I knew which areas required more study and where I should be confident with my state of knowledge. This self-assessment text provides all of that for the readers with no effort on their part. Its six 105-question examinations will test the readers' knowledge across a wide range of topics. Not only does the self-assessment include all aspects of clinical neurology but also basic science, ethics, and interpersonal skills. Such an offering is vital to high-quality patient care and professional requirements such as in-service examinations, board examinations, and maintenance of certification testing. The range of the questions' difficulty will be valuable for everyone interested in the field of neurology, from medical students to seasoned practitioners.

The ability to examine a question, consider the answers, make a selection, and then quickly refer to the answer is consistent with the long-known neuroscience principle that a stimulus and its response, when quickly rewarded, reinforces the information. This text provides exactly that stimulus-response exercise. That the answers are referenced to *Bradley's Neurology in Clinical Practice* further provides the user with the opportunity to read in more depth about a topic, particularly if that person has answered incorrectly.

The trio has done a masterful job in providing a comprehensive set of 630 questions that will challenge the readers and allow for a thorough self-assessment of their knowledge base. As one of the co-editors of *Bradley's Neurology in Clinical Practice*, I speak on behalf of the four of us in complimenting Drs. Jordan, Mayans, and Soileau on their very successful self-assessment text.

John C. Mazziotta, MD, PhD

for the editors of *Bradley's Neurology in Clinical Practice*

Robert B. Daroff, MD

Joseph Jankovic, MD

Scott L. Pomeroy, MD, PhD

Preface

The field of neurology is more exciting and rapidly advancing today than ever before, and as new light is shed on the etiology of disease, effective and revolutionary therapies follow close behind. This translates to improved quality of care for patients and improved satisfaction for neurologists.

As our drive for scientific progress continues, neurologists should make every effort to maintain a firm understanding of available data in order to provide the best care possible for patients. This necessity is not only apparent in daily practice, but also in professional requirements including in-service examinations, board examinations, and maintenance of certification. It was in this context that we three approached *Neurology Self-Assessment*.

Not only are the six 105-question examinations a tool for assessing one's strengths and weaknesses, but they also provide a valuable resource for exam studying, with in-depth explanations for both correct and incorrect answers, as well as further reading suggestions from *Bradley's Neurology in Clinical Practice*. Questions are written in a style similar to full examinations, with a strong representation of clinical vignettes and images. The depth of knowledge required to perform well on these examinations is likely more than sufficient to pass professional examinations, although should not be beyond the grasp of medical students.

On the whole, we believe that *Neurology Self-Assessment* will become a strong tool in the development and maintenance of neurologic expertise for practitioners at all levels.

Justin T. Jordan, MD

David R. Mayans, MD

Michael J. Soileau, MD

Test One

QUESTIONS

1. A 23-year-old female presents to the clinic for evaluation of a headache. She is currently 14 weeks pregnant. She complains of a holocephalic headache for the last week, which is worsening in intensity. The headache is worse at night and causes blurry vision. Her neurological examination is remarkable for bilateral papilledema. The sagittal T1 magnetic resonance image (MRI) is shown here. Which of the following is the most likely diagnosis?

   A. Pseudotumor cerebri
   B. Meningioma
   C. Venous sinus thrombosis
   D. Preeclampsia
   E. Optic neuritis

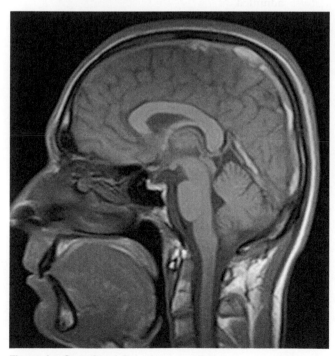

Figure for Question 1.1.

2. In reference to the patient in the previous question, which of the following would be the most appropriate treatment?

   A. Diamox
   B. Acetaminophen and rest
   C. Magnesium
   D. Warfarin
   E. Enoxaparin

3. Which of the following is *not* a means by which autoimmunity occurs?

   A. Genetic predisposition
   B. Failure of self-tolerance
   C. Molecular mimicry
   D. Major histocompatibility failure
   E. Environmental factors

4. Dopamine beta hydroxylase converts dopamine to which of the following?

   A. Epinephrine
   B. L-Dopa
   C. Tyrosine
   D. Serotonin
   E. Norepinephrine

5. Which of the following is *not* a standard component of a patient handoff between care providers?

   A. Identification
   B. Family history
   C. Diagnoses
   D. Treatment plan
   E. Code status

6. Convulsive seizures during pregnancy can have all of the following effects on the developing fetus *except*?

   A. Fetal bradycardia and asphyxia
   B. Fetal increased risk of epilepsy
   C. Increased risk of lower verbal IQ
   D. Blunt trauma to the fetus
   E. Large for gestational age

7. The following section is obtained at autopsy from a 60-year-old woman who died of sepsis. What is the cause of the lesion seen in the photomicrograph?

    A. Autopsy artifact

    B. Amyloid plaque

    C. Viral infection

    D. Contusion

    E. Infarct

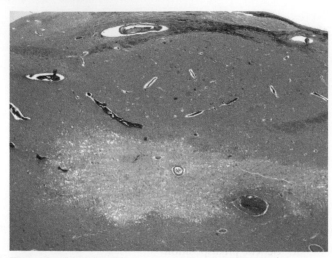

Figure for Question 1.7.

8. Which of the following suggests that a patient's vertigo is from a brainstem or cerebellar lesion, as opposed to a peripheral cause?

    A. Nystagmus worse with visual fixation

    B. Decreased hearing in one ear

    C. Ear pain

    D. Tinnitus in one ear

    E. Acute onset

9. A 55-year-old female presents to your office with a complaint of weakness which came on gradually over the last several months. She has difficulty raising her arms and walking up stairs. Her examination demonstrates significant proximal arm and leg weakness with forearm flexors spared. Creatine kinase is 2500. She has a rash around her eyes and on her knuckles. Electromyography demonstrates small motor units with ample fibrillations and positive sharp waves seen in proximal muscles and paraspinal muscles. What pattern of abnormalities would be expected on this patient's muscle biopsy?

    A. Endomysial inflammatory infiltrate with CD8 T-cells

    B. Endomysial inflammatory infiltrates with cytoplasmic inclusions and rimmed vacuoles

    C. Nests of angular atrophic muscle fibers with fiber type grouping

    D. Perimysial infiltrate with perifascicular atrophy

    E. Ragged red fibers that stain COX– and SDH+

10. A 26-year-old female patient is diagnosed with an astrocytoma. In childhood, she also suffered from osteosarcoma. Her family history is notable for several cancers in her maternal lineage, including both breast and brain tumors in her mother. Which of the following is the most likely underlying problem?

    A. Li-Fraumeni syndrome

    B. Neurofibromatosis 1

    C. Retinoblastoma

    D. Multiple endocrine neoplasia type 1

    E. Von Hippel-Lindau

11. Which of the following is an N-methyl-D-aspartate (NMDA) receptor antagonist?

    A. Rivastigmine

    B. Vigabatrin

    C. Memantine

    D. Donepezil

    E. Entacapone

12. A 64-year-old woman presents to the emergency room with confusion and difficulty walking. Her examination shows nystagmus, limited ocular movements on lateral gaze, and ataxia. Given her daughter's report of chronic alcoholism, intoxication is suspected. Labs return showing a blood alcohol content of zero and slight hyponatremia. What is the next best step?

    A. Give intravenous (IV) thiamine 500 mg tid × 3–5 days followed by maintenance thiamine thereafter.

    B. Continue metabolic workup as the patient is admitted.

    C. Rule out infectious causes of her altered mental status.

    D. Obtain an electroencephalogram.

    E. Obtain GQ1b antibody testing.

13. On average, what is the resting membrane potential of most neurons?

    A. +60 mV

    B. +60 μV

    C. 0 mV

    D. −60 mV

    E. −60 μV

14. A 63-year-old female presented to the emergency room with an acute aneurysmal subarachnoid hemorrhage (SAH) and underwent a clipping procedure on admission. She has since been recovering in the intensive care unit. On the tenth postoperative day, she was noted to have slurred speech, worsening right facial droop, and right arm weakness. She was more difficult to rouse. Noncontrast head computed tomography (CT) and four-vessel angiogram are shown. Which of the following is the best treatment for her condition?

    A. Intravenous (IV) tissue plasminogen activator (tPA)

    B. Intraarterial calcium channel blockers

    C. IV fosphenytoin load

    D. Placement of extraventricular drain

    E. IV mannitol

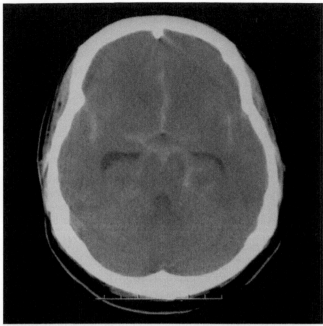

Motor nerve	Location	Latency (ms)	Amplitude (mV)	Velocity (m/s)
Radial	Elbow	2.0	14.0	
	Midarm	6.0	7.0	30

Sensory nerve	Location	Latency (ms)	Amplitude (mV)	Velocity (m/s)
Median (D2)	Wrist	3.0	40	55
Ulnar (D5)	Wrist	2.5	25	52
Radial	Forearm	Not recordable	Not recordable	Not recordable

Which of the following best explains the patient's symptoms?

A. Posterior cord brachial plexopathy

B. Posterior interosseus neuropathy

C. Ulnar neuropathy at the elbow

D. Radial neuropathy at the spiral groove

E. C7 nerve root avulsion

16. A 9-year-old left-handed boy presents to the clinic with his parents due to concerns over school performance. He previously hit all milestones and was an average student in school. Over this past school year, he had progressive difficulty with reading, but did not display behavioral problems at school or at home. His neurological examination and mental status examination are normal and show that he is able to write a simple paragraph in clinic. An electroencephalogram (EEG) is normal in the awake and sleep states. Which of the following is the most likely diagnosis?

A. Infarct of the splenium of the corpus callosum and left occipital lobe

B. Landau-Kleffner syndrome

C. Developmental dyslexia

D. Mild intellectual disability

E. Attention-deficit/hyperactivity disorder

17. A 17-year-old girl arrived to class immediately after cross-country running practice. While sitting at her desk, she felt sweaty, warm all over, and nauseated. She then slumped forward with fast, jerklike movements of her arms and legs. Her teacher rushed over to lower her to the floor, and she quickly began to rouse. She initially appeared confused but was able to answer questions appropriately. She had some urinary incontinence during the episode but no tongue trauma. She returned to her baseline mental status within a few minutes of the episode but was taken to the emergency room nonetheless. What is most likely the diagnosis?

A. Complex partial seizure

B. Convulsive syncope

C. Nonepileptic spell

D. Absence seizure

E. Generalized seizure

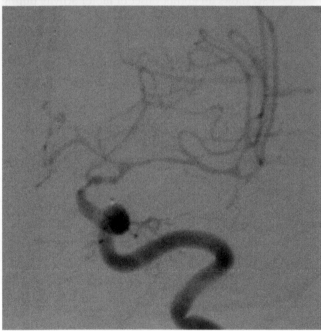

Figure for Question 1.14.

15. A 17-year-old male who suffered a broken humerus during a football game noticed a wrist drop in his right arm with preserved triceps strength ever since the cast was removed. The following nerve conduction study was performed.

TABLE FOR QUESTION 1.15

Motor nerve	Location	Latency (ms)	Amplitude (mV)	Velocity (m/s)
Median	Wrist	3.5	6.0	
	Forearm	7.0	5.8	55
Ulnar	Wrist	2.5	9.0	
	Below elbow	7.9	8.8	53
	Above elbow	9.5	8.6	52

18. Which sensory organ/receptor type is most closely linked with perception of temperature?
    A. Pacinian corpuscles
    B. Merkel disks
    C. Meissner corpuscles
    D. Free nerve endings
    E. Ruffini endings

19. A 63-year-old woman presents with left shoulder pain and gait difficulty for the last 1 year. Her husband states that she does not swing her left arm when she walks and has had difficulty using this hand to manipulate buttons. The patient also reports constipation and falling out of bed during vivid dreams for 6 years before the onset of gait difficulty. She denies history of tremor. What is the most likely diagnosis?
    A. Rotator cuff injury
    B. Cervical myelopathy
    C. Idiopathic Parkinson disease
    D. Vascular parkinsonism
    E. Peripheral neuropathy

20. Which examination finding is typical early in the disease for the correct diagnosis discussed in the previous question?
    A. Severe orthostatic hypotension
    B. Postural instability
    C. Suboptimal response to levodopa
    D. Hypophonia
    E. Symmetrical bradykinesia and rigidity

21. What is the most likely imaging finding seen with this diagnosis for the patient in Question 1.19?
    A. Normal magnetic resonance imaging (MRI) of the brain
    B. Increased uptake of dopamine on a dopamine transporter (DAT) scan
    C. Contrast enhancement of basal ganglia on MRI of the brain
    D. Bilateral T2 hyperintensities in the periventricular white matter
    E. Cervical cord compression from disc protrusion

22. What would be the treatment of choice for the patient in Question 1.19?
    A. High-volume lumbar puncture
    B. Surgical decompression
    C. Arthroscopic surgical repair of shoulder
    D. Aggressive medical treatment of vascular risk factors
    E. Trial of carbidopa/levodopa

23. Which of the following combinations is *not* correctly paired with the corresponding nucleus in the hypothalamus?
    A. Suprachiasmatic nucleus—appetite function
    B. Arcuate nucleus—dopaminergic neurons that inhibit prolactin
    C. Posterior nucleus—lesions produce hypothermia
    D. Anterior nucleus—lesions produce hyperthermia
    E. Paraventricular nucleus—secretes corticotropin-releasing hormone (CRH) and thyrotropin-releasing hormone (TRH)

24. An 83-year-old male with a history of Parkinson disease presents to clinic for a follow-up appointment. His wife has noticed that he is not sleeping well. At night he appears restless, yells, and seems to be running in his sleep. She has been kicked on several occasions, so she sleeps in the next room. Which of the following is true of this condition?
    A. First-line treatment is amitriptyline.
    B. Polysomnogram (PSG) shows rapid eye movement (REM) sleep without atonia.
    C. PSG shows an abrupt onset of motor activity during slow wave sleep.
    D. Genetic testing for mutations in *CHRNA2* would be positive.
    E. First-line treatment is ropinirole.

25. Which of the following is an example of declarative memory?
    A. Tying one's shoe
    B. Predicting the weather based on environmental clues
    C. Recalling a word when a related word is presented
    D. Recalling a birthday
    E. Expecting food when the oven timer ends

26. An 8-year-old boy presents with frequent staring episodes while in class. Based on the electroencephalogram (EEG) shown, which of the following is the most appropriate medication for this patient?
    A. Valproic acid
    B. Ethosuximide
    C. Phenytoin
    D. Levetiracetam
    E. Carbamazepine

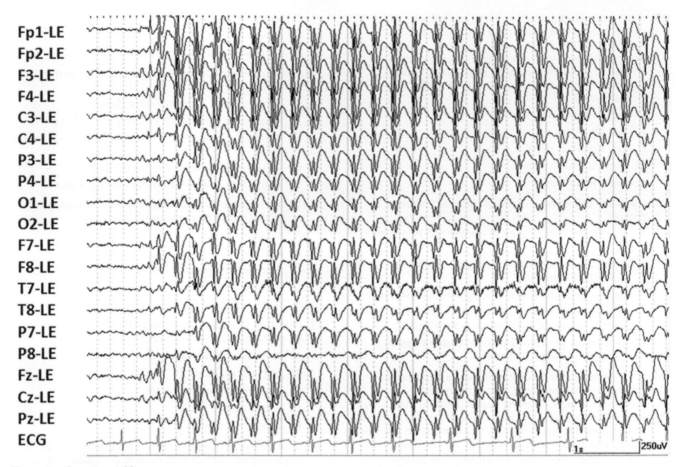

Fp1-LE
Fp2-LE
F3-LE
F4-LE
C3-LE
C4-LE
P3-LE
P4-LE
O1-LE
O2-LE
F7-LE
F8-LE
T7-LE
T8-LE
P7-LE
P8-LE
Fz-LE
Cz-LE
Pz-LE
ECG

1s   250uV

Figure for Question 1.26.

27. A 72-year-old female smoker was active and independent, taking hormone replacement as her only medication. She spent all weekend in her yard pulling weeds in the warm summer sun. The next day, she complained of headaches, but declined an appointment with her physician. Her headache worsened, and she became confused then sleepy over the next 2 days. She passed away at home alone and was later found by her daughter. An image of her brain taken at autopsy is shown. Which of the following would have been appropriate therapy had she sought emergency care?

    A. Triple H therapy

    B. Intravenous tissue plasminogen activator therapy

    C. Platelets and clotting factors

    D. Unfractionated heparin and intravenous fluids

    E. Normotension and observation

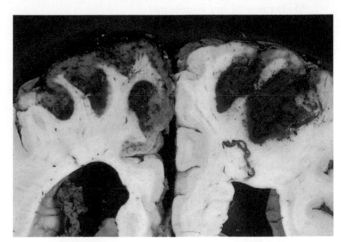

Figure for Question 1.27.

28. A 42-year-old man develops vertical diplopia, which seems worst when watching television from bed. On examination, he has left hypertropia, which is exacerbated with downward gaze of an adducted left eye. If he tilts his head to the right, the vision improves. Which of the following is the affected cranial nerve?

    A. Right oculomotor nerve

    B. Left abducens nerve

    C. Left trochlear nerve

    D. Right trochlear nerve

    E. Right abducens nerve

29. All of the following are true of informed consent except?

    A. Patient has the capacity to understand information presented.

    B. Physician must disclose risks and benefits of potential treatment.

    C. Patient decision is made freely without coercion.

    D. Detailed document outlining all potential complications of a procedure is provided.

    E. Treatments performed without consent can be considered assault or battery.

30. A 43-year-old female with a history of depression presents to the emergency department with unresponsiveness. Over the past 3 days, she had been increasingly somnolent, such that her family could no longer wake her up at home. On examination she was difficult to arouse with sternal rub. She moaned, but did not speak. She withdrew all limbs to painful stimulation. A computed tomography scan of her head without contrast is normal. A basic metabolic panel reveals a sodium level of 115 mmol/L (normal 135–145 mmol/L). Which of the following is the most likely cause of her symptoms?

    A. Nortriptyline

    B. Trazodone

    C. Citalopram

    D. Aripiprazole

    E. Phenelzine

31. A 68-year-old man with stage IV renal failure is receiving erythropoietin with a target hemoglobin of 14 g/dL. Which is the most directly increased risk as a result of this therapy?

    A. Peripheral neuropathy

    B. Ischemic stroke

    C. Seizures

    D. Dementia

    E. Headaches

32. An 8-year-old male is brought into the clinic by his mother because of problems with his behavior. He never follows his mother's rules and won't complete his chores, which causes significant family stress. He argues with his parents constantly (which is very different from his siblings), and has even stolen from a babysitter. He doesn't feel there is a problem, but merely thinks his parents' requests are unreasonable. The patient denies a poor mood or sleep difficulties. Which of the following is the most likely diagnosis?

    A. Oppositional defiant disorder (ODD)

    B. Antisocial personality disorder

    C. Major depressive disorder

    D. Autism

    E. Narcissistic personality disorder

33. Which of the following is an example of negative reinforcement?

    A. Paying money for completing chores

    B. Nagging a child for not cleaning his or her room

    C. Promising a trip to a theme park for making honor roll

    D. Taking away video games for cursing

    E. Yelling at a child for running into the street

34. Which of the following tumors is most commonly associated with opsoclonus-myoclonus?

    A. Neuroblastoma

    B. Medulloblastoma

    C. Juvenile pilocytic astrocytoma

    D. Ependymoma

    E. Wilms tumor

35. Olfactory sensation travels from the olfactory bulb to all of the following structures, except?

    A. Anterior olfactory nucleus

    B. Prepyriform cortex

    C. Posterior entorhinal cortex

    D. Amygdala

    E. Superior colliculus

36. A 63-year-old man presents to the neurology clinic for burning pain in both feet, causing discomfort while walking. He also feels as if something is stuck in his shoe at times. His examination is notable for normal vibration, pin prick, and temperature sensation, although he complains of tenderness to palpation of his feet. His deep tendon reflexes are normal. Which of the following is *not* true regarding the most likely diagnosis?

    A. The diagnosis is often made on skin biopsy.

    B. Nerve conduction studies are usually normal.

    C. Disorders of glucose dysregulation cause the majority of cases.

    D. This condition most often affects myelinated $A\delta$ and unmyelinated C-fibers.

    E. Examination usually shows impaired proprioception and light touch.

37. A 4-month-old baby is brought to the emergency room by his grandmother, who is visiting for the weekend. He has been inconsolable for many hours. His general medical examination reveals a crying child, but is otherwise unrevealing. His neurological examination reveals slightly decreased movements in the right arm and leg compared with the left. Further, his ophthalmological examination is abnormal, shown here. A computed tomography (CT) on the head is performed and also shown here. Which of the following is the next most appropriate action?

    A. Renal consult for malignant hypertension

    B. Neurosurgery consult for tumor resection

    C. Genetics consult for Tay-Sachs disease

    D. Hematology consult for coagulopathy

    E. Child protective services notification for abuse

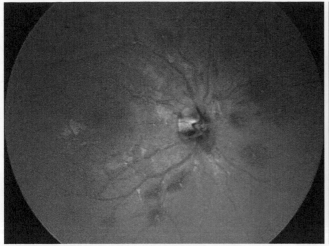 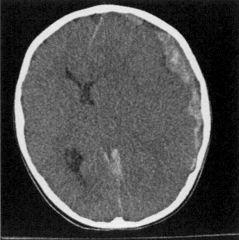

Figure for Question 1.37.

38. A 24-year-old woman with asthma has several years' history of recurrent headaches that are severe, pulsatile, and holocephalic in nature, with associated nausea. The headaches occur at least twice per week and tend to last about half a day, after which she feels "worthless" for the remainder of the day. She refused a trial of oral birth control pills due to religious beliefs. Based on the suspected headache diagnosis, which of the following would be appropriate first-line daily therapy?

    A. Sumatriptan

    B. Topiramate

    C. Amitriptyline

    D. Valproic acid

    E. Propranolol

39. Which of the following proteins is involved in the initial step in light absorption in the vision pathway?

    A. Rhodopsin

    B. Cyclic guanosine monophosphate

    C. Retinal

    D. Beta-carotene

    E. Volt-gated calcium channel

40. A 64-year-old woman with a history of poorly controlled diabetes, hypertension, and tobacco use is admitted 6 hours after acutely developing right hemiparesis, visual field deficit on the right, and expressive aphasia. Workup for stroke etiology reveals no evidence of atrial fibrillation, normal transthoracic echo, and a computed tomography angiogram that shows 80% stenosis of the left common carotid artery and 60% stenosis of the right common carotid artery. Which of the following is the next best step?

    A. Treat the patient medically with an antiplatelet agent

    B. Treat the patient medically with anticoagulation

    C. Perform a left carotid endarterectomy (CEA)

    D. Perform a right CEA

    E. Perform a right carotid artery stent (CAS)

41. Which of the following is *not* associated with trisomy 21?

    A. Abnormally low alpha fetoprotein (AFP) and abnormally high beta–human chorionic gonadotropin (HCG) levels in maternal blood screening during pregnancy

    B. Increased tone at birth

    C. Small white/brown spots on the outer iris

    D. Atrioventricular (AV) septal defect

    E. Increased risk of leukemia

42. Which of the following organizations accredits healthcare facilities, a process that is linked to payments from Medicaid and Medicare?

    A. American Medical Association (AMA)

    B. Centers for Medicare and Medicaid Services (CMS)

    C. Food and Drug Administration (FDA)

    D. American Hospital Association (AHA)

    E. Joint Commission on Accreditation of Health Care Organizations (JACHO)

43. A 55-year-old man presents with a 3-month history of progressive right hemiparesis. A contrast-enhanced magnetic resonance image of the brain was obtained in the emergency room and is shown here. What is the most likely diagnosis for the lesion shown?

    A. Meningioma

    B. Glioblastoma

    C. Central nervous system (CNS) lymphoma

    D. Ependymoma

    E. Metastasis

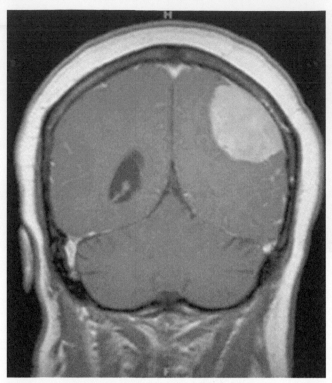

Figure for Question 1.43.

his neck the day before. In completing a full neurological examination, the emergency room physician additionally notes the abnormality shown here. Which of the following is the most likely test to demonstrate the etiology of the patient's symptoms?

A. Magnetic resonance imaging (MRI) of the brain

B. Chest x-ray

C. Electroencephalogram

D. Edrophonium test

E. Magnetic resonance angiogram of the neck

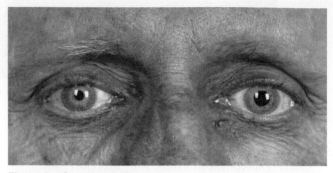

Figure for Question 1.47.

44. Which of the following is the mainstay of therapy for meningioma?

A. Stereotactic radiotherapy

B. Whole-brain radiotherapy

C. Chemotherapy

D. Observation

E. Resection

45. During resection of a right vestibular schwannoma, brainstem auditory evoked potentials (BAEPs) were monitored. Near the end of the surgery, there was loss of wave III and wave V, but wave I remained on the right side. These waves did not recover by the end of the surgery. BAEP on the left remained normal. What is the clinical significance of this change?

A. Significant right-sided hearing loss

B. Transient right-sided hearing loss

C. Right pontine infarct

D. Displacement of acoustic stimulator

E. No significant neurological injury

46. Which of the following is different between the prion protein PrP^c associated with sporadic Creutzfeldt-Jakob disease and the normal prion protein PrP^{Sc}?

A. Amino acid sequence

B. Three-dimensional structure

C. N-terminal charge

D. Splice variants

E. No difference

47. A 45-year-old man presents to the emergency room with 1 day of headache and several hours of left arm heaviness. He notes that he fell off a ladder and hurt

48. A 26-year-old man is brought to your office by his spouse who complains that her husband's behavior has changed in the last 8 months. They will frequently argue, as he insists that she is cheating on him with one of his friends. She feels he is often not logical as he moves from one topic to the next, and she often finds him responding to "the voices." Lately, his personal hygiene has declined, leaving him unable to work. She worries that he is becoming depressed like his father. Assuming no drug or substance use, which is most likely the diagnosis?

A. Brief psychotic disorder

B. Schizophrenia

C. Bipolar disorder

D. Schizophreniform disorder

E. Delusional disorder

49. Which of the following is the most common cause of early-onset autosomal-dominant Alzheimer disease?

A. Amyloid precursor protein

B. Presenilin 1

C. Presenilin 2

D. ApoE4

E. SEPT9

50. A patient presents to the emergency department with acute horizontal binocular diplopia and left hemiparesis. Examination reveals mild ptosis and mydriasis on the right, as well as weakness of the medial rectus, superior rectus, inferior rectus, and inferior oblique muscles on the right. Which of the following is the most likely location of this stroke?

A. Midbrain tegmentum

B. Lateral medulla

C. Cerebral peduncle

D. Angular gyrus

E. Medial medulla

51. Neurology is consulted for an infant in the nursery with abnormal movements. Continuous electroencephalograph (EEG) monitoring shows frequent seizures associated with a decreased level of alertness. A general medical workup includes a lumbar puncture that shows no white or red blood cells, normal protein, and a glucose level of 22 mg/dL (serum glucose 102 mg/dL). Central nervous system imaging is normal. Which of the following is not true regarding this condition?

    A. The *SLC2A1* gene is defective.

    B. Paroxysmal exertional dyskinesia can occur with this condition.

    C. A ketogenic diet is an absolute contraindication.

    D. The most common inheritance is autosomal dominant.

    E. Microcephaly is often present.

52. A 23-year-old woman enjoys playing golf on the weekends with her friends. However, for the last month she has not wanted to go, creating various excuses. She is frequently tearful, and her boyfriend often finds her crying in bed wishing she were dead. Also in the last month, her appetite has decreased, and she feels as if she has no energy. Her boyfriend states that she had a similar episode about 6 months ago. Which of the following diagnoses best applies in this case?

    A. Major depressive disorder

    B. Major depressive episode

    C. Dysthymic disorder

    D. Bipolar 2 disorder

    E. Seasonal affective disorder

53. Which of the following is the approximate rate of cerebrospinal fluid (CSF) production in an adult?

    A. 20 mL/hr

    B. 50 mL/hr

    C. 2 mL/hr

    D. 0.5 mL/hr

    E. 100 mL/hr

54. All of the following are causes of mental retardation in the pediatric population except?

    A. Toxoplasmosis

    B. Alcohol exposure in utero

    C. Radiation exposure in utero

    D. Maternal rhinovirus infection

    E. Maternal malnutrition

55. Which portion of the circuit of Papez is injured in Korsakoff syndrome?

    A. Hippocampus

    B. Anterior thalamic nucleus

    C. Entorhinal cortex

    D. Fornix

    E. Mammillary bodies

56. Which of the following is true of mood-stabilizing agents?

    A. Lithium can cause hyponatremia.

    B. Valproic acid is not commonly used as a mood stabilizer.

    C. They are used to treat major depressive disorder.

    D. Lithium is contraindicated in patients with sick sinus syndrome.

    E. They are not used in treating schizoaffective disorder.

57. The posterior cord gives rise to which of the following nerves?

    A. Medial pectoral nerve

    B. Thoracodorsal nerve

    C. Long thoracic nerve

    D. Musculocutaneous nerve

    E. Suprascapular nerve

58. A 6-month-old was brought to the emergency room with eye movement abnormalities and head bobbing, which were thought to represent seizure. On examination, the patient appears to be comfortable and in no apparent distress. He has nystagmus, which is primarily horizontal, and head nodding. Additionally, his neck intermittently turns to the left. Brain imaging is normal, as is the remainder of the patient's neurological examination. Which of the following is the most likely diagnosis?

    A. Congenital nystagmus

    B. Seizure

    C. Chiari malformation

    D. Spasmus nutans

    E. Benign paroxysmal torticollis of infancy

59. Which of the following medications slows the metabolism of dopamine in the central nervous system?

    A. Rivastigmine

    B. Trihexyphenidyl

    C. Carbidopa

    D. Entacapone

    E. Amantadine

60. A 36-year-old male with a history of gastric bypass surgery developed numbness in his legs over the last 2 months. Three weeks ago he started having falls. He presented to the emergency department because he could no longer void on his own. His neurological examination shows prominent loss of sensation to vibration and proprioception in his lower extremities along with mild weakness in his legs. He seems to have maintained strength and sensation in his arms. He has brisk reflexes at the knees, but his reflexes at his ankles are absent. Which of the following is the most likely diagnosis?

    A. Vitamin E deficiency

    B. Vitamin D deficiency

    C. Vitamin B6 toxicity

    D. Vitamin A toxicity

    E. Vitamin B12 deficiency

61. At what age does the Moro reflex disappear in normal children?

    A. 2 months

    B. 4 months

    C. 6 months

    D. 9 months

    E. 12 months

62. A colleague presents to the office with her husband for an evaluation. He is a 56-year-old male cardiologist with no significant medical history whose wife is concerned about recent changes in his behavior, including gambling and inappropriate sexual comments at work. His wife has also noticed that he mixes up the names of medications, but he insists there is nothing wrong. His neurological examination is unremarkable, and he scores 28/30 on the mini mental state examination. He was able to name seven animals in 1 minute. Laboratory work is normal, including a complete blood count, metabolic panel, liver enzymes, urine drug screen, vitamin B12, thyroid-stimulating hormone, and rapid plasma reagin. Magnetic resonance imaging (MRI) of his brain is also unremarkable. Which of the following is true of this condition?

    A. Fluorodeoxyglucose–positron emission tomography (FDG-PET) scan shows hypometabolism of the posterior temporoparietal region.

    B. This is caused by buildup of amyloid protein.

    C. Lithium is commonly used for behavioral control.

    D. Obsessions and hoarding are common behaviors.

    E. Histopathological hallmarks include neurofibrillary tangles.

63. A 45-year-old man has recently moved from Mexico. He suffers a focal seizure followed by secondary generalization. He denies symptoms of active infection and has not suffered any recent trauma. His neurological examination has returned to normal in the emergency room. A magnetic resonance image (MRI) of the brain is shown. Which of the following is the next best step in management?

    A. Levetiracetam and albendazole

    B. Levetiracetam and acyclovir

    C. Lacosamide and a biopsy of the largest lesion

    D. Lacosamide, vancomycin, and cefepime

    E. Fosphenytoin and methylprednisolone

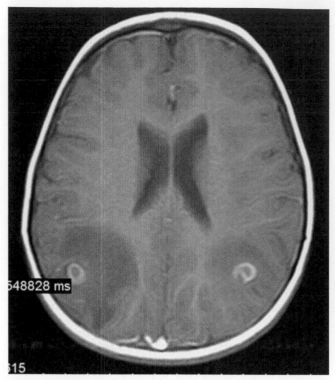

Figure for Question 1.63.

64. Which of the following is an example of availability bias?

    A. Recent missed diagnosis of amyotrophic lateral sclerosis (ALS) leads to ALS diagnosis in a second patient

    B. Assuming a patient has ALS and not changing diagnoses despite contrary information

    C. Finding fasciculations on electromyogram confirming suspicion of ALS

    D. Concluding a diagnosis of ALS without any testing

    E. Treating a patient with a prior diagnosis of ALS without confirming the diagnosis

65. Which of the following is a direct thrombin inhibitor?

    A. Rivaroxaban

    B. Apixaban

    C. Dabigatran

    D. Cilostazol

    E. Ticlopidine

66. A 57-year-old alcoholic was found unresponsive behind a gas station. A head computed tomography was negative for hemorrhage. Complete blood count and basic metabolic profile were normal. His examination demonstrates a somnolent male who wakes up briefly to painful stimulation, grunts, and moves all of his extremities equally. He is afebrile, and no nuchal rigidity is noted. The electroencephalogram (EEG) is shown here. Which of the following is the most likely diagnosis?

    A. Herpes encephalitis

    B. Nonconvulsive status epilepticus

    C. Hepatic encephalopathy

    D. Ischemic stroke

    E. Meningitis

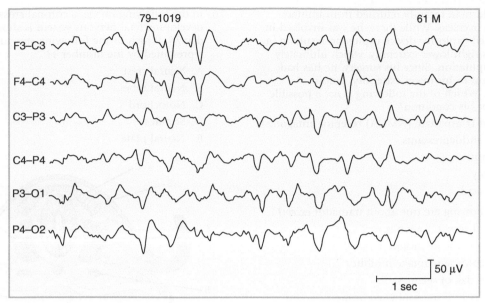

Figure for Question 1.66.

67. A 26-year-old man with a history of Tourette syndrome presents for new symptoms that are causing great distress with maintaining a job. He is often late for work because he feels the need to check the lock on his front door five times each morning. If he forgets or is distracted, he feels the need to start over and recheck the door five times. Another example he provides includes stepping up on curbs three times and tapping the wall four times before walking through a doorway. What is the most likely diagnosis?

    A. Manifestations of his Tourette syndrome

    B. Panic disorder with agoraphobia

    C. Obsessive-compulsive disorder (OCD)

    D. Obsessive-compulsive personality disorder (OCPD)

    E. Paranoid personality disorder

68. A 32-year-old female who is 27 weeks pregnant presents to your office for evaluation of abnormal movements. She cannot sit still and is always fidgeting. Her husband says her arms always move but this stops when she goes to sleep. She has no urge to move and does not get a sense of relief with movements. There is no family history of movement disorders, and she is not taking any medications. Her neurological examination is normal except for abnormal movements of her arms that seem to flow from body part to body part. They do not interrupt her ability to reach for objects or keep her from walking. Laboratory work, including a complete blood count, metabolic panel, liver function tests, thyroid-stimulating hormone, and ceruloplasmin, were normal. Which of the following is true of this condition?

    A. There is a high risk of recurrence with future pregnancies.

    B. Her child has a 50% chance of inheriting this disorder.

    C. Treatment with haloperidol is necessary.

    D. Slit lamp examination would demonstrate Kayser-Fleischer rings.

    E. Treatment with clonidine is helpful.

69. Which part of the autonomic nervous system and which neurotransmitter are responsible for activation of sweat glands?

    A. Postganglionic sympathetic fibers and norepinephrine

    B. Postganglionic sympathetic fibers and acetylcholine

    C. Postganglionic parasympathetic fibers and norepinephrine

    D. Preganglionic parasympathetic fibers and acetylcholine

    E. Preganglionic sympathetic fibers and epinephrine

70. After a prolonged course of steroids for reactive airway disease, a 30-year-old woman develops fatigue, generalized muscle weakness, and weight loss. Which of the following is the most likely source of her symptoms?

    A. Low serum cortisol

    B. High serum cortisol

    C. Low serum T4

    D. High serum T4

    E. Low serum glucose

71. The Wisconsin Card Sorting Test is helpful in determining functional abnormalities in which domain of cognitive function?

    A. Language

    B. Visuospatial function

    C. Declarative memory

    D. Executive function

    E. Intelligence

72. A 43-year-old man recently returned from military deployment overseas. While there, he was involved in an improvised explosive device explosion resulting in injury to his right lower extremity, which ultimately required amputation. Since his surgery, he has had increased pain in his lower extremity, despite amputation. Which of the following is *not* a possible treatment for his condition?

    A. N-methyl-D-aspartate (NMDA) receptor antagonists
    B. Tricyclic antidepressants
    C. Gabapentin
    D. Rhizotomy
    E. Valproic acid

73. All of the following are true about tramadol *except*?

    A. Mu-opioid receptor agonist
    B. Serotonin reuptake inhibitor
    C. Norepinephrine reuptake inhibitor
    D. Decreases risk of seizures
    E. Increases risk of serotonin syndrome

74. A 62-year-old female with a history of poorly controlled diabetes presents with left leg weakness. This initially began with severe left hip pain. Over the course of several weeks, she had weakness in her left leg and loss of muscle mass in the left thigh. She has minimal numbness, but has noted significant weight loss. Her examination demonstrates weakness of left hip flexion, knee flexion, and knee extension, but normal foot plantar flexion and dorsiflexion. Left patellar and ankle reflexes were absent. There was no incontinence. Magnetic resonance imaging of her lumbar spine and lumbosacral plexus were normal. Laboratory work, including complete blood count, complete metabolic panel, sedimentation rate, and C-reactive protein (CRP) were normal. Which of the following is true of this condition?

    A. Standard treatment involves 1 gram of intravenous methylprednisolone over 5 days.
    B. Standard treatment involves physical therapy.
    C. Sural nerve biopsy is necessary for the diagnosis.
    D. Genetic testing for *SEPT9* gene should be performed.
    E. Long-term immunosuppression is needed to prevent recurrence.

75. After an 18-hour delivery, a 26-year-old woman with a history of relapsing remitting multiple sclerosis gives birth to her first child. After her epidural wears off, the patient goes for a walk in the hall and notices that both feet slap the floor more loudly than before. There is tingling on the lateral aspect of both lower legs, but otherwise intact strength and sensation throughout. Which is the most likely mechanism of her problem?

    A. Side effect of oxytocin
    B. Lumbosacral plexopathy resulting from pelvic trauma
    C. Uhthoff phenomenon after strenuous labor
    D. Side effect of epidural anesthesia
    E. Compressive neuropathy of bilateral common peroneal (fibular) nerves

76. In the following image, a coronal cross-section of a developing fetal nervous system is shown at around day 25. Which of the following structures is represented by the number 1?

    A. Neural crest
    B. Neural tube
    C. Notochord
    D. Somites
    E. Neural plate

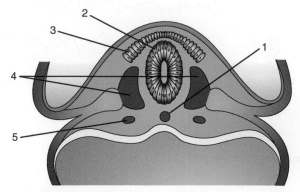

Figure for Question 1.76.

77. An 8-year-old boy has a history of developmental delay with an intelligence quotient (IQ) of 45. His pediatrician also notes that he has an elongated face with protuberant ears and enlarged testicles. His family has a long history of mental retardation. Which of the following is true regarding his condition?

    A. He has mild mental retardation.
    B. He has moderate mental retardation.
    C. He has severe mental retardation.
    D. He has the least common inherited cause of mental retardation.
    E. Women do not manifest symptoms of this condition.

78. A 25-year-old woman presents with a history of left arm automatisms and lip smacking, followed by a generalized convulsion. Her history is also remarkable for recurring headaches previously attributed as migraines. An axial magnetic resonance image (MRI) is shown. Which of the following is considered the most likely diagnosis?

    A. Developmental venous anomaly
    B. Cavernous malformation
    C. Cerebral aneurysm
    D. Arteriovenous malformation
    E. Capillary telangiectasia

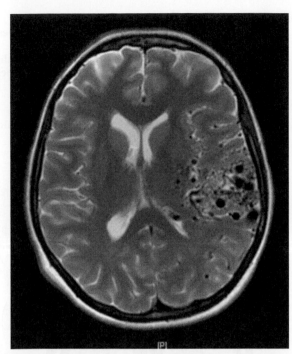

Figure for Question 1.78.

79. According to the Carotid Revascularization Endarterectomy vs. Stenting Trial (CREST), which is associated with a periprocedural increased risk of stroke?
    A. Carotid endarterectomy
    B. Carotid stenting
    C. Clopidogrel load
    D. Catheter angiography
    E. Cardiac stenting

80. A 33-year-old woman presents with an inability to sit still and difficulty sleeping, which have developed gradually over 3 years. On examination, there are subtle choreiform movements involving both the trunk and the distal upper extremities. She also has delayed initiation of saccades, as well as tongue impersistence. She is adopted, but knows that her mother committed suicide after years of abusing drugs. Her magnetic resonance image (MRI) is shown. What is the most likely diagnosis?
    A. Stroke
    B. Sydenham chorea
    C. Anti–N-methyl-D-aspartate (anti-NMDA) encephalitis
    D. Huntington disease
    E. Cocaine intoxication

81. Which of the following hormones is released from the posterior pituitary (neurohypophysis)?
    A. Oxytocin
    B. Follicle-stimulating hormone (FSH)
    C. Adrenocorticotropic hormone (ACTH)
    D. Thyroid-stimulating hormone (TSH)
    E. Prolactin

82. Which of the following results from excess endolymphatic fluid?
    A. Meniere disease
    B. Benign paroxysmal positional vertigo
    C. Mal de debarquement syndrome
    D. Opsoclonus-myoclonus
    E. Labyrinthitis

83. A 42-year-old male presents with memory loss over the last several months. He notes antecedent arthralgia, low-grade fevers, skin hyperpigmentation, and frequent diarrhea. On examination he has mild rigidity in his upper extremities, and concurrent slow pendular movements of the eyes and contraction of the masseter. Which of the following is the most likely diagnosis?
    A. Wilson disease
    B. Neurosyphilis
    C. Whipple disease
    D. Early-onset Alzheimer disease
    E. Human immunodeficiency virus dementia

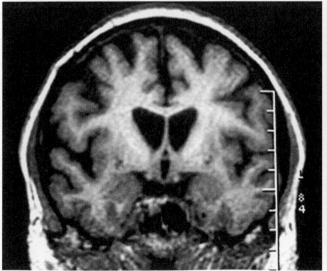
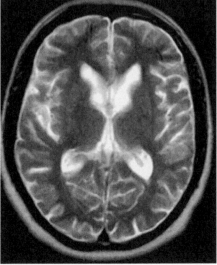

Figure for Question 1.80.

84. A 17-year-old male presents to your office for evaluation of excessive sleepiness. He falls asleep frequently in class and even fell asleep while giving a speech in class. His mother notes that when he is angry, he will drop objects or become "weak in the knees." He will frequently wake in the morning but be unable to move or speak for 3 minutes before he can get out of bed. Which of the following would be seen in this condition?

    A. Apnea-Hypopnea Index (AHI) of 15

    B. Electroencephalogram (EEG) with continuous slow wave and spikes during sleep

    C. Sleep latency of 20 minutes

    D. Frequently associated with hyperphagia and hypersexuality

    E. Low cerebrospinal fluid hypocretin level

85. A 16-year-old male suffers sharp, stabbing pain across his entire head each time he coughs. The pain is severe, but resolves quickly after coughing. Which of the following should be done?

    A. Daily antihistamine

    B. Amitriptyline

    C. Pulmonary function tests

    D. Cranial magnetic resonance imaging (MRI)

    E. Nothing; the pain is too brief for therapy

86. Which of the following layers of the retina does light first encounter after passing through the lens?

    A. Retinal ganglion cell layer

    B. Optic nerve layer

    C. Inner plexiform layer

    D. Photoreceptor layer

    E. Retinal pigment epithelium

87. A 50-year-old man experiences frequent recurrent pain on the left side of his throat, near his tonsils. He says that this feels like a hot poker. Assuming a radiographic evaluation is unrevealing, which of the following is the appropriate first-line therapy?

    A. Carbamazepine

    B. Amitriptyline

    C. Levetiracetam

    D. Phenytoin

    E. Oxycodone

88. In posterior tibial somatosensory evoked potentials (SSEPs), the P37 peak corresponds with which anatomical location?

    A. Lumbar plexus

    B. Lumbar roots

    C. Cerebral cortex

    D. Dorsal columns

    E. Medial lemniscus

89. Which day during embryogenesis does the distal neural tube pore close?

    A. Day 7

    B. Day 13

    C. Day 27

    D. Day 40

    E. Day 60

90. A 6-year-old girl presents with involuntary jerking movements of her right arm. She had several episodes of this that would last for hours before stopping spontaneously. In the last 2 weeks, the patient's mother has noted that she seems unaware during parts of these episodes and may have had shaking in her right leg and right side of her face. Her speech has been regressing. Electroencephalogram reveals left hemispheric spikes. A magnetic resonance image (MRI) of her brain is shown. Which of the following is the best treatment for this condition?

    A. Carbamazepine

    B. Hemispherectomy

    C. Vagal nerve stimulator

    D. Valproic acid

    E. Intravenous (IV) immunoglobulin

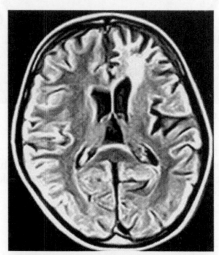

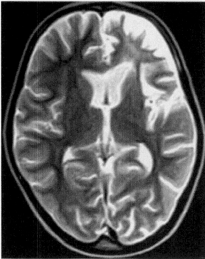

Figure for Question 1.90.

91. Spelling "world" backward in a mental status examination most closely tests which of the following?

    A. Attention

    B. Concentration

    C. Abstraction

    D. Executive function

    E. Memory

92. Select the most common bacterial cause of meningitis for neonates (<1 year old).
    A. Group B streptococci
    B. *Listeria monocytogenes*
    C. *Neisseria meningitidis*
    D. *Pseudomonas aeruginosa*
    E. *Staphylococcus aureus*

93. Which of the following is *not* structurally responsible for movement of cargo along the axon?
    A. Kinesin
    B. Neurolemma
    C. Dynein
    D. Neurofilaments
    E. Microtubules

94. Which of the following is *not* true regarding the clinical syndrome depicted?
    A. Diagnosis is made radiographically when one or both cerebellar tonsils are below the foramen magnum by ≥5 mm.
    B. Treatment involves surgical decompression if findings are present on magnetic resonance imaging (MRI), regardless of symptoms.
    C. Syringomyelia is a common association with type 1 malformation.
    D. Type I malformations do not have neural tube defects such as a myelomeningocele.
    E. Syringomyelia is the most common presentation of type II malformations.

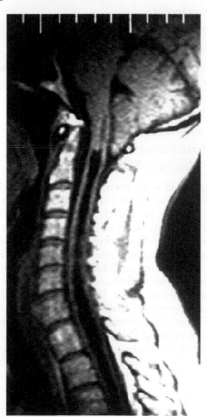

Figure for Question 1.94.

95. For an action to be considered ethical in accordance with the principle of nonmaleficence, all of the following must be present except?
    A. The nature of the act/intervention must not be intrinsically wrong.
    B. The intention is for good effect even if side effects are probable.
    C. The bad effects are not a means to the good effects.
    D. The action must be approved by the ethics committee.
    E. The good effects must outweigh the bad effects.

96. After a bat bite, a rural farmer suffers from flu-like symptoms. Over the following days he develops diffuse weakness and confusion and is dead within 1 month. The following image was taken from autopsy. What is the name of the pathognomonic findings indicated by the arrows?
    A. Negri bodies
    B. Cowdry type A
    C. Cowdry type B
    D. Howell-Jolly bodies
    E. Rosenthal fiber

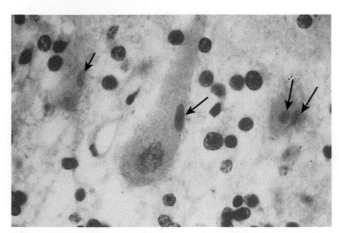

Figure for Question 1.96.

97. A 6-year-old boy is brought to the emergency department by his parents for 3 weeks of headache, 2 weeks of increasing ataxia, and 2 days of headache and vomiting. A magnetic resonance image is obtained, and postcontrast T1 sagittal imaging is shown. Based on the most likely diagnosis, which of the following is the best first treatment?
    A. Intravenous antibiotics
    B. Surgical resection
    C. Embolization
    D. Intravenous chemotherapy
    E. Craniospinal radiation

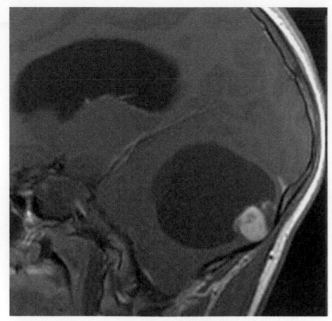

Figure for Question 1.97.

98. A 42-year-old diabetic woman develops maxillary pain and rhinorrhea. Four days later, she notes epistaxis, diplopia, and retroorbital pain. On presentation to the emergency room, she is noted to have a dark mass in each nostril. Further, she has bilateral ptosis, numbness in V1 and V2 distributions, and bilateral ophthalmoplegia. There is no proptosis. Which of the following is the most likely etiology for her symptoms?

A. Tolosa-Hunt syndrome

B. Idiopathic intracranial hypertension

C. Pituitary adenoma

D. Mucormycosis infection

E. Carotid-cavernous fistula

99. All of the following are true about cocaine use *except*?

A. It can lead to development of chorea.

B. Headache is the most common side effect on presentation at emergency room.

C. Paranoia, hallucinations, and agitation are common side effects.

D. It blocks synaptic reuptake of dopamine.

E. It causes pupillary constriction.

100. Which of the following is Food and Drug Administration (FDA) approved for secondary progressive multiple sclerosis?

A. Teriflunomide

B. Fingolimod

C. Dimethyl fumarate

D. Glatiramer acetate

E. Mitoxantrone

101. Which of the following is least likely to improve multiple sclerosis–related fatigue?

A. Pemoline

B. Modafinil

C. Memantine

D. Amantadine

E. Dalfampridine

102. A 53-year-old female presents to your outpatient clinic with 3 months of pain in the left arm. She describes a burning and tingling pain in the lateral aspect of her forearm and her left thumb. Examination reveals normal strength and normal cranial nerves. She has reduced sensation over the lateral aspect of her forearm and her entire left thumb, but no sensory loss in other parts of the hand. Her biceps and brachioradialis reflexes are reduced. Which of the following muscles would most likely show electromyography (EMG) abnormalities?

A. First dorsal interosseous and abductor pollicis brevis

B. Flexor pollicis longus and flexor carpi ulnaris

C. Brachioradialis and pronator teres

D. Triceps and extensor indicis proprius

E. Biceps and adductor pollicis

103. A 33-year-old male recently started a migraine preventive medication. Two weeks later he presents to the emergency department with severe abdominal pain, nausea, and vomiting. His complete blood count has normal white blood cells and hemoglobin, and a mildly low level of platelets. A complete metabolic panel is normal, including liver enzymes. Amylase and lipase are both elevated. Which of the following is the most likely cause of his condition?

A. Valproic acid

B. Topiramate

C. Propranolol

D. Amitriptyline

E. Verapamil

104. The gamma aminobutyric acid B (GABA$_B$) receptor is which of the following?

A. A voltage-gated sodium channel

B. A ligand-gated chloride channel

C. A metabotropic receptor

D. A ligand-gated sodium channel

E. A voltage-gated potassium channel

105. A 63-year-old male presents to the clinic with memory problems. Over the last several months he developed problems with his speech. He frequently calls objects by the wrong name or cannot come up with the words he wants to say. His neurological examination is normal, and magnetic resonance imaging (MRI) of his brain shows temporal lobe atrophy. On mental status examination he is alert and oriented. His speech is clear and he can repeat, but he has difficulty with naming objects. He frequently replaces words with either nonsensical words or the wrong words. He is able to remember three words at 3 minutes, draw intersecting pentagons, and draw a clock accurately. In 1 minute he was only able to name four animals. Which of the following is the most likely diagnosis?

A. Alzheimer disease

B. Dementia with Lewy bodies

C. Primary progressive aphasia

D. Mild cognitive impairment

E. Vascular dementia

ANSWERS

1. **C.** This patient presents with worsening headaches and features of increased intracranial pressure with worsening headaches at night and papilledema. In pregnant patients, there should be immediate concern for venous sinus thrombosis (VST). Pregnancy-induced pseudotumor is possible, but VST must be ruled out first. Pregnant patients are at higher risk of VST because pregnancy creates a hypercoagulable state often worsened by dehydration. MRI and magnetic resonance venography are the first-line tests for determining whether there is a VST because both can be done without contrast. The provided image is a noncontrast T1-weighted image. This demonstrates a hyperintense T1 signal in the sagittal sinus and the great vein of Galen, which is consistent with an acute VST. Papilledema could be seen additionally in preeclampsia and optic neuritis. The image provided does not show signs of optic neuritis because the optic nerves are not in the imaging plane. Optic neuritis would show hyperintense optic nerves on T2 imaging along with contrast enhancement. Preeclampsia has no radiographic findings. Meningiomas are not hyperintense on T1 imaging without contrast. However, they do homogeneously enhance with contrast (*see* Bradley's NiCP, Ch. 112, pp. 1973–1991). Figure from Yildiz OK, Cevik S, Cil G, Oztoprak I, Bolayir E, Topaktas S 2012 Cerebral venous sinus thrombosis presenting as transient ischemic attacks in a case with homozygous mutations of MTHFR A1298C and CG677T. *Journal of Stroke and Cerebrovascular Diseases* 21(1): 75–77, with permission.

2. **E.** The patient has a cerebral venous sinus thrombosis. Anticoagulation is recommended, even in the case of intracranial hemorrhage, to prevent propagation of the clot. Enoxaparin is the preferred agent in pregnancy, although heparin could be used. Warfarin is pregnancy category X and is not recommended; however, outside of pregnancy warfarin is the standard anticoagulant used. Diamox would be a treatment for pseudotumor and is pregnancy class C. Acetaminophen can be used for tension-type headaches and other pain during pregnancy. Magnesium is used to treat eclampsia (*see* Bradley's NiCP, Ch. 112, pp. 1973–1991).

3. **D.** Major histocompatibility (MHC) factors are key antigen-presenting components of the immune system. Although overactive MHC may cause autoimmunity, a lack of activity would lead to immune suppression. Other common pathways to autoimmunity include genetic predisposition, failure of self-tolerance, molecular mimicry, and environmental factors (*see* Bradley's NiCP, 7th edn, Ch. 51, pp. 676–695).

4. **E.** Dopamine is a monoamine neurotransmitter that is vital to normal neurological function. Dopamine is formed from L-dopa (through the action of dopa decarboxylase), and L-dopa is formed from tyrosine (through the action of tyrosine hydroxylase). Dopamine is metabolized to norepinephrine (through the action of beta hydroxylase), which is metabolized to epinephrine (through the action of phenylethanolamine N-methyltransferase). Serotonin is also a monoamine created from tyramine through two enzymatic steps, including tryptophan hydroxylase and aromatic L-amino acid decarboxylase. The figure demonstrates the pathway from tyrosine to epinephrine.

Figure for Answer 1.4 *(from Weimer JM, Benedict JW, Elshatory YM, et al. 2007 Alterations in striatal dopamine catabolism precede loss of substantia nigra neurons in a mouse model of juvenile neuronal ceroid lipofuscinosis. Brain Research 1162: 98–112, with permission.)*

5. **B.** Patient handoffs are an important component of transitioning care between hospital shifts or between medical facilities. Although there are many verbal and/or written handoff systems in place across institutions, most include patient identification, diagnosis, treatment plan, and code status as a minimum amount of information. Family history is an important consideration in an initial diagnostic consultation with patients, but is not generally of high importance for passing off the care of a patient.

6. **E.** Convulsive seizures can have significant effects on the fetus and are felt to be of higher risk than of antiepileptic medications. They can also cause maternal trauma, which can even lead to death. The fetus can be injured with blunt trauma, or seizures can cause placental abruption. The fetus can have bradycardia and asphyxia during and after a seizure. Children with epileptic mothers not on medications during pregnancy have twice the risk of developing epilepsy compared with children born to epileptic mothers well controlled on medications. Repeated convulsive seizures can lead to miscarriage, stillbirth, prematurity, smallness for gestational age, and an increased risk of

major malformations. Fortunately, a single uncomplicated seizure during the first trimester does not seem to have an increased risk for fetal malformations (*see* Bradley's NiCP, Ch. 112, pp. 1973–1991).

7. E. The image demonstrates a sharply outlined region of pallor with scalloped edges and "spongy" center, which are classic for cerebral infarction. Although there are a few classic artifacts in autopsy evaluation of the brain, such as "Swiss cheese" artifact from gaseous buildup or flattening artifact from resting on the bottom of a bucket during fixation, parenchymal pallor is not a common artifact. Amyloid plaques are within the parenchyma, but do not represent a change in the parenchyma itself. Viral infection generally requires a much higher power to identify inclusions. Contusion does not generally cause pallor, as blood extravasates into adjacent tissues (*see* Bradley's NiCP, 7th edn, Ch. 65, pp. 920–967). Figure from Camelo-Piragua S, Hedley-White ET 2010, Infections of the Nervous System. In: Kradkin RL (ed.) *Diagnostic Pathology of Infectious Disease*, pp. 483–518, Elsevier, with permission.

8. A. Differentiating peripheral from central causes of vertigo is an important, albeit challenging, component to caring for the vertiginous patient. Peripherally associated vertigo may have other signs indicating ear involvement, including tinnitus, hearing loss, or ear pain. Vertigo can be acute onset with either peripheral or central lesions. Nystagmus can be present in either central or peripheral lesions, but tends to improve with visual fixation in peripheral lesions, and worsen with visual fixation in brainstem or cerebellar lesions (*see* Bradley's NiCP, 7th edn, Ch. 46, pp. 583–604).

9. D. Dermatomyositis (DM) is differentiated from polymyositis (PM) clinically by the presence of a rash, although in darker-skinned patients the rash may be difficult to see. On biopsy, DM involves perimysial infiltrates with perifascicular atrophy. PM involves endomysial inflammation with CD8 cells. Inclusion body myositis (IBM) has a different pattern of weakness than PM or DM, involving the forearm flexors and quads before other weakness developing. On biopsy, IBM has inclusions and rimmed vacuoles. Angular atrophic fibers with fiber type grouping would be seen in a neuropathic, not myopathic, condition. Ragged red fibers in combination with a COX– and SDH+ stain is highly suggestive of a mitochondrial disorder (*see* Bradley's NiCP, 7th edn, Ch. 110, pp. 1915–1956).

10. A. Li-Fraumeni syndrome is an autosomal-dominant disorder caused by a loss of function mutation in the *p53* tumor suppressor gene. Patients are at significantly increased risk of childhood sarcomas, early breast cancers, and brain tumors. Neurofibromatosis 1 (NF1) is an autosomal-dominant disorder caused by a loss of function mutation in the *NF1* gene, the loss of which leads to constitutive activation of cellular growth pathways, including RAS/RAF/MEK/ERK. Individuals with NF1 are at increased risk of developing multiple nerve sheath tumors (neurofibromas), malignant peripheral nerve sheath tumors, gastrointestinal stromal tumors, and breast cancer. Retinoblastoma is a cancer of the retina that is associated with autosomal-dominant inactivation of the *Rb* tumor suppressor gene in 40% of patients. The other 60% of patients develop retinoblastoma spontaneously. Multiple endocrine neoplasia type 1 is a syndrome of cancers in the pituitary, parathyroid, and pancreas associated with autosomal-dominant mutation in the tumor suppressor gene *MEN1*. Von Hippel-Lindau is an autosomal-dominant syndrome associated with mutations in the *VHL* gene that leads to hemangioblastomas of the brain, clear cell carcinomas of the kidneys, and pancreatic neuroendocrine tumors (*see* Bradley's NiCP, 7th edn, Chs. 71 and 75, pp. 1018–1025 and 1065–1083).

11. C. Memantine is an NMDA receptor antagonist used in the treatment of moderate-to-severe Alzheimer disease. Rivastigmine and donepezil are acetylcholinesterase inhibitors used in the treatment of Alzheimer disease. Vigabatrin is a gamma aminobutyric acid (GABA) metabolism inhibitor used to increase GABA activity in the central nervous system. Entacapone is a catechol-O-methyl transferase inhibitor used as an adjunct in the treatment of Parkinson disease (*see* Bradley's NiCP, 7th edn, Ch. 95, pp. 1422–1461).

12. A. The most likely diagnosis in this woman with chronic alcoholism who presents with encephalopathy, nystagmus, ophthalmoparesis, and ataxia is Wernicke encephalopathy secondary to thiamine deficiency. Chronically, Wernicke encephalopathy can develop into Korsakoff syndrome, manifested by anterograde amnesia. Magnetic resonance imaging most often shows petechial hemorrhages in the mammillary bodies, hypothalamus, medial thalami, and periaqueductal gray matter. Before any glucose is given to this patient, IV thiamine should be supplemented first and foremost, as glucose metabolism further depletes thiamine. Given that this patient is symptomatic from thiamine deficiency, treatment doses should be administered preferably with the IV formulation. Obtaining GQ1b antibodies (often helpful in Miller-Fisher syndrome) should be considered in cases of ataxia and ophthalmoparesis, but is not the best answer in this case because there is no mention of peripheral neuropathy. The other choices mentioned are also reasonable in anyone with altered mentation, but it is important to recognize the syndrome and treat with thiamine early and first.

13. D. −60 mV is the average resting membrane potential of most neurons. At rest the membrane is most permeable to chloride, so the resting potential of neurons resides near the Nernst potential of chloride (*see* Bradley's NiCP, 7th edn, Ch. 34–35, pp. 349–391).

14. B. The patient is suffering from postsubarachnoid hemorrhage vasospasm. This is a common complication that can occur in the first 14 days after SAH, and can lead to further neurological deficits or even death if not quickly recognized and treated. The main emergent therapy remains intraarterial administration of calcium channel blockers and angioplasty. IV tPA would not be indicated, even if this patient had an ischemic stroke, because of her recent hemorrhage and cranial surgery. Although seizures are a possible cause of reduced level of alertness, new focal findings in the setting of an SAH should prompt an evaluation for vasospasm, which the angiogram shows. The CT shown does not demonstrate hydrocephalus, so an extraventricular drain is not necessary. There is no indication of severe increased intracranial pressure, so mannitol is not necessary (*see* Bradley's NiCP, 7th edn, Ch. 40, pp. 459–485 and Ch. 67, pp. 981–995). Figure from Rabinstein AA, Resnick SJ 2009 *Practical*

Neuroimaging in Stroke, 1st edn, Elsevier, with permission.

15. D. This patient suffered a radial neuropathy at the spiral groove, a relatively common occurrence with humeral fractures because the nerve passes through the spiral groove on the posterior portion of the humerus. Associated symptoms include numbness on the posterior portion of the hand between the thumb and second digit and loss of strength in radial-innervated muscles distal to the spiral groove (the triceps is spared). If the triceps is also weak, the injury must be more proximal (radicular injury or plexopathy). The tables show normal median and ulnar motor and sensory studies. The radial motor response has a drop in amplitude of 50% with proximal stimulation compared with distal stimulation and reduction in velocity to the demyelinating range, indicating a conduction block, likely at the spiral groove. An absent radial sensory response indicates this is a neuropathic lesion, not a radicular or isolated posterior interosseus lesion (*see* Bradley's NiCP, 7th edn, Ch. 35, pp. 366–390).

16. C. Developmental dyslexia, also known as *specific reading disorder*, is an unexpected difficulty in learning to read despite normal intelligence. It is usually associated with a normal neurological examination, and is without structural abnormalities on imaging. It is more common in left-handed males with a family history of dyslexia. An infarct of the splenium of the corpus callosum and left occipital lobe could cause alexia without agraphia, but this should come on acutely, unlike the progressive course in this case. Landau-Kleffner syndrome is an acquired epileptic aphasia in which children slowly lose previous verbal language and can have electrographic status epilepticus of sleep seen on EEG. Mild intellectual disability involves deficits in language, reading, memory, social skills, and executive function, and is associated with an intelligence quotient between 50 and 70. Attention-deficit/hyperactivity disorder can lead to school problems in this age group, but typically these patients present with complaints of inattention, hyperactivity, or impulsivity, which can result in disciplinary problems at school or home (*see* Bradley's NiCP, 7th edn, Ch. 90, pp. 1301–1323).

17. B. The case is consistent with convulsive syncope, based on the history of recent vigorous exercise, a prodrome of nausea and diaphoresis, and loss of consciousness. Additional components of her presentation that suggest a syncopal etiology rather than seizure include the brevity of her loss of consciousness, the brevity of the postictal confusion, and the fast, jerklike movements that were likely myoclonus. Note that there was no mention of repetitive or stereotyped movement before losing consciousness that would suggest automatisms or tonic/clonic activity. There was a loss of bladder control during the episode, but this can occur with any alteration in consciousness. There is nothing in the question stem that would indicate a nonepileptic spell. The diagnostic workup for syncope would generally include orthostatic vital signs, an electrocardiogram, Holter monitor, and/or transthoracic echocardiogram if there is a high suspicion of a cardiac etiology. If events are recurrent, an electroencephalogram may also be considered in case of an atypical seizure presentation. Treatment for the case presented would likely include volume resuscitation, with no other definitive therapy

indicated unless there are abnormalities on evaluation. If the patient suffers recurrent syncope, both conservative measures (i.e. compression stockings, abdominal binders, liberalization of salt intake, moving legs before standing) and pharmacological measures (i.e. fludrocortisone, midodrine, droxidopa, pyridostigmine) may be considered (*see* Bradley's NiCP, 7th edn, Ch. 2, pp. 8–16).

18. D. Free nerve endings are associated with sensation of temperature and pain. Pacinian corpuscles are responsible for the sensation of pressure and vibration. Merkel disks sense light touch and pressure and are slowly adaptive. Meissner corpuscles are the most sensitive to vibration and are rapidly adaptive. Ruffini endings are sensitive to stretch and mechanical changes, with little or no adaptation.

19. C. The patient has shoulder pain and gait difficulty for the last 1 year with decreased arm swing when walking and loss of dexterity in the left hand. These historical clues point toward bradykinesia and rigidity, two of the cardinal features of idiopathic Parkinson disease (PD). Note that tremor is not part of the diagnostic criteria of PD, as one can have the akinetic/rigid subtype. The physical examination would, of course, confirm these examination findings. It is not uncommon for patients to complain of joint pains likely from dystonia or rigidity, some of which persist after operations for orthopedic issues. Constipation and falling out of bed during vivid dreams (rapid eye movement [REM] sleep behavior disorder) are two nonmotor features of PD that often precede the diagnosis by up to 10 years, pointing further toward a neurodegenerative alpha-synucleinopathy. Although shoulder injuries such as a rotator cuff injury could certainly cause decreased arm swing, other historical points with the constipation and REM sleep behavior disorder make this less likely. The same is also true for cervical myelopathy. Vascular parkinsonism would also not have these nonmotor features and would present predominately with lower extremity involvement and gait difficulty much more than asymmetric upper extremity involvement. A peripheral neuropathy is not likely given the constellation of other symptoms presented (*see* Bradley's NiCP, 7th edn, Ch. 23, pp. 223–249).

20. D. Hypophonia is often appreciated along with micrographia in idiopathic Parkinson disease (PD). The other choices are red flags that the diagnosis is *not* idiopathic PD. Severe orthostatic hypotension is a common symptom of a Parkinson-plus syndrome such as multiple system atrophy (MSA). Postural instability early in the course is often a sign of progressive supranuclear palsy (PSP); idiopathic PD is usually associated with late postural instability. Both a suboptimal response to levodopa and symmetrical bradykinesia and rigidity are typical of Parkinson-plus syndromes, including PSP and MSA. Remember that idiopathic PD typically presents with asymmetric onset of rigidity and/or bradykinesia (*see* Bradley's NiCP, 7th edn, Ch. 23).

21. A. Idiopathic Parkinson disease typically has no abnormalities on MRI imaging, including no evidence of contrast enhancement. Although not relevant to this case, symptomatic parkinsonism may stem from structural lesions in the contralateral basal ganglia. A DAT scan measures the presynaptic activity of dopamine in the striatum (caudate and putamen) and would demonstrate decreased uptake with idiopathic

Parkinson disease. Bilateral T2 hyperintensities are typical findings in patients with vascular risk factors such as hypertension, hyperlipidemia, and tobacco use, indicating vascular parkinsonism. Cervical cord compression from a disc protrusion would cause a compressive myelopathy with upper motor neuron signs, including spasticity, hyperreflexia, and weakness rather than parkinsonism (*see* Bradley's NiCP, 7th edn, Ch. 23, pp. 223–249).

22. E. A trial of carbidopa/levodopa would be the treatment of choice for this patient. Levodopa eventually becomes dopamine once it passes the blood–brain barrier and presents itself for storage into the brain. Carbidopa prevents the breakdown of levodopa in the periphery, outside of the blood–brain barrier. In this particular age group, carbidopa/levodopa is considered the gold standard for treatment of Parkinson disease. Other options (not listed), depending on disease severity, would include dopamine agonists, monoamine oxidase-B inhibitors, or catechol-O-methyl transferase inhibitors. A high-volume lumbar puncture would be a treatment option for patients with normal pressure hydrocephalus, which typically presents with gait apraxia, urinary incontinence, and cognitive decline. Surgical decompression would be indicated if a patient had weakness and pain from a compressive myelopathy, such as would occur with a bulging disc. Aggressive medical treatment of vascular risk factors would be indicated for vascular parkinsonism. An arthroscopic surgical repair could be considered if there were no features of parkinsonism and the decreased arm swing and pain were found to be due to orthopedic injury (*see* Bradley's NiCP, 7th edn, Ch. 96, pp. 1422–1460).

23. A. The suprachiasmatic nucleus of the hypothalamus receives input from the retina and helps to control circadian rhythm. In contrast, the hypothalamus has two nuclei that control appetite. The lateral nuclei contain the "feeding center," which stimulates appetite. A lesion here would lead to decreased oral intake. The ventromedial nuclei serve as the "satiety center," where a lesion here would lead to obesity and savage behavior. The arcuate nucleus produces a number of hormones that affect pituitary function, including gonadotropin-releasing hormone, growth hormone–releasing hormone, and dopamine, which later inhibits the release of prolactin. Both the anterior and posterior nuclei serve to regulate temperature. The paraventricular nucleus releases three major hormones that control the pituitary function. First, it releases CRH, which stimulates adrenocorticotropic hormone. It also releases TRH, which releases thyroid stimulation hormone. Finally, it releases somatostatin, which acts to inhibit release of growth hormone (useful in the treatment of acromegaly from growth hormone excess). Not mentioned is the supraoptic nucleus, which sits above the optic chiasm and helps to produce vasopressin (antidiuretic hormone). A lesion here would lead to diabetes insipidus (*see* Bradley's NiCP, 7th edn, Ch. 52, pp. 696–712).

24. B. This patient presents with REM sleep behavior disorder (RBD). This is a disorder that generally starts in middle age or in the elderly and is more common in men. It is typically seen in association with neurodegenerative conditions like Parkinson disease, progressive supranuclear palsy, multiple system atrophy, and various dementias. This disorder involves the loss of REM atonia, resulting in patients acting out their dreams. This involves talking, yelling, kicking movements, arm movements, or walking. It can result in injury to the patient or the bed partner, as well as result in very vivid dreams often confused with hallucinations. PSG is not necessary for the diagnosis, although if performed, it would demonstrate increased electromyogram activity during REM sleep. PSG findings of an abrupt onset of motor activity during slow wave sleep are consistent with night terrors, not RBD. Amitriptyline, other tricyclics, sedative-hypnotics, and anticholinergics can cause or exacerbate this disorder. *CHRNA2* mutations are common in autosomal-dominant frontal lobe epilepsy. RBD can be confused with frontal seizures due to the occurrence at night and odd behaviors (*see* Bradley's NiCP, 7th edn, Ch. 102, pp. 1615–1685).

25. D. Recalling a birthday is an example of declarative (or explicit) memory, which is localized to the medial temporal lobe and hippocampi. The other items listed in the question are examples of nondeclarative (or implicit) memories. Tying one's shoe is a procedural memory, receiving input from the basal ganglia and frontal lobes. Predicting the weather based on cues is an example of probabilistic learning, which is localized to the basal ganglia. Recalling a word when an associated word is presented is called *priming*, and is localized to the neocortex. Expecting an event with a certain stimulus is called *classical conditioning*, and is a cerebellar and amygdala function (*see* Bradley's NiCP, 7th edn, Ch. 7, pp. 57–65).

26. B. The EEG demonstrates the typical 3-Hz spike and wave pattern seen in absence epilepsy. The best medication for absence epilepsy is ethosuximide. Valproic acid is also used in absence epilepsy, but typically if there are generalized tonic-clonic seizures in addition to staring episodes. Phenytoin and carbamazepine have the potential to worsen generalized epilepsy. Levetiracetam is also a good option for generalized epilepsy, but is not the best choice listed (*see* Bradley's NiCP, 7th edn, Ch. 101, pp. 1563–1614). Figure from Daroff RB, Jankovic J, Mazziotta JC, Pomeroy SL 2016 *Bradley's Neurology in Clinical Practice*, 7th edn, Elsevier, with permission.

27. D. The case and image are classic for cerebral venous thrombosis. The woman was prothrombotic due to smoking and estrogen use and likely became hypovolemic in the sun. The pathology image demonstrates thrombosed cortical veins as well as superficial hemorrhage. The best treatment for cerebral venous thrombosis is volume expansion and anticoagulation, usually with unfractionated heparin. Triple H therapy (hypertension, hypervolemia, hemodilution) is appropriate for subarachnoid hemorrhage. Platelets and clotting factors are appropriate for intracerebral hemorrhage if there is history of antiplatelet or anticoagulant use or laboratory evidence of clotting cascade insufficiency. Normotension and observation would not be appropriate for cerebral venous thrombosis (*see* Bradley's NiCP, 7th edn, Ch. 65, pp. 920–967). Figure from Ellison D, Love S, Chimelli L, et al. 2013 *Neuropathology*, 3rd edn, Elsevier, with permission.

28. C. The trochlear nerve innervates the superior oblique muscle, whose job is to abduct, depress, and intort the eye. With trochlear nerve palsy, patients generally have vertical diplopia that is worsened by looking down the

nose—watching television from bed or descending stairs. Resting gaze tends to have hypertropia ipsilateral to the affected eye. The Bielschowsky head tilt test may also help localize the affected nerve, as tilting the head away from the affected eye leads to globe extorsion and correction of the diplopia. Individuals with chronic trochlear nerve palsy may have a chronic head tilt as an unconscious compensatory movement (*see* Bradley's NiCP, 7th edn, Ch. 104, pp. 1720–1735).

29. D. Informed consent is the process by which medical decisions are made. This involves a conversation between the physician, the patient, and any medical decision makers about risk, benefits, and expected results of a medical intervention. The discussion should be in a manner which they can understand, and the patient should have the capability to understand those risks and benefits. The patient's decision should be made free of coercion, manipulation, or undue influence. Informed consent does not require a signed legal document outlining potential complications, although these are helpful in malpractice cases. In most states, treatments given against consent or without consent can be considered assault or even battery.

30. C. Citalopram is a selective serotonin reuptake inhibitor, which is known for causing hyponatremia. Although a nortriptyline overdose would cause somnolence, it would not cause hyponatremia. Tricyclic antidepressant overdoses can cause fatal cardiac arrhythmias. Trazodone overdose would cause somnolence, but would not cause hyponatremia. Aripiprazole is a partial dopamine agonist and causes sedation, akathisia, and extrapyramidal symptoms. Phenelzine is a nonselective monoamine oxidase inhibitor that can precipitate a hypertensive crisis if used in the setting of other serotonin-enhancing medications or if the diet is high in tyramine (*see* Bradley's NiCP, 7th edn, Ch. 84, pp. 1209–1225).

31. B. Administration of erythropoiesis-stimulating agents (ESA) to patients with renal impairment has come under scrutiny in recent years. Whereas historical treatment goals were to obtain normal hemoglobin levels, recent evidence from large randomized trials has demonstrated an increased cardiovascular and stroke risk in patients treated to normal hemoglobin values. Peripheral neuropathy risk is increased with chronic uremia, but not by ESA administration. Seizure risk may be increased with electrolyte disarray or severe uremia, but is generally not increased with ESA administration. Dementia risk is increased by both chronic renal failure and cerebrovascular events, but not directly from ESA. Headaches may relate to polycythemia, but are otherwise not directly related to ESA administration (*see* Bradley's NiCP, 7th edn, Ch. 65, pp. 920–967).

32. A. ODD is marked by consistent hostility and defiance of authority figures out of proportion to what is generally accepted. Notably, children with ODD do not have associated depression, anxiety, or substance abuse. Oppositional defiance is considered disordered (e.g. ODD) when the defiant behavior causes significant personal, family, or societal stress, or if it leads to potentially dangerous or criminal behaviors. Depression in younger children usually presents with sadness, worry, and hopelessness, whereas in teenagers it involves anger, anxiety, or withdrawal. A diagnosis of major depressive disorder involves a depressed mood or anhedonia for at least 2 weeks, with a significant impact on social functioning and can include changes in sleep, appetite, energy levels, interest in activities, and feelings of guilt or hopelessness. Antisocial personality disorder involves a pattern of disregard for authority, failure to conform to social norms, deception, impulsivity, aggressiveness, and lack of remorse. This personality disorder is diagnosed in patients above the age of 15 and is usually comorbid in patients with ODD. Narcissistic personality disorder involves a grandiose self-opinion, preoccupation with success or power, arrogance, envy of others, and often lack of empathy. Autism is a disorder with impairments in social functioning, communication, and imagination. Often these patients display stereotypes or other repetitive behaviors. Impaired social interaction can lead to oppositional behaviors, but they are not usually devious.

33. B. A negative reinforcement is an aversive event that is removed when a desired behavior transpires. In the question, the nagging is the negative reinforcer, and cleaning the room is the desired outcome. A positive reinforcement is a desired event that occurs as a result of a desired behavior, such as paying money for completing chores or taking a child to Disneyland. Positive punishment is when an unwanted behavior is answered by an unwanted consequence, such as yelling at a child for running into the street. A negative punishment is when a desired stimulus is removed due to unwanted behavior, such as taking away video games.

34. A. Opsoclonus-myoclonus is a rare, disabling disorder in which a patient has rapid, involuntary, conjugate fast eye movements paired with diffuse myoclonus. This condition is most common in children, with about 50% paraneoplastic presentations related to neuroblastoma, and about 50% autoimmune (often parainfectious). Opsoclonus-myoclonus may present in adults as well, either as autoimmune or as an anti-Ri (also known as *anti-ANNA2*)–mediated paraneoplastic disorder related to small cell lung cancer, gynecological cancers, or breast cancers. There are no paraneoplastic disorders commonly associated with the other pediatric tumors listed (*see* Bradley's NiCP, 7th edn, Ch. 81, pp. 1187–1195).

35. E. Olfaction involves transmission of sensory information through the olfactory bulb to the anterior olfactory nucleus, prepyriform cortex, amygdala, and posterior entorhinal cortex, which has extensive interactions with the hippocampus. This allows for elements of smell to be broken down into different components and even have smells associated with event memory and emotional memory. The superior colliculus is involved in vision, particularly orienting the eyes and head to different stimuli (*see* Bradley's NiCP, 7th edn, Ch. 19, pp. 190–196).

36. E. This case discusses the most common scenario of an early peripheral polyneuropathy. He has a normal neurological examination with no evidence of large-fiber nerve dysfunction, although he is symptomatic because his small peripheral nerve fibers are affected (myelinated Aδ and unmyelinated C-fibers). Given that he has normal vibration and pin prick on his examination, his A-alpha and A-beta fibers are likely unaffected. Typically, proprioception and light touch are also normal. Many patients report the feeling of a wrinkle in their sock or small pebbles in their shoe. They also may report coldlike pain, tingling, or pins

syndrome (ipsilateral tongue weakness, contralateral weakness and sensory loss to vibration and proprioception) is related to a medial medullary lesion, where the hypoglossal nucleus, pyramidal tract, and medial lemniscus are adjacent. This generally results from occlusion of the anteromedial artery (off the vertebral artery) or from basilar artery perforators (*see* Bradley's NiCP, 7th edn, Ch. 104, pp. 1720–1735).

51. C. The case describes an infant with deficiency of glucose transporter type I (GLUT1), which facilitates glucose transport across the blood–brain barrier. The GLUT1 protein is encoded by the *SLC2A1* gene, the same gene that is mutated in paroxysmal exertional dyskinesia. GLUT1 deficiency often leads to an epileptic encephalopathy with infantile-onset seizures, developmental delay, complex movement disorders, and microcephaly. Evaluation shows a remarkably low cerebrospinal fluid glucose level. Imaging is often normal, and EEG typically shows epileptiform activity that is improved with the ketogenic diet (*see* Bradley's NiCP, 7th edn, Ch. 111, pp. 1956–1972).

52. A. The described symptoms of anhedonia (loss of interest), sadness, worthlessness, decreased appetite, and decreased energy all point toward depression. The presence of symptoms for at least 2 weeks, nearly every day, along with a change from her previous state, is classified as major depressive episode. However, given recurrent episodes more than 2 months apart, she meets criteria for major depressive disorder. Other common symptoms of depression include SIG-E-CAPS: sleep disturbance (insomnia or hypersomnia), loss of interest, guilt, loss of energy, loss of concentration, appetite change (increased or decreased), psychomotor agitation or retardation, and suicidal ideation. Depression affects 10%–25% of women and 5%–12% of men and is more likely to occur when there is a family history, recent stressor, substance abuse, medical issues, pregnancy, or poor social support. Treatment involves both medicinal and nonmedicinal modalities, including a combination of selective serotonin reuptake inhibitors or serotonin-norepinephrine reuptake inhibitors, as well as psychotherapy. In this case dysthymic disorder is the incorrect answer because the patient's symptoms are more severe, cause disruption in her social and occupational function, and the onset was more acute. There is no indication that the patient has any symptoms of hypomania. Finally, there is no indication that the patient's symptoms had a temporal onset with a season change or that it remitted at a different time of year.

53. A. CSF, produced by the choroid plexus, is produced at approximately 20 mL/hr. This means that the entire volume of CSF in an adult is replaced approximately four times per day (*see* Bradley's NiCP, 7th edn, Ch. 88, pp. 1261–1278).

54. D. Maternal rhinovirus infection has not been associated with mental retardation (MR) in the pediatric patient. MR can be classified as mild (IQ = 50–70), moderate (IQ = 35–49), severe (IQ = 20–34), and profound (IQ ≤ 20). The potential etiologies are broad, including infections (congenital toxoplasmosis, cytomegalovirus, rubella), environmental (alcohol exposure leading to fetal alcohol syndrome), genetic (trisomy 21, fragile X syndrome), acquired (hemorrhage, near-drowning), and metabolic (hypothyroidism). Diagnosing the underlying cause

of MR is performed by neurocognitive testing, as well as a good prenatal and perinatal history, evaluation for speech and language delays, evaluation of dysmorphic features, and evaluation of growth curves. Depending on the level of severity, patients may be able to fully care for themselves or require maximal assistance.

55. E. The circuit of Papez is a major pathway involved in memory. The circuit includes the hippocampus, fornix, mammillary bodies, mammillothalamic tract, anterior thalamic nucleus, cingulum, and the entorhinal cortex. In Korsakoff syndrome frequently there is damage to the mammillary bodies, which interrupts this pathway, disrupting the ability to learn new information or retrieve recent memories (*see* Bradley's NiCP, 7th edn, Ch. 7, pp. 57–65).

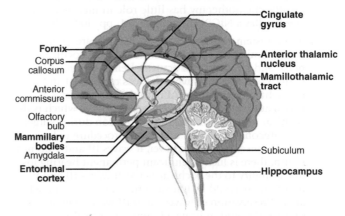

Figure for Answer 1.55 *The components of the Papez circuit are in bold font, from Beh SC, Frohman TC, Frohman EM 2013 Isolated mammillary body involvement on MRI in Wernicke's encephalopathy. Journal of the Neurological Sciences 334(1–2): 172–175, with permission.*

56. D. Mood stabilizers consist of lithium, valproic acid, lamotrigine, carbamazepine, oxcarbazepine, and even some atypical antipsychotics. Lithium works by inhibiting inositol and glycogen synthase kinase 3 signal pathways. Serum drug levels should be frequently monitored, and side effects include weight gain, nausea, vomiting, tremor, thyroid dysfunction, nephrogenic diabetes insipidus (leads to hypernatremia), and negative chronotropic effect on the heart (contraindicated in sick sinus syndrome). Valproic acid is an anticonvulsant with mood-stabilizing properties through enhancing GABAergic action. Side effects include tremor, thrombocytopenia, hair loss, nausea, and neural tube defects if taken while pregnant. Oxcarbazepine and carbamazepine both are sodium channel inhibitors that are used as anticonvulsants, but also have mood-stabilizing properties. Oxcarbazepine has a slightly different chemical structure than carbamazepine, and has theoretically less metabolism by the liver, as well as fewer side effects, such as agranulocytosis and hyponatremia. Fatigue and ataxia can occur with higher drug levels. Lamotrigine acts, in part, by inhibiting serotonin reuptake and does not require monitoring serum levels. The most well-known side effects (although not the most common) are life-threatening rashes such as Stevens-Johnson syndrome or toxic

epidermal necrolysis. Other mood stabilizers include topiramate and gabapentin.

57. B. Nerves branching directly from the posterior cord include the upper subscapular nerve, the lower subscapular nerve, and the thoracodorsal nerve. The terminal branches of the posterior cord are the radial and axillary nerves. The medial pectoral nerve branches directly from the medial cord. The long thoracic nerve is derived from C5, C6, and C7 nerve roots before the brachial plexus forms. The musculocutaneous nerve is a terminal branch of the lateral cord. The suprascapular nerve comes directly off of the superior trunk. See the representation of the brachial plexus (*see* Bradley's NiCP, 7th edn, Ch. 106, pp. 1766–1790).

58. D. The patient has spasmus nutans, which is a triad of pendular nystagmus, head nodding, and cervical dystonia. Most cases begin between 4 and 12 months of age and are sporadic, although rarely patients with spasmus nutans may be found to have structural causes such as tumors in the optic pathway. The nystagmus can be horizontal, vertical, or rotatory and is usually pronounced more in one eye than the other. Further, the nystagmus is almost never synchronized between the two eyes, and most often is associated with a dysconjugate gaze. The head motion associated with spasmus nutans is usually oblique with both nodding and shaking and is usually a compensatory measure that suppresses nystagmus. The cervical dystonia is not always present, but occurs in up to 30% of the patients

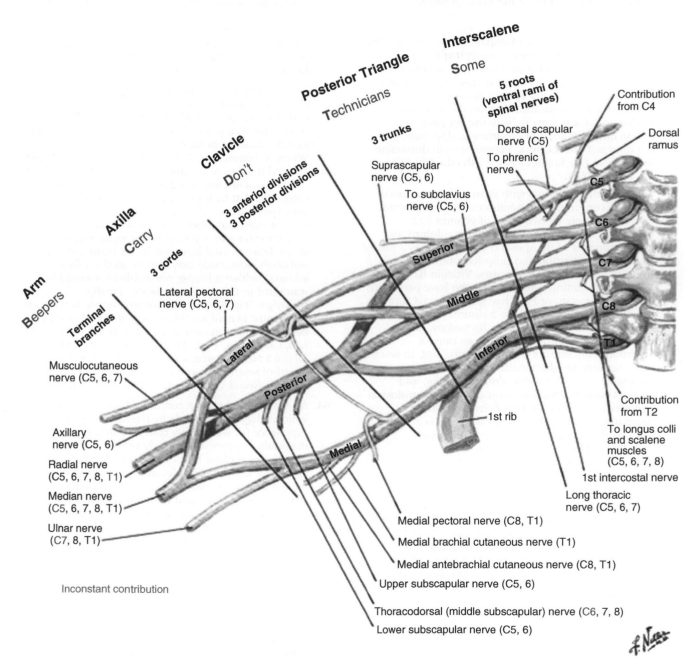

Figure for Answer 1.57 (*from Mikityansky I, Zager EL, Yousem DM, Loevner LA 2012 MR Imaging of the brachial plexus.* Magnetic Resonance Imaging Clinics of North America 20(4): 791–826, with permission.)

with spasmus nutans. Idiopathic spasmus nutans is considered self-limiting and transient, lasting only a few months to years. Alternatively, congenital nystagmus almost always begins at less than 6 months old and is not associated with head nodding or cervical dystonia. In addition, congenital nystagmus has a larger amplitude, slower frequency, and does not usually resolve. Seizures are typically associated with forced gaze deviation or head deviation rather than nystagmus or nodding. A Chiari malformation may have downward nystagmus but without the association of head nodding or cervical dystonia. Benign paroxysmal torticollis may have intermittent episodes of cervical dystonia, but does not have nystagmus (*see* Bradley's NiCP, 7th edn, Ch. 44, pp. 528–572).

59. D. Entacapone is a catechol-O-methyl transferase inhibitor, which is one of the main enzymes responsible for the breakdown of dopamine in the central nervous system. The other main enzymes are monoamine oxidase B and dopamine beta hydroxylase (which converts dopamine to norepinephrine). Rivastigmine is an acetylcholinesterase inhibitor used in the treatment of Alzheimer disease and dementia with Parkinson disease. Trihexyphenidyl is an anticholinergic medication used in the treatment of dystonia. Carbidopa reduces the peripheral destruction of L-dopa (a precursor to dopamine), but does not affect central nervous system dopamine metabolism (*see* Bradley's NiCP, 7th edn, Ch. 96, pp. 1422–1460).

60. E. This patient presents with signs and symptoms of subacute combined degeneration of the spinal cord, which is a severe consequence of vitamin B12 deficiency, which affects the posterior columns and lateral columns of the spinal cord. This causes a loss of sensation to vibration and proprioception and can result in weakness in severe cases. Vitamin B12 deficiency is common in patients who have pernicious anemia, are vegan, or have had gastric bypass surgery. Vitamin E deficiency leads to a clinical picture of a spinocerebellar ataxia. Vitamin B6 toxicity, usually doses of more than 200 mg/day, can cause a predominantly sensory polyneuropathy and, in severe cases, sensory ganglionopathy. Vitamin A toxicity is associated with dry pruritic skin, joint pain, and pseudotumor cerebri. The most common neurological presentation of vitamin D deficiency is a mild myopathy with proximal leg weakness. It is also associated with diffuse bone pain and muscle pain (*see* Bradley's NiCP, 7th edn, Ch. 85, pp. 1237–1253).

61. B. The Moro reflex is a primitive reflex seen in the newborn until the age of 4 months, and its presence later could indicate developmental delay. The reflex is elicited by a quick movement of the head or a startle, which causes the hands to extend upwards with simultaneous neck extension; then the hands are brought back together and the child cries. Other primitive reflexes include the rooting reflex in which stroking the cheek will cause the newborn to rotate the head ipsilaterally; this usually disappears after 1 month of age. The tonic neck reflex (previously known as the *Galant reflex*) is elicited by turning the head to one side, which causes the ipsilateral arm to extend while the contralateral arm bends and the patient appears to be in a "fencing" posture. This should disappear by 6 months of age. The extensor plantar reflex is present

until 1 year old or until the child begins walking (*see* Bradley's NiCP, 7th edn, Ch. 111, pp. 1956–1972).

62. D. The patient presents with behavioral variant frontotemporal dementia (FTD), which is marked by early behavioral changes, including impulsivity, hypersexuality, obsessions, and compulsions. Other common features include difficulty with planning, early loss of speech, and apathy. MRI may show anterior temporal and frontal atrophy. FDG-PET scans show anterior temporal and frontal lobe hypometabolism, whereas posterior temporoparietal hypometabolism is seen in Alzheimer disease. FTD is caused by a buildup of tau protein, which can be seen histologically as Pick bodies, whereas neurofibrillary tangles are seen in Alzheimer disease. Frequently trazodone, selective serotonin reuptake inhibitors, and antipsychotics are used for behavioral control. Lithium is used in the treatment of bipolar disorder. Although he has some impulsivity and hypersexuality, the presence of memory loss and language dysfunction points to FTD rather than a manic episode (*see* Bradley's NiCP, 7th edn, Ch. 95, pp. 1380–1421).

63. A. The clinical presentation and MRI findings are classic for neurocysticercosis, a tapeworm infection with *Taenia solium*, which is often related to ingestion of undercooked pork. This disease is commonly seen in individuals from Mexico and South America. Whereas treatment with an antihelminth may be safely avoided in cases of completely calcified cysts, the cysts on this patient's MRI appear active with a scolex, suggesting that treatment may be beneficial in reducing subsequent seizure risk. As such, treating with both levetiracetam and albendazole is warranted. Levetiracetam and acyclovir is not suggested, as there is no evidence of viral infection in the history or on MRI. Although lacosamide may also be used for focal seizures, neither a biopsy nor antibiotics would be warranted in this patient currently. Finally, methylprednisolone would not necessarily provide any therapeutic benefit for this patient in the absence of edema or inflammatory disease (*see* Bradley's NiCP, 7th edn, Ch. 79, pp. 1147–1158). Figure from Del Brutto OJ 2013 Neurocysticercosis in infants and toddlers: report of seven cases and review of published patients. *Pediatric Neurology* (48)6: 432–435, with permission.

64. A. Availability bias is a common diagnostic error in which a diagnosis is made by referring to a recent experience (or what easily comes to mind) to make a diagnosis. If a provider recently missed a diagnosis of ALS, this may cause him or her to be hypersensitive and quick to diagnose it (even if incorrectly) in a second patient. Anchoring bias occurs when a diagnosis is assumed and not changed despite identifying contrary evidence. Confirmation bias is using a test to prove a diagnosis rather than using tests to rule out alternative diagnoses. Diagnosis momentum involves accepting a prior diagnosis without confirming the diagnosis.

65. C. Dabigatran is a direct thrombin inhibitor approved for the prevention of stroke in the setting of nonvalvular atrial fibrillation. Rivaroxaban and apixaban are factor Xa inhibitors also used for stroke prevention in the setting of nonvalvular atrial fibrillation. Cilostazol is a phosphodiesterase inhibitor that blocks platelet aggregation, and is rarely used in thrombotic stroke prevention. Ticlopidine is an

adenosine diphosphate receptor inhibitor that acts similar to clopidogrel, but is rarely used in thrombotic stroke prevention (*see* Bradley's NiCP, 7th edn, Ch. 65, pp. 920–967).

66. C. The EEG demonstrates triphasic waves, which are classically seen in hepatic encephalopathy, but they can be seen in other metabolic or toxic encephalopathies. The patient's history of alcoholism should also point to hepatic encephalopathy. The EEG in herpes encephalitis would show temporal periodic lateralized epileptiform discharges (PLEDs). The EEG in nonconvulsive status epilepticus would show rhythmic discharges with spikes and slow waves, which can be confused with triphasic waves. The EEG in acute strokes is frequently normal, but focal slowing or even focal PLEDs can be seen in some cases. Meningitis does not have any characteristic EEG findings, but seizures and various levels of encephalopathy can be seen (*see* Bradley's NiCP, 7th edn, Ch. 84, pp. 1209–1225). Figure from Daroff RB, Jankovic J, Mazziotta JC, Pomeroy SL 2016 *Bradley's Neurology in Clinical Practice*, 7th edn, Elsevier, with permission.

67. C. OCD often coexists with Tourette syndrome. Obsessions are recurring ideas or thoughts that are intrusive, causing great anxiety and stress. Compulsions are repetitive behaviors such as counting, checking, or repeating actions. Most patients realize that the obsessions or compulsions are unreasonable and excessive. OCD can be very time consuming, often affecting school or workplace performance. Treatment involves selective serotonin reuptake inhibitors, tricyclic antidepressants, and psychotherapy involving various forms of behavioral therapy. Imaging usually shows decreased caudate size and hypermetabolism in the frontal cortex. Although OCD can coexist with Tourette syndrome, there is no indication that these are motor tics, as there is no indication of preceding urge or sense of relief after. Panic disorder is less likely, as there is no mention of panic attacks. OCPD is incorrect, as the obsessions and compulsions in this case are seen as unhealthy and unwanted, which tend to go with OCD rather than OCPD. In OCPD, they are often rational and desirable. There is no indication of paranoia such as distrust or suspiciousness to suggest paranoid personality disorder.

68. A. This patient presents with movements concerning for chorea. These can be described as movements that flow from one part of the body to the next without interrupting overall movements. Patients are able to walk, but have a "lurching" gait. They can reach for objects, but may have extra movements on the way to that object. Chorea gravidarum is not uncommon and typically starts in the second to fifth month of pregnancy and typically resolves within a few months of delivery without needing treatment. There is a high risk of recurrence with future pregnancies. Low doses of haloperidol or similar dopamine antagonists can be useful if treatment is needed, but these are rarely required and not necessary in most patients. Without a family history and given her pregnancy status, an autosomal-dominant disorder like Huntington disease is less likely. Wilson disease would show Kayser-Fleischer rings on slit lamp examination, but this patient's ceruloplasmin and liver function tests are normal. Her movements are not tics because there is no urge to move, no sense of relief with the movements, and cannot be suppressed. Clonidine is helpful with tics but not chorea (*see* Bradley's NiCP, Ch. 112, pp. 1973–1991).

69. B. Sweat glands are activated by postganglionic sympathetic fibers releasing acetylcholine to muscarinic receptors. This is the only part of the sympathetic system that releases acetylcholine. The adrenal medulla is innervated by preganglionic sympathetic fibers resulting in the release of epinephrine and norepinephrine. The parasympathetic system only releases acetylcholine—it does not innervate sweat glands (*see* Bradley's NiCP, 7th edn, Ch. 108, pp. 1867–1895).

70. A. Prolonged corticosteroid use may suppress natural cortisol production by the adrenal glands. Sudden discontinuation of exogenous corticosteroids may, therefore, leave a patient with acutely low cortisol availability. As such, steroid taper is generally preferred if exposure has been sufficiently long to warrant it. Symptoms of low cortisol include fatigue, generalized muscle weakness, weight loss, diarrhea, vomiting, and low blood pressure. High serum cortisol, as seen with Cushing syndrome, may cause weight gain, lipodystrophy, thinning of the skin, insulin insensitivity, immunosuppression, and agitation. Low serum T4 is associated with hypothyroidism, and may cause weight gain, fatigue, constipation, and edema. High serum T4 is associated with hyperthyroidism and may cause weight loss, tremor, anxiety, palpitations, or excessive sweating. Low serum glucose is generally related to exogenous insulin use with inadequate food intake, and may acutely cause sweating, palpitations, confusion, or loss of consciousness.

71. D. Executive function includes problem solving, planning, organization, selective attention, and inhibition, which are evaluated with a variety of tests, including the Wisconsin Card Sorting Test and Trail Making Test. The Wisconsin Card Sorting Test involves a patient given a set of cards and told to make matches with the cards. The patient is not told what are considered matches but only told when the match is correct or incorrect, and a score is based off of the

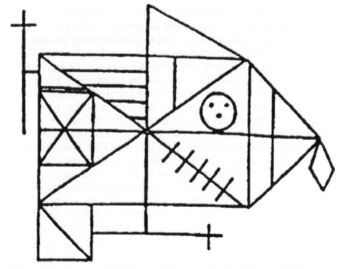

Figure for Answer 1.71 (*from Schouten D, Hendriksen JGM, Aldenkamp AP 2008 Performance of children with epilepsy on the Rey-Osterrieth complex figure test: is there an effect of localization or lateralization? Epilepsy Research 83(2–3): 184–189, with permission.*)

ability to make a match and how quickly the patient is able to do so. Language is evaluated with a variety of tests, often including the Boston Naming Test. Visuospatial function is evaluated simply with the Clock Draw Test or the Rey-Osterrieth complex (see the figure). Memory is assessed with multiple tests, but the Wechsler Memory Scale is a typical tool used. Intelligence is tested using an IQ test, commonly the Wechsler Adult Intelligence Scale (*see* Bradley's NiCP, 7th edn, Ch. 43, pp. 511–527).

72. E. The patient has phantom limb pain, a condition that commonly follows amputation. The onset of pain is often early, but may be delayed for months or years. It is most common in patients who suffered pain before their amputation. Pain is described as sharp, stabbing, shooting, or squeezing, and patients may also have vivid feelings of the previously amputated limb (phantom limb sensation). The exact pathophysiology is unknown, but many factors may contribute to phantom limb pain, such as vascular etiology for amputation, lower limb amputation, prior use of prosthesis, and prior history of stump pain. Treatment can include opiates, tricyclic antidepressants, antiepileptics such as carbamazepine (not calcium channel blockers), lidocaine, and NMDA receptor antagonists such as memantine or ketamine, as well as beta-blockers. Nonmedicinal treatments can also be of benefit, such as acupuncture, biofeedback, and massage. Finally, surgical treatments may provide benefit in refractory cases, including surgical dorsal root entry zone lesions, rhizotomies, or sympathectomies (*see* Bradley's NiCP, 7th edn, Ch. 54, pp. 720–741).

73. D. Tramadol is a mu-opioid receptor agonist that can also block reuptake of both serotonin and norepinephrine. This increases the risk of serotonin syndrome when combined with selective serotonin reuptake inhibitors or serotonin and norepinephrine reuptake inhibitors. Tramadol increases the risk of seizures at high doses due to gamma aminobutyric acid A inhibition and delta opioid antagonism (*see* Bradley's NiCP, 7th edn, Ch. 54, pp. 720–741).

74. B. This patient has diabetic radiculoplexopathy, formerly known as *diabetic amyotrophy*. This is a condition usually occurring in patients over the age of 50, usually during times of uncontrolled diabetes. Initially, it presents with severe hip, back, or leg pain for a few days and is followed by weight loss and muscle atrophy in the proximal leg that eventually stabilizes. Over the course of several months, most have improvement in their strength. This can be a similar presentation to a vasculitic neuropathy; but with normal sedimentation rate and CRP, vasculitis is unlikely. A sural biopsy would be normal because the pathological abnormality is in the lumbosacral plexus. In cases of vasculitis, findings are more widespread, so biopsies can be helpful. *SEPT9* mutations are seen in hereditary neuralgic amyotrophy, which typically affects the upper extremities. Diabetic radiculoplexopathy is generally a single event and does not require long-term immunosuppression (*see* Bradley's NiCP, 7th edn, Chs. 106 and 107, pp. 1766–1867).

75. E. The common peroneal (fibular) nerve passes over the fibular head superficially. In prolonged childbirth, if a woman holds back her legs around the knees or malpositions her legs in the stirrups, she may compress these nerves and lead to temporary peroneal neuropathy. Generally the symptoms of weakness and numbness will resolve spontaneously within weeks, although the patient may benefit from an ankle–foot orthotic to prevent falls as her strength returns. Neither oxytocin nor epidural anesthesia causes mononeuropathies. A lumbosacral plexopathy may result from pelvic trauma, but would present with more widespread symptoms. Although the risk of multiple sclerosis relapse is thought to increase during the first few postpartum months, there is little study of Uhthoff phenomenon after delivery. Further, although foot drop may be seen with either a multiple sclerosis flare or Uhthoff phenomenon (assuming prior symptom thereof), this is most likely to result from a central nervous system lesion and therefore would not have concurrent sensory loss in the same peripheral nerve distribution (*see* Bradley's NiCP, 7th edn, Ch. 107, pp. 1791–1866).

76. C. The notochord is represented by the number 1. This will later become the nucleus pulposus of the spinal cord. The neural tube, represented by the number 2, is formed by the neural plate bending and folding (neural folds) into a tube. It will later develop into the brain and spinal cord. The neural crest, represented by the number 3, initially forms the roof of the neural tube. Subsequently, these cells differentiate into multiple mesenchymal cells, including glia, melanocytes, smooth muscle cells, cartilage, and bone. The somites are labeled 4 in this drawing. These represent pairs of mesodermal tissue that develop along the axis of the developing embryo. The neural tube develops between the pairs of somites; fusion of the neural tube begins at the fifth somite; and the ultimate division between brain and spinal cord is at the fourth somite. The neural plate is not present in this drawing. The neural plate becomes the neural tube and neural crest cells after folding in on itself (temporarily becoming the neural folds). Figure from Moore KL, Persaud TVN, and Torchia MG 2013 Nervous system. In: *The Developing Human*, 9th edn, pp. 389–427, Figure 17-1, Elsevier, with permission.

77. B. The patient has moderate mental retardation (MR) based on his IQ of 45. Normal IQ is >70, mild MR has an IQ range of 55–70, moderate MR has a range of 40–55, and severe MR has a range of 25–40. Based on the included description of his habitus along with a strong family history of MR, fragile X syndrome is most likely. This is the most commonly inherited form of MR and is due to a CGG expansion in *FMR1* on the X chromosome. Common physical signs include elongated face, high forehead, protuberant ears, and enlarged testicles. There is often a strong family history of MR, and men are most often affected (due to the dysfunction of a single X chromosome). Females may also be affected by fragile X syndrome due to X inactivation (lyonization) of the normal X copy. Their phenotype is generally less severe, though it often includes premature ovarian failure. Other causes of MR include chromosomal abnormalities such as Down syndrome (trisomy 21), Rett syndrome, Prader-Willi syndrome, Angelman syndrome, toxic disturbances, metabolic disturbances, and pre/perinatal birth injuries or infections.

78. D. The most likely diagnosis is a complex partial seizure with secondary generalization from an

arteriovenous malformation (AVM, seen in the MRI). AVMs are arteriovenous connections without capillary networks, usually with gliotic brain tissue within the AVM. These often present with hemorrhages, headaches, or seizures. Typically, AVMs are observed if unruptured, but several factors are taken into consideration when determining whether or not to intervene: age, surgical risk, location, gender, and lifetime hemorrhage risk. Treatment options include surgical resection, radiosurgery, endovascular embolization, or a multimodal approach (especially if >3 cm). The Spetzler-Martin grading system is a scale of 1–5 that helps estimate the risk of surgical repair of AVMs. A developmental venous anomaly is a congenital malformation of veins that drain normal brain and is considered one of the most common cerebral vascular malformations. On imaging, it appears as a curvilinear enhancing structure best seen on contrast sequences or susceptibility weighted imaging. A cavernous malformation is a collection of vessels without elastic tissue and has no normal brain parenchyma between the hyalinized vessels. They typically appear as a "popcorn kernel" on T2 imaging. An aneurysm is a weakening of a vessel wall that creates either a saccular aneurysm or a fusiform aneurysm. Capillary telangiectasias are capillary-sized vessels that have normal brain tissue in between them and are typically found in the pons. They often appear as ill-defined areas of focal enhancement (*see* Bradley's NiCP, 7th edn, Chs. 40, pp. 459–485 and 56, pp. 758–783). Figure from Murray AL, Dally M, Jeffreys A, Hwang P, Anderson JFI 2014 Neuropsychological outcomes of stereotactic radiotherapy for cerebral arteriovenous malformations. *Journal of Clinical Neuroscience* 21(4): 601–606, with permission.

79. B. Although the outcome of the CREST trial demonstrated no difference in the composite risk of stroke, myocardial infarction, or death between carotid stenting or carotid endarterectomy, it did demonstrate a periprocedural increased risk of stroke among patients who underwent carotid stenting, and a periprocedural increased risk of myocardial infarction among patients who underwent carotid endarterectomy (*see* Bradley's NiCP, 7th edn, Ch. 65, pp. 920–967).

80. D. Huntington disease (HD) is an autosomal-dominant condition resulting from an expansion of CAG repeats of the HD gene on chromosome 4. Generally, HD appears with more than 40 CAG repeats, and tends to be earlier onset with greater numbers of repeats, known as *genetic anticipation*. From a psychiatric perspective, patients can have depression, irritability, psychosis, obsessive-compulsive disorder, or even suicide. Many times, patients will complain of difficulty with sleep initiation as well. The examination will often show parkinsonism, especially in young-onset HD. Other examination findings include dystonia and chorea (either facial, truncal, distal extremities, or generalized). Imaging will often show atrophy or absence of the caudate, resulting in "box-car ventricles." In this case, the gradual onset (rather than acute) of both motor and psychiatric symptoms in the setting of family history of suicide and drug use makes HD high on the differential. Even if family history is unknown or reportedly negative, genetic testing should still be completed. A stroke of the subthalamic nucleus can also lead to choreiform movements, but the onset

is usually acute and leads to unilateral chorea. There is nothing in the question stem indicating a recent streptococcal infection that would point toward Sydenham chorea. Anti-NMDA receptor encephalitis has been associated with chorea, but would not show an absence of caudate nuclei. Substance abuse resulting in dopamine release, such as cocaine intoxication, can also lead to chorea, but usually has an acute onset and would not have absent caudate nuclei (*see* Bradley's NiCP, 7th edn, Ch. 96, pp. 1422–1460). Figure from, Perkin DG, Miller DC, Lane RJM, Patel MC, Hochberg FH 2010 *Atlas of Clinical Neurology*, 3rd edn, Saunders, with permission.

81. A. Oxytocin and vasopressin are produced in the supraoptic and paraventricular nuclei of the hypothalamus, then stored in and secreted from the posterior pituitary gland (neurohypophysis). It drives many physiological functions, including the "letdown reflex" involved with breastfeeding and uterine contractions during labor. The other hormones listed in the question are released from the anterior pituitary gland and can be remembered by the mnemonic *FLAT PiG* including FSH, luteinizing hormone (LH), ACTH, TSH, prolactin, and growth hormone (*see* Bradley's NiCP, 7th edn, Ch. 52, pp. 696–712).

82. A. Meniere disease is caused by excess endolymph in the inner ear, also known as *endolymphatic hydrops*. The exact cause of the fluid buildup is not known. Symptoms include episodic vertigo, progressive hearing loss in one or both ears, tinnitus, and aural pressure. This disease may uncommonly run in families. Benign paroxysmal positional vertigo is associated with sudden, severe bursts of vertigo with head movement, usually lasting seconds, and is often thought to be associated with otolith malpositioning. It may improve with otolith repositioning maneuvers such as the Epley maneuver. Mal de débarquement syndrome is a vertigo syndrome of a persistent sense of rocking or swaying movement felt after a cruise or turbulent flight. This syndrome often resolves spontaneously with time. Opsoclonus-myoclonus is a rare syndrome in which patients have continuous, involuntary, conjugate, random movements of the eyes, as well as jerking movements of the axial skeletal muscles. Other symptoms include ataxia, mutism, and developmental delay. Opsoclonus-myoclonus is felt to be autoimmune, and may be associated with neuroblastoma or ovarian cancer as a paraneoplastic syndrome. Labyrinthitis, most commonly associated with a viral infection or less frequently with medications or trauma, is associated with vertigo, hearing loss, and tinnitus (*see* Bradley's NiCP, 7th edn, Ch. 46, pp. 583–604).

83. C. Whipple disease is caused by an infection with *Tropheryma whippelii*, leading to low-grade fevers, arthralgia, diarrhea, muscle wasting, and hyperpigmentation. Neurological symptoms include extrapyramidal symptoms, limitations of vertical gaze, and characteristic oculomasticatory myorhythmia (pendular oscillations of the eyes with rhythmic contractions of the masticatory muscles). Wilson disease is an autosomal-recessive disorder resulting in accumulation of copper resulting in liver disease, movement disorders, and dementia. Fever and oculomasticatory myorhythmia are not present in Wilson disease. Neurosyphilis causes psychosis,

necessary for pilocytic astrocytomas. Finally, intravenous antibiotics would only be necessary if the lesion were an abscess, along with surgical draining (*see* Bradley's NiCP, 7th edn, Ch. 75, pp. 1065–1083). Figure from Grant LE, Griffin N 2013 *Grainger and Allison's Diagnostic Radiology Essentials*, Churchill Livingstone, with permission.

98. D. Mucormycosis classically affects diabetic patients, involving invasion of the cavernous sinuses. Tolosa-Hunt syndrome is an idiopathic, recurrent, steroid-responsive granulomatous disease that usually affects the cavernous sinuses. Idiopathic intracranial hypertension may cause abducens palsy due to tension on the nerve, but is not associated with cavernous sinus syndrome. Pituitary adenomas may invade the cavernous sinuses and cause compressive cranial neuropathies. However, the rapidity of symptom onset, epistaxis, and nasal mass noted in the question stem make this less likely. Rather than cavernous sinus symptoms, carotid-cavernous fistulae more commonly present with pain, pulsatile proptosis, ocular injection, progressive vision loss, and an ocular bruit on careful auscultation (*see* Bradley's NiCP, 7th edn, Chs. 79, pp. 1147–1158 and 104, pp. 1720–1735).

99. E. Cocaine is the most commonly abused illegal stimulant. With acute use, cocaine typically causes pupillary dilation, tachycardia, and hypertension. Headaches are the most common reason for patients to seek medical attention after using cocaine, but many other neurological side effects are possible, including hemorrhagic or ischemic strokes, seizures, chorea, tics, paranoia, and hallucinations. It is believed that hallucinations, paranoia, and agitation are a result of cocaine blocking dopamine reuptake in the nucleus accumbens, causing psychiatric symptoms and promoting addiction through stimulation of reward centers (*see* Bradley's NiCP, 7th edn, Ch. 87, pp. 1254–1260).

100. E. Mitoxantrone is an infused drug that is technically classified as an antineoplastic therapy, suppressing T-cells, B-cells, and macrophages. This drug is FDA approved for secondary progressive multiple sclerosis. Teriflunomide is an oral pyrimidine synthetase inhibitor, an enzyme required by lymphocytes for proliferation. It is FDA approved for relapsing multiple sclerosis. Fingolimod is an oral sphingosine 1-phosphage receptor modulator that keeps lymphocytes in lymph nodes (and therefore out of the blood or brain). It is FDA approved for relapsing multiple sclerosis. Dimethyl fumarate is an oral

medication whose mechanism of action is unclear, other than the fact that it inhibits immune cells and may have protective antioxidant properties in the brain and spine. It is FDA approved for relapsing forms of multiple sclerosis. Glatiramer acetate is an injectable synthetic protein that is thought to simulate myelin basic protein and block myelin-damaging T-cells, although the mechanism of its efficacy is poorly understood. It is FDA approved for relapsing multiple sclerosis (*see* Bradley's NiCP, 7th edn, Ch. 80, pp. 1159–1186).

101. C. Memantine is an N-methyl-D-aspartate antagonist used to treat cognitive impairment related to various conditions, but it is not used to treat fatigue. Notably, however, a placebo-controlled trial of memantine did not show improvement of cognitive impairment related to multiple sclerosis. Pemoline, modafinil, amantadine, and dalfampridine all have been shown to improve multiple sclerosis–related fatigue (*see* Bradley's NiCP, 7th edn, Ch. 80, pp. 1159–1186).

102. C. This patient has a C6 radiculopathy on the left side. She has dermatomal sensory loss in a pattern consistent with a C6 radiculopathy. The area of sensory loss is innervated by the lateral antebrachial cutaneous nerve, superficial radial sensory, and median nerve. The only area in which these nerves all meet is at the C6 root. EMG should show abnormalities in muscles with significant C6 innervation, like the biceps, brachioradialis, triceps, pronator teres, and brachialis (see Table 1.102).

103. A. Valproic acid has been shown to have a slight, but significant, risk of pancreatitis, among many other side effects, including hepatoxicity, thrombocytopenia, teratogenicity, and milder effects like tremor and weight gain. Topiramate has an increased risk of teratogenicity, metabolic acidosis, nephrolithiasis, anhydria, and cognitive slowing. Propranolol has an increased risk of worsening depression, cardiac arrhythmias, and worsening asthma. Amitriptyline has an increased risk of depression, QT prolongation, and other cardiac arrhythmias. Verapamil has an increased risk of cardiac arrhythmias, hepatotoxicity, and paralytic ileus (*see* Bradley's NiCP, 7th edn, Ch. 101, pp. 1563–1614).

104. C. $GABA_B$ receptors are metabotropic receptors that cause a downstream efflux of potassium leading to hyperpolarization. $GABA_A$ receptors are ligand-gated chloride channels leading to an influx of chloride and hyperpolarization.

TABLE FOR ANSWER 1.102

C5	C6	C7	C8	T1
Rhomboids	**Biceps**	**Triceps**	**Extensor indicis proprius**	**Abductor pollicis brevis**
Infraspinatus	**Brachialis**	**Pronator teres**	**Flexor pollicus longus**	*First dorsal interosseus*
Supraspinatus	**Pronator teres**	**Extensor carpi radialis**	**Extensor digitorium communis**	*Pronator quadratus*
Deltoid	**Triceps**	**Flexor carpi radialis**	**Pronator quadratus**	*Adductor pollicis*
Biceps	**Brachioradialis**	**Anconeus**	**First dorsal interosseus**	*Adductor digiti minimi*
Brachialis	*Anconeus*		**Adductor digiti minimi**	
	Deltoid		**Adductor pollicis**	
	Supra/infraspinatus		**Flexor digitorium profundus**	
	Extensor carpi radialis		**Flexor carpi ulnaris**	

Adapted from AANEM Minimonograph #32. Bolded muscles indicate major root contribution. Italicized muscles indicate minor contribution from the root.

105. C. Primary progressive aphasia is a subclass of frontotemporal dementia that involves progressive loss of speech to the point of mutism. This patient presents with normal memory and orientation but has paraphasic errors. Memory and visuospatial function should be normal. Early in the disease this disorder may not be appreciated unless testing of verbal fluency is performed, including categorical fluency (naming as many animals as possible in 1 minute, or naming as many words starting with the letter "S" as possible in 1 minute) or more formal testing like the Boston Naming Test. Alzheimer disease would present with short-term memory loss and visuospatial dysfunction, in addition to anomic aphasia. Dementia with Lewy bodies presents with well-formed visual hallucinations, fluctuating levels of alertness, memory loss, and parkinsonism. Mild cognitive impairment is a disorder of mild memory impairment that is isolated and not significant enough to affect daily life. Although this patient's language dysfunction is isolated, the speech abnormalities are significant and abnormalities are noted on imaging. Vascular dementia is the second most common type of dementia and results from cerebral ischemia, usually progressing in a stepwise fashion, related to either large or small infarcts. This often results in poor short-term memory and slow processing, and can appear similar to Alzheimer disease except the MRI shows multiple ischemic lesions. This disorder should be recognized because with stroke risk reduction measures, the underlying process of this type of dementia can be slowed (*see* Bradley's NiCP, 7th edn, Ch. 95, pp. 1422–1461).

Test Two

QUESTIONS

1. A 45-year-old female with a history of hyperlipidemia, hypertension, and gout presents with a 2-week history of progressive pain in her shoulders and hips. She has difficulty reaching objects in her tall kitchen cabinets and has noticed the need to use her arms when rising from a chair. Which of the following medications is not associated with this condition?

   A. Colchicine

   B. Lisinopril

   C. Atorvastatin

   D. Labetalol

   E. Niacin

2. A 12-year-old boy presents to the office for evaluation of weakness. With exercise, he gets cramps and fatigue in his legs to the extent that he is unable to keep up with his peers during gym class. Cramps usually occur within minutes of starting exercise, and he seems to get a "second wind" if he is able to rest for a few minutes after the cramps begin. He denies dark urine. His neurological examination is normal. Serum creatine kinase (CK) level is elevated at 650 IU/L (normal is usually 50–200 IU/L). An exercise forearm test is performed and shows a normal rise in ammonia, but no rise in the lactate. The patient's most likely diagnosis is caused by which of the following?

   A. Alpha-glucosidase deficiency

   B. Myophosphorylase deficiency

   C. *PMP22* duplication

   D. Absence of muscular dystrophin

   E. Debranching enzyme deficiency

3. Which of the following is *not* a type of multiple sclerosis?

   A. Relapsing-remitting

   B. Primary progressive

   C. Secondary progressive

   D. Progressive relapsing

   E. Intermittent progressive

4. Which of the following is the primary source of energy production in the human body?

   A. Urea cycle

   B. Krebs cycle

   C. Beta-oxidation

   D. Malate-aspartate shuttle

   E. Anaerobic metabolism

5. A 62-year-old woman presents with gradually progressive cognitive decline, along with stiffness, slowness, and intermittent jerks of her right upper extremity. Her speech has become monotone, slurred, and slow. On examination, she has dystonic posturing of the right arm with increased rigidity and bradykinesia. There is also intermittent myoclonus when the right arm is held up. When speaking, the patient's right arm will seemingly rise on its own accord, and she will use the left arm to pull it back down. Her family feels that she often neglects the right side of her body. The patient's MRI is shown in the figure below. Which of the following is typical of this diagnosis?

   A. Tau deposition

   B. Alpha-synuclein deposition

   C. Levodopa-responsive rigidity

   D. Autonomic dysfunction

   E. Prominent hallucinations

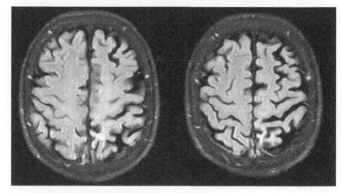

Figure for Question 2.5.

6. Which of the following medications has the highest risk of fetal malformation?

   A. Carbamazepine

   B. Valproic acid

   C. Phenytoin

   D. Phenobarbital

   E. Lamotrigine

7. Which is the most prevalent bloodborne inflammatory cell type within infarcted tissue at 1 hour poststroke?

   A. Neutrophils

   B. Macroglia

   C. Lymphocytes

   D. Eosinophils

   E. Dendritic cells

8. Which is the key distinction between vestibular neuritis and labyrinthitis?

   A. Direction of nystagmus

   B. Sensation of rotating vs. undulating ground

   C. Hearing loss

   D. Fever

   E. Loss of balance

9. A 15-year-old male presents to your office with a complaint of falls. This has been occurring over the last several months. His examination demonstrates bilateral foot drop, loss of sensation to the midshin in both legs, absent reflexes, and high arched feet with atrophy in his feet. Nerve conduction studies demonstrate motor conduction velocities at 20 m/s in all nerves without conduction blocks and absent sensory responses. Electromyography shows neurogenic units in the distal leg. Which genetic mutation is most likely responsible for this patient's symptoms?

   A. *PMP22* deletion on chromosome 17

   B. *MFN2* mutation on chromosome 3

   C. *PMP22* duplication on chromosome 17

   D. *SOD1* mutation on chromosome 21

   E. GAA triplet repeat on chromosome 9

10. Mutation in which of the following is *not* associated with an increased risk of Alzheimer disease (AD)?

    A. Amyloid precursor protein

    B. Presenilin-1

    C. Presenilin-2

    D. Apolipoprotein E4

    E. Gamma secretase

11. Which of the following is the most likely cause of the magnetic resonance imaging (MRI) finding demonstrated here?

    A. Intracranial hypertension

    B. Motion artifact

    C. Subdural hemorrhage

    D. Wegener granulomatosis

    E. Glioblastoma

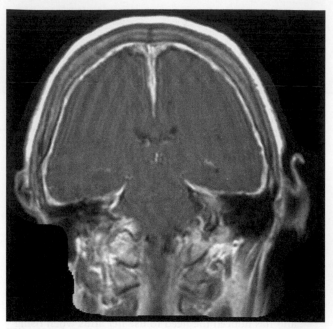

Figure for Question 2.11.

12. A 45-year-old woman presents for evaluation of severe major depressive disorder that is refractory to treatment with multiple serotonergic agents, adjunct therapy with mood stabilizers, and antipsychotics. Electroconvulsive therapy (ECT) is considered. All of the following is true regarding ECT *except*?

    A. Electroconvulsive therapy is for the treatment of catatonia.

    B. Anterograde amnesia is a possible side effect of ECT.

    C. Electroconvulsive therapy has been shown to be a safe but effective treatment for depression.

    D. Recent myocardial infarction is a relative contraindication to ECT.

    E. A space-occupying brain lesion is a relative contraindication to ECT.

13. At rest, neuronal membranes are most permeable to which ion?

    A. Sodium

    B. Chloride

    C. Potassium

    D. Calcium

    E. Magnesium

14. A 53-year-old female presents to the emergency department with fevers, confusion, and severe headache. On neurological examination she has a stiff neck, papilledema, and a temperature of 103.6°F. Computed tomography scan of her head is unremarkable. A lumbar puncture is performed and demonstrates a white blood cell count of 400 (with a predominance of neutrophils), protein of 90, and glucose of 10. Which of the following is the most appropriate empiric treatment?

    A. Vancomycin, ampicillin, and ceftriaxone

    B. Vancomycin and ceftriaxone

    C. Vancomycin, metronidazole, and ceftriaxone

    D. Isoniazid, rifampin, and ethambutol

    E. Vancomycin and metronidazole

15. A 63-year-old female who is on her seventh day of a hospital stay for a subarachnoid hemorrhage (SAH) acutely develops right arm weakness and slurred speech. The following transcranial Doppler (TCD) of her left middle cerebral artery (MCA) is shown. Which of the following is the best treatment for this condition?

    A. Oral nimodipine
    B. IV tissue plasminogen activator (tPA)
    C. IV mannitol
    D. Extraventricular drain placement
    E. Intraarterial calcium channel blocker

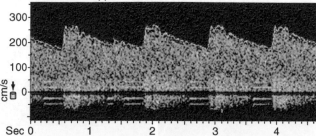

Figure for Question 2.15.

16. A 7-year-old left-handed boy presents for evaluation of poor grades. The patient previously hit all developmental milestones, and in his first 2 years of school he progressed with the other children. In the last 4 months he has developed significant difficulty with his math class to the extent that he is now well behind his peers. However, he maintains average grades in his other classes. Neurological examination is normal, and electroencephalogram (EEG) in both the awake and sleep state is normal. Which of the following is the most likely diagnosis?

    A. Mild intellectual disability
    B. Dyscalculia
    C. Gerstmann syndrome
    D. Attention-deficit/hyperactivity disorder (ADHD)
    E. Metachromatic leukodystrophy

17. A 17-year-old girl with a history of anxiety and migraines is evaluated for dizzy spells. Each episode seems to occur upon standing, and is associated with lightheadedness, palpitations, and the perception of falling, although she has never lost consciousness. Increased fluid intake has not improved the symptoms, and electroencephalogram is normal. A tilt-table test reveals an increase of heart rate by 40 beats per minute without change in blood pressure. Although tachycardic on the tilt-table, she experiences a typical spell of dizziness. Which of the following would *not* be considered part of the workup for this condition?

    A. Supine plasma norepinephrine levels
    B. Standing plasma norepinephrine levels
    C. Holter monitor
    D. Magnetic resonance image (MRI) of the brain
    E. Plasma metanephrines

18. Which of the following hypothalamic nuclei controls the circadian rhythm?

    A. Supraoptic nucleus
    B. Lateral nucleus
    C. Anterior nucleus
    D. Suprachiasmatic nucleus
    E. Arcuate nucleus

19. An otherwise healthy 68-year-old woman presents with 1 week of difficulty reading and right-sided clumsiness. Routine blood work, including complete blood count, was normal. Her brain magnetic resonance image is shown, including T1 postcontrast and the apparent diffusion coefficient (ADC) images. Which of the following is the most likely cause of her symptoms?

    A. Glioblastoma
    B. Meningioma
    C. Metastatic lung cancer
    D. Central nervous system (CNS) lymphoma
    E. Progressive multifocal leukoencephalopathy (PML)

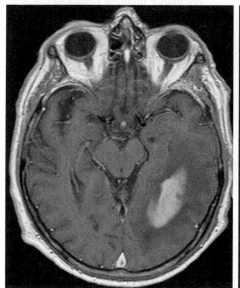
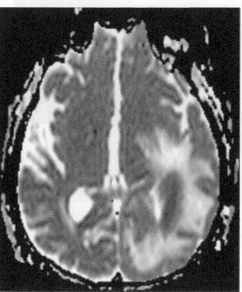

Figure for Question 2.19.

28. A 67-year-old woman with a long history of smoking presents with new horizontal diplopia and headache. On examination, her right eye is deviated inferiorly and laterally, she has mild right ptosis, and she has marked right mydriasis with no reaction to light. Which of the following is the most important next step in her care?
    A. Antiplatelet therapy
    B. Cerebral angiography
    C. Hemoglobin A1C
    D. Ophthalmology consult
    E. Brain computed tomography (CT)

29. Despite return of circulation and respiratory function, an 82-year-old patient has been declared brain dead after suffering an anoxic injury from cardiac arrest. The patient's family is requesting that the patient have a percutaneous endoscopic gastrostomy and tracheostomy placed for long-term nutrition and ventilation. Which of the following is the most appropriate response?
    A. Refuse to perform any further procedures.
    B. Transfer the patient to a different hospital.
    C. Comply with family requests.
    D. Consult the ethics committee.
    E. Contact organ donation services.

30. Which of the following antipsychotics should be avoided in patients with obesity?
    A. Olanzapine
    B. Aripiprazole
    C. Clozapine
    D. Haloperidol
    E. Ziprasidone

31. After a night without her continuous positive airway pressure (CPAP; usually set at 20 cm positive end-expiratory pressure [PEEP]), a morbidly obese woman is noticeably more drowsy and confused than usual. Which of the following is the likely etiology?
    A. Hyperventilation
    B. Hyperammonemia
    C. Hypoxia
    D. Hypercarbia
    E. Uremia

32. A 22-year-old female presents for evaluation of arm numbness. Over the last year, she has experienced numbness in both hands and forearms, which waxes and wanes throughout the day. She was previously seen by three other neurologists and had normal magnetic resonance images (MRIs) of her neck and head; normal electromyography and nerve conduction studies; and normal blood work looking for metabolic, inflammatory, and toxic exposures. She is preoccupied with the idea that she may have multiple sclerosis (MS), despite reassurances of multiple normal MRIs. She has even joined a local MS support group. Which of the following is the most likely diagnosis?
    A. Conversion disorder
    B. Malingering
    C. Illness anxiety disorder
    D. Factitious disorder
    E. Generalized anxiety disorder

33. By what age should a child be able to produce two-word sentences?
    A. 6 months
    B. 12 months
    C. 18 months
    D. 24 months
    E. 36 months

34. Which of the following is primarily responsible for switching from a urinary storage state to a urinary voiding state?
    A. Sympathetic outflow
    B. Pontine micturition center
    C. Thalamic nuclei
    D. Local spinal reflex
    E. Motor cortex

35. Taste receptors on the fungiform papillae are innervated by which cranial nerve (CN)?
    A. V
    B. VII
    C. IX
    D. X
    E. XII

36. A 43-year-old man who recently received chemotherapy presents with sharp and stabbing pain in the left T4 dermatome. Approximately 4 months before his visit, he was diagnosed with acute herpes zoster infection in the same dermatome, which has now resolved. The present pain is much more severe than the original rash. On examination, there is scarring from his prior eruption, along with a decrease in sensation to temperature and pin prick in the left T4 dermatome. Which of the following is true regarding this condition?
    A. The condition affects only peripheral pain receptors.
    B. Young age is a risk factor for developing this condition.
    C. This condition always occurs after a vesicular rash.
    D. The location of the preceding virus does not affect the risk of developing this condition.
    E. An immunocompromised state is a risk factor for developing this condition.

37. Assuming a nonfatal injury and medical stability, which of the following is an important component to patient care after a gunshot wound to the right parietal lobe?
    A. Urgent removal of bullet fragments
    B. Angiography to rule out pseudoaneurysms
    C. Broad-spectrum antibiotics to prevent abscess formation
    D. Magnetic resonance imaging (MRI) of the brain to identify the extent of tissue damage
    E. Early transcranial magnetic stimulation for rehabilitation

38. A 16-year-old female suffers with recurrent severe, lateralized, pulsatile headaches with light and sound sensitivity. These tend to occur during her menses and may last for up to 3 days at a time. Which of the following would be the best choice for a first-line therapeutic trial?
    A. Hydrocodone as needed
    B. Perimenstrual scheduled naproxen
    C. Perimenstrual scheduled propranolol
    D. Valproic acid as needed
    E. Perimenstrual magnesium oxide and riboflavin

39. A patient is asked to show how to use a hammer. The patient acts out cutting with a saw instead of using a hammer. Which of the following correctly identifies this condition?
    A. Ideomotor apraxia
    B. Ideational apraxia
    C. Conceptual apraxia
    D. Limb-kinetic apraxia
    E. Dissociation apraxia

40. A 33-year-old previously healthy woman has an acute onset of neck pain, headache, and decreased vision on the right field. She also complains of heaviness in her right arm and difficulty speaking. Her examination shows nonfluent aphasia, a right homonymous hemianopsia, and right hemiparesis. Magnetic resonance imaging confirms the suspected etiology of her symptoms, from which a key T1 fat-saturated image is shown. Otherwise, workup is negative. What is the most likely etiology of her condition?
    A. Venous sinus thrombosis
    B. Hypercoagulable state from neoplasm
    C. Atrial fibrillation
    D. Oral contraception pills
    E. Arterial dissection

41. Which syndrome is associated with a surprisingly good verbal and social capacity despite a mildly diminished intelligence quotient (IQ), often referred to as having a "cocktail party" personality?
    A. Asperger syndrome
    B. Down syndrome
    C. Fragile X syndrome
    D. Williams syndrome
    E. Angelman syndrome

42. Which of the following insurance programs is available to Americans over the age of 65 who have paid Medicare tax, or to a person of any age with a diagnosis of end-stage renal disease or amyotrophic lateral sclerosis?
    A. Medicaid
    B. Medicare
    C. Affordable Care Act
    D. Aetna
    E. Tricare

43. A 40-year-old woman underwent muscle biopsy for progressive weakness, among other symptoms. Which of the following is her most likely diagnosis based on the image shown?
    A. Emery-Dreifuss muscular dystrophy
    B. Dermatomyositis
    C. Polymyositis
    D. Conversion disorder
    E. Inclusion body myositis

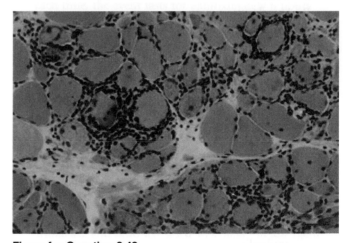

Figure for Question 2.43.

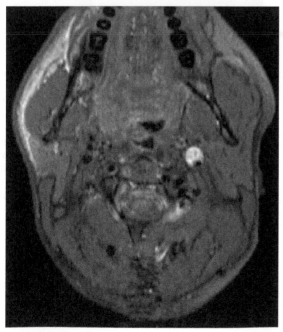

Figure for Question 2.40.

60. The magnetic resonance image (MRI) of the lumbar spine shown here demonstrates which abnormality?

    A. Syringomyelia
    B. Transverse myelitis
    C. Subacute combined degeneration
    D. Diastematomyelia
    E. Congenital spinal stenosis

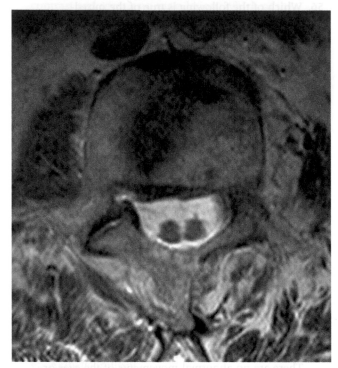

Figure for Question 2.60.

61. All of the following are appropriate uses of social media by physicians except?

    A. Separate profiles for private and professional use
    B. Using high privacy settings to protect personal information
    C. Reporting unprofessional content by colleagues
    D. Communication with patients about their medical conditions
    E. Messaging a patient to start a romantic relationship

62. The brain photomicrograph shown here is suggestive of which condition?

    A. Herpes simplex virus (HSV) encephalitis
    B. Dementia with Lewy bodies
    C. Creutzfeldt-Jakob disease
    D. Alzheimer disease
    E. Oligodendroglioma

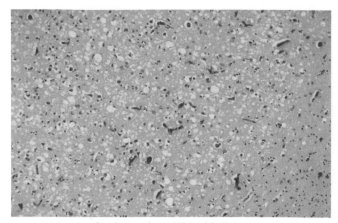

Figure for Question 2.62.

63. A 50-year-old man with acquired immunodeficiency syndrome (AIDS) presents to the hospital with several days of confusion, followed by a decline in level of consciousness. A computed tomography scan of the brain demonstrates diffuse atrophy, but no acute findings. A lumbar puncture is performed, and opening pressure is 60 cm (normal is <20 cm). The spinal fluid further demonstrates a glucose of 10 mg/dL (normal is 45–80 mg/dL), protein of 140 mg/dL (normal is 15–45 mg/dL), normal red blood cells, and 9 white blood cells/mL (normal is <5 cells/mL) with a lymphocytic predominance. Based on your suspected diagnosis and while awaiting further studies, which of the following is the best course of action after removing a large volume of cerebrospinal fluid (CSF)?

    A. Emergent ventriculoperitoneal shunt
    B. Initiate amphotericin B and flucytosine
    C. Initiate antituberculous therapy
    D. Initiate acetazolamide
    E. Initiate vancomycin and rifampin therapy

64. A 22-year-old female presents to the office with an episode of left arm weakness. The suspected diagnosis is multiple sclerosis (MS), and the only test ordered is a magnetic resonance imaging (MRI) of the brain to help confirm that suspicion. It shows a single small subcortical white matter hyperintense fluid attenuated inversion recovery (FLAIR) lesion. Treatment for MS is started. Which cognitive bias is shown by this example?

    A. Availability bias
    B. Confirmation bias
    C. Anchoring bias
    D. Premature closure
    E. Diagnosis momentum

65. All of the following are true about rod cells in the retina *except*?

    A. Predominantly in the peripheral portion of the retina
    B. Sensitive to low levels of illumination
    C. Contains chromatic photopigments
    D. More easily activated by light
    E. Contain more photopigment than cones

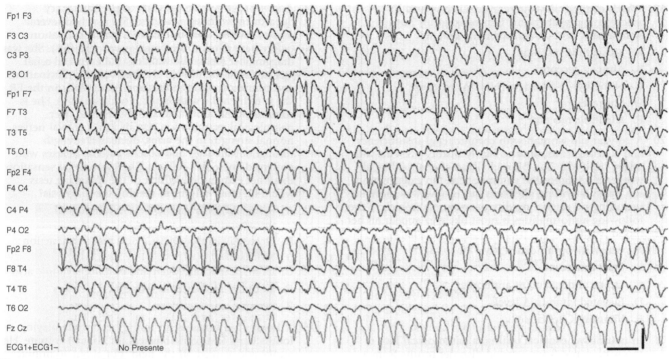

Figure for Question 2.66.

66. A 61-year-old male was admitted to the hospital with sepsis from pneumonia. He was intubated in the intensive care unit (ICU) while being stabilized. On his fourth day of admission his vital signs had normalized, but he would not wake up off of sedation. The electroencephalogram (EEG) shown here was obtained. Which of the following is the most likely diagnosis?

    A. Herpes encephalitis

    B. Nonconvulsive status epilepticus

    C. Hepatic encephalopathy

    D. Medication-induced encephalopathy

    E. Bacterial meningitis

67. Since witnessing his younger brother drown in a pool, a 20-year-old man has panic attacks and recurring dreams of drowning. Now each time he closes his eyes, he has flashbacks of attempting to jump into the pool to save his brother, which results in poor sleep. These flashbacks are vivid and are often hard to distinguish from reality. He has also avoided vacations to the beach with friends due to a fear of swimming. What is the most likely diagnosis?

    A. Panic disorder

    B. Posttraumatic stress disorder (PTSD)

    C. Rapid eye movement (REM) sleep behavior disorder

    D. Generalized anxiety disorder

    E. Bereavement

68. A 27-year-old female who is currently 25 weeks pregnant presents to the emergency department with double vision. She recently started an oral magnesium supplement because of headaches. Double vision started 1 week ago and has been intermittent during this time. Today on awakening, the patient could not open her left eye. Her neurological examination demonstrates left-sided ptosis, and her left eye is adducted at rest. She has limited movements of the left eye and cannot look upward for more than a few seconds with the right eye before her right eye closes. She has no pupillary abnormalities, and she has mildly nasal speech. Magnetic resonance imaging and magnetic resonance angiography of the head were both normal. All of the following are true of this condition during pregnancy *except*?

    A. Exacerbations can be precipitated by the use of magnesium, fluoroquinolones, macrolides, and certain anesthetics.

    B. Prednisone is the first-line treatment during pregnancy.

    C. Poor feeding and respiratory weakness can persist in the child for 6 weeks after delivery.

    D. Intravenous immunoglobulin (IVIG) is a treatment option during pregnancy.

    E. This disorder is transmitted to the child in an autosomal-dominant manner.

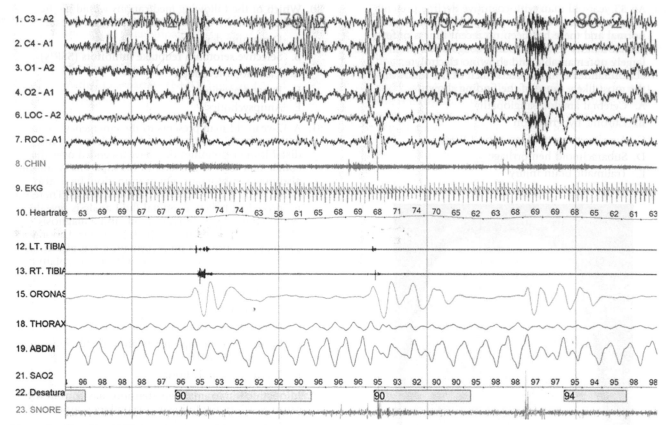

Figure for Question 2.84.

84. The figure below shows a 120-second segment from an overnight polysomnogram. Which of the following is demonstrated in the picture?

    A. Mixed apnea
    B. Obstructive apnea
    C. Central apnea
    D. Paradoxical breathing
    E. Cheyne-Stokes breathing

85. A 48-year-old woman awakens with a severe "thunderclap" headache and a stiff neck and is taken to the emergency room. A computed tomography (CT) scan of the brain reveals no evidence of hemorrhage. Which of the following is the next best step?

    A. Lumbar puncture
    B. Angiogram
    C. Ergotamine therapy
    D. Nimodipine therapy
    E. Venography

86. In comparison to type II muscle fibers, type I muscle fibers include which of the following qualities?

    A. Fast-twitch fibers
    B. Easy fatigability
    C. Higher contractile strength
    D. Higher amount of mitochondria
    E. Anaerobic respiration

87. Which of the following may be problematic after blunt-force neck injury?

    A. Hearing
    B. Ocular alignment
    C. Sense of smell
    D. Heart rate
    E. Articulation

88. In median nerve somatosensory evoked potentials, the N13 peak corresponds with which anatomical location?

    A. Medial meniscus
    B. Cerebral cortex
    C. Thalamus
    D. Cervical spinal cord
    E. Erb's point

89. A magnetic resonance image (MRI) of a newborn infant is shown here. Which of the following defects is demonstrated?
    A. Lissencephaly
    B. Pachygyria
    C. Encephalocele
    D. Porencephaly
    E. Schizencephaly

90. The electroencephalogram (EEG) of a 7-year-old boy during wakefulness and sleep is shown in the figure below. He presented with speech delay. Which of the following is the most likely diagnosis?
    A. Childhood absence epilepsy
    B. Lennox-Gastaut syndrome
    C. Juvenile myoclonic epilepsy
    D. Autosomal-dominant nocturnal frontal lobe epilepsy
    E. Landau-Kleffner syndrome

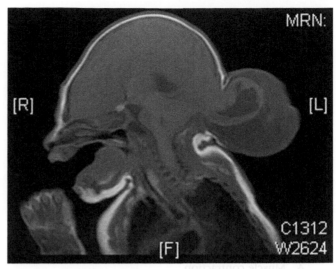

Figure for Question 2.89.

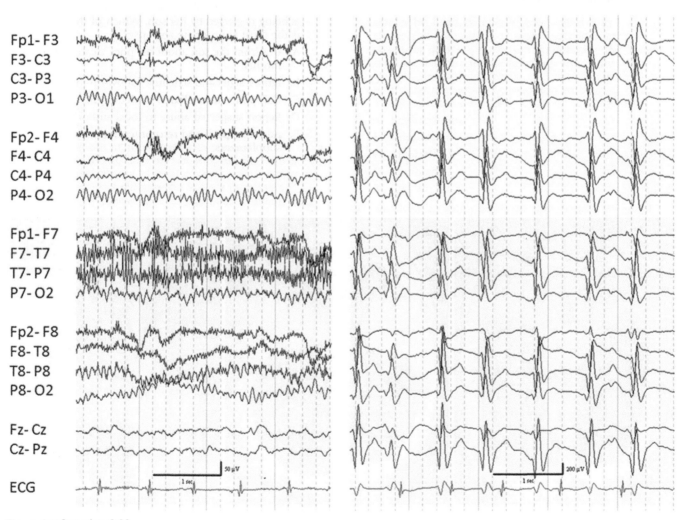

Figure for Question 2.90.

102. All of the following medications can precipitate a myasthenic crisis except?

    A. Lisinopril

    B. Prednisone

    C. Magnesium

    D. Propranolol

    E. Ciprofloxacin

103. Which of the following antiepileptic medications is a strong hepatic enzyme inhibitor?

    A. Phenytoin

    B. Valproic acid

    C. Carbamazepine

    D. Levetiracetam

    E. Zonisamide

104. Which statement about voltage-gated sodium channels is false?

    A. The activation gate is closed at resting membrane potential and rapidly opens upon depolarization.

    B. The inactivation gate is open at resting membrane potential and closes slowly upon depolarization.

    C. Opening of the activation gate leads to an influx of sodium and resting membrane hyperpolarization.

    D. The inactivation gate remains closed until repolarization has occurred.

    E. Voltage-gated sodium channels cluster in the nodes of Ranvier.

105. A 75-year-old male presents with an acute stroke. On examination he has mild right arm and face weakness. He has spontaneous speech with occasional paraphasic errors. He can understand and follow commands. Repetition is severely impaired. Which of the following best explains his speech pattern?

    A. Broca aphasia

    B. Transcortical aphasia

    C. Anomic aphasia

    D. Conduction aphasia

    E. Wernicke aphasia

ANSWERS

1. B. Lisinopril does not cause a toxic myopathy, whereas colchicine, statin medications, niacin, and labetalol are all known for causing toxic myopathies. Other common substances that can lead to toxic myopathy include zidovudine, propofol, alcohol, and corticosteroids, to name a few (*see* Bradley's NiCP, 7th edn, Ch. 110, pp. 1915–1955).

2. B. McArdle disease, also known as *myophosphorylase deficiency* or *type V glycogenosis*, is an autosomal-recessive disorder resulting in a deficiency of myophosphorylase. This is the most common disorder of carbohydrate metabolism. Patients typically present in childhood with exercise intolerance, cramps, and pain induced by brief intense activity. CK may be elevated. Often a phenomenon known as *second wind* is seen with McArdle disease, which involves a return of strength and reduction in pain after a short rest due to mobilization of blood glucose as a muscle energy source rather than relying on breakdown of glycogen. An exercise forearm test can identify a disorder of glycogen metabolism by measuring levels of ammonia and lactate. In this test, baseline ammonia and lactate levels are drawn, followed by intense exercise of the hand with levels of ammonia and lactate drawn at serial intervals. Glycogen metabolism disorders show a normal elevation of ammonia, but a lack of rise in lactate. The diagnosis is confirmed with a muscle biopsy that shows a lack of uptake to a myophosphorylase stain. Alpha-glucosidase deficiency is also known as *Pompe disease*. The most common form of this condition presents in childhood with hypotonia, cardiomegaly, and hepatomegaly. The juvenile form presents with progressive proximal muscle weakness, lumbar lordosis, and a waddling gait, which can appear similar to Duchenne muscular dystrophy (DMD). An adult form presents in the 40s, with proximal muscle weakness similar to polymyositis. Pompe disease is diagnosed with an assay for alpha glucosidase activity or muscle biopsy. *PMP22* duplication is the genetic defect seen in Charcot-Marie-Tooth disease type 1A, which is an autosomal-dominant hereditary demyelinating neuropathy. Absence of dystrophin on muscle biopsy makes a diagnosis of DMD, which presents with progressive weakness, pseudohypertrophy of the gastrocnemii, and a Gower's sign typically in young males. There is no "second wind" phenomenon in DMD. Debranching enzyme deficiency is a rare glycogenosis that presents in the third to fourth decade and causes severe weakness and atrophy of muscles, often mimicking amyotrophic lateral sclerosis. Liver failure can also occur, but there is no "second wind" phenomenon (*see* Bradley's NiCP, 7th edn, Ch. 110, pp. 1915–1955).

3. E. The four types of multiple sclerosis are named for the pattern of their clinical presentation. The image shows the typical pattern of progressive disability with these disease types, (**A**) relapsing-remitting (the most common), (**B**) secondary progressive, (**C**) primary progressive, and (**D**) progressive relapsing (*see* Bradley's NiCP, 7th edn, Ch. 51, pp. 676–695).

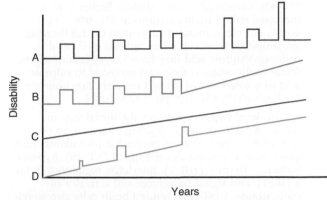

Figure for Answer 2.3 *(from Greenberg BM 2009 Multiple sclerosis. In: Waldman SA, Terzic A (eds.)* Pharmacology and Therapeutics: Principles to Practice, *Elsevier, with permission.)*

4. B. The Krebs cycle (also known as the *citric acid cycle* or the *tricarboxylic acid cycle*) produces the majority of energy in the human body in the form of adenosine triphosphate (ATP). In the Krebs cycle, acetate from carbohydrates, lipids, and proteins is oxidized to produce 38 ATP per glucose molecule. The urea cycle is a pathway for turning ammonia into urea. Beta-oxidation refers to the breakdown of fatty acid molecules for the production of acetate (which later enters the Krebs cycle). The malate shuttle is a shunt of electrons across the inner membrane of the mitochondrion for use during oxidative phosphorylation. Anaerobic metabolism occurs when no oxygen is available, and pyruvate is broken down in the cytoplasm (rather than mitochondrion), leaving a waste product of lactic acid. Anaerobic metabolism produces 2 ATP per molecule of glucose.

5. A. This case is a typical clinical scenario for corticobasal ganglionic degeneration (CBGD). This is a progressive neurodegenerative disease characterized by tau deposition and a number of clinical findings, including motor apraxia, cortical sensory loss, sensory neglect, myoclonus, tremor, rigidity, and dystonia. Typically, the onset begins asymmetrically and may look clinically similar to idiopathic Parkinson disease (PD). However, CBGD is usually unresponsive to levodopa, and is associated with more cortical findings than is typical for idiopathic PD. Occasionally patients will have one limb that will slowly rise and "have a mind of its own," known as *alien limb syndrome*. Although CBGD may have some clinical overlap with progressive supranuclear palsy or frontotemporal dementia, magnetic resonance imaging will often differentiate with asymmetric parietal lobe atrophy. Alpha-synuclein deposits are commonly associated with multiple system atrophy (MSA), idiopathic PD, and dementia with Lewy bodies, but not with CBGD. Typically, autonomic dysfunction is found in MSA. Prominent hallucinations are found in dementia with Lewy bodies (*see* Bradley's NiCP, 7th edn, Ch. 96, pp. 1422–1460). Figure from Lize J, Jong FJ, van Swieten J 2013 An unusual case of logopenic progressive aphasia associated with corticobasal syndrome. *Alzheimer's & Dementia: The Journal of the Alzheimer's Association* 9(4.S): 23, with permission.

6. B. Valproic acid is the anticonvulsant with the highest risk of fetal malformations, in the range of 9%–10%, whereas other antiepileptics are in the range of

3%–5%. Lamotrigine has a slightly higher-than-average increased risk of malformations at 5%–6%. Valproic acid is not recommended in women of childbearing age unless there are no other options to control epilepsy. Valproic acid may have longer-lasting effects. Some studies suggest that fetal exposure to valproic acid may lower verbal IQ and memory function (*see* Bradley's NiCP, Ch. 112, pp. 1973–1991).

7. A. Localized hypoxia prompts the initial step in poststroke inflammation, leading to activation of second-messenger systems expressing proinflammatory genes such as nuclear factor kappaB (NF-κB), hypoxia-inducible factor 1 (HIF-1), interferon regulatory factor 1 (IRF1), and signal transducer and activator of transcription 3 (STAT3). Injured brain cells also secrete platelet-activating factor (PAF), tumor necrosis factor alpha (TNF-α), and interleukin 1-beta (IL-1β). These reduce the stability of the blood–brain barrier and allow for cellular infiltration. Neutrophils are the first cells to invade the infarcted tissue within 30 minutes to a few hours after stroke and peak by 1–3 days. By 4–6 hours postinfarct, astrocytes become hypertrophic and microglia activate. Lymphocytes, dendritic cells, monocytes, and macrophages follow thereafter. Macrophages become the predominant cell type by 5–7 days postinfarction (*see* Bradley's NiCP, 7th edn, Ch. 65, pp. 920–967).

8. C. Labyrinthitis and vestibular neuritis are both peripheral vertigo syndromes, usually caused by viral infection. The key distinction between the two is that labyrinthitis affects both the cochlear and vestibular nerves and, therefore, causes hearing loss in addition to vertigo, whereas vestibular neuritis affects the vestibular nerve and only causes vertigo. Either of these viral syndromes can lead to fever or loss of balance. The type of perceived movement and the direction of nystagmus are not specifically helpful in determining the affected nerves in these conditions (*see* Bradley's NiCP, 7th edn, Ch. 46, pp. 583–604).

9. C. This patient has a hereditary, not acquired, demyelinating neuropathy, as evidenced by slow nerve conduction velocities without conduction block. The most common hereditary demyelinating neuropathy is Charcot-Marie-Tooth (CMT) type 1a, which is caused by a *PMP22 duplication* on chromosome 17. *PMP22 deletion* causes the syndrome of hereditary neuropathy with liability to pressure palsies. *MFN2* is a common abnormality in CMT2a, which typically causes an axonal neuropathy more than a demyelinating neuropathy. *SOD1* on chromosome 21 is involved in autosomal dominant motor neuron disease. GAA triplet repeat on chromosome 9 is involved in Friedrich ataxia (*see* Bradley's NiCP, 7th edn, Ch. 107, pp. 1791–1867).

10. E. Gamma secretase is an amyloid-cleaving enzyme. Excessive gamma secretase activity has been associated with AD development, though there is no causative genetic mutation known for this. Autosomal-dominant mutations in amyloid precursor protein, presenilin-1, and presenilin-2 are all causative of early-onset AD. Apolipoprotein E4 is an isoform associated with an increased risk of AD development, though it has not been proven to be causative (*see* Bradley's NiCP, 7th edn, Ch. 95, pp. 1380–1421).

11. D. The MRI shown is a postcontrast T1 image demonstrating diffuse enhancement of the meninges called *pachymeningitis*, which is seen in intracranial hypotension, Wegener granulomatosis, Sjögren disease, temporal arteritis, rheumatoid arthritis, carcinomatosis, and several infections, including Lyme disease, syphilis, tuberculosis, and various fungal infections. Although motion artifact is present on this scan, the most significant finding is pachymeningeal enhancement (*see* Bradley's NiCP, 7th edn, Ch. 105, pp. 1736–1765). Figure from Mayans D, personal collection, with permission.

12. B. Electroconvulsive therapy is considered a safe and effective treatment (in up to 80% of patients) of many conditions, including medically unresponsive depression, highly suicidal patients, mania, catatonia, neuroleptic malignant syndrome, and acute schizophrenia. Electroconvulsive therapy is also used in severely depressed patients who are also pregnant. Many times, ECT must be repeated for seven to eight sessions. Absolute contraindications are unclear, but relative contraindications include unstable coronary disease with recent infarction, congestive heart failure, poorly controlled hypertension, seizure disorder, and space-occupying lesions. Possible side effects include memory impairment such as retrograde amnesia for the time surrounding the hospitalization, autonomic instability, headache, nausea, and confusion after ECT.

13. B. At rest the membrane is most permeable to chloride (*see* Bradley's NiCP, 7th edn, Ch. 34–35, pp. 349–391).

14. A. This patient presents with bacterial meningitis, which is diagnosed by her lumbar puncture showing an elevated white cell count with a neutrophil predominance, elevated protein, and low glucose. A lymphocytic pleocytosis in the cerebrospinal fluid with relatively normal glucose indicates a viral infection. Empiric treatment depends on age and predisposing factors. Recommendations are shown in the following table. In this patient, because she is over the age of 50, ampicillin must be added for empiric coverage of *Listeria* (*see* Bradley's NiCP, 7th edn, Ch. 79, pp. 1147–1158).

TABLE FOR ANSWER 2.14 Empiric Antibiotics for Bacterial Infections of the CNS

Disease entity	Organisms	Empiric antibiotics
Bacterial meningitis		
Age <50 and no risk factors for *Listeria*	*S. pneumoniae*, *N. meningitidis*	Vancomycin + ceftriaxone *or* cefotaxime or cefepime
Age >50 and/or risk factors for *Listeria*	As noted earlier + *L. monocytogenes*	As noted earlier + ampicillin
Sinusitis, mastoiditis, or otitis predisposing cause of meningitis	As noted earlier (depending on age and risk factors) + anaerobes	As noted earlier (depending on age and risk factors) + metronidazole
Brain abscess	*S. aureus*, aerobic and anaerobic streptococci, oral and gastrointestinal flora (including *Bacteroides* spp.)	Vancomycin + ceftriaxone *or* cefotaxime or cefepime + metronidazole
	Nocardia	Trimethoprim-sulfamethoxazole
Spinal epidural abscess	*Staphylococcus* spp., *Streptococcus* spp., enteric gram-negative bacilli	Vancomycin + ceftriaxone *or* cefotaxime *or* cefepime
Any of the above	*M. tuberculosis* (high suspicion)	Four-drug therapy (isoniazid, rifampin, ethambutol, pyrazinamide)

From Bradley's NiCP, 7th edn, Table 53C.2.

15. E. TED should be used on patients with subarachnoid hemorrhage (SAH) for at least the first 14 days after the hemorrhage to assess for vasospasm. When mean flow velocities reach 200 m/s (and our case is 215 m/s), this indicates severe vasospasm. The patient clinically has symptoms of ischemia that correspond to the artery that has velocities indicating vasospasm. Emergent treatment with intraarterial calcium channel blockers and angioplasty should be performed to prevent further ischemia. Oral nimodipine is used in SAH to prevent vasospasm, but would not be useful in the acute setting. Although the patient appears to have cerebral ischemia based on clinical exam, IV tPA would not be indicated because of the recent SAH and because the mechanism for ischemia is vasospasm rather than thrombosis. Increased intracranial pressure is common in patients with SAH and should be a consideration. TCD in increased intracranial pressure typically shows a high-resistance waveform, normal or low velocities, and low diastolic flow, whereas the waveform in the figure demonstrates an elevated velocity with elevated diastolic flow (*see* Bradley's NiCP, 7th edn, Ch. 40, pp. 459–485). Figure from Winn H 2011 *Youmans Neurological Surgery*, Saunders, with permission.

16. B. Dyscalculia is the inability to manipulate numeric information, learn arithmetic facts, or execute arithmetic procedures in the setting of a normal neurological examination and normal cognitive function. Dyscalculia is common in patients with ADHD, but this patient does not show impulsivity, impaired attention, distractibility, or hyperactivity. Generally patients with ADHD have problems in all of their classes rather than a specific subject. Mild intellectual disability involves deficits in multiple cognitive domains, including language, executive function, memory, reading, and social skills, and is associated with an IQ between 50 and 70. These patients do not develop normally, and impairments are usually known before starting school. Gerstmann syndrome involves left–right dissociation, finger agnosia, dyscalculia, and constructional apraxia due to a lesion in the dominant inferior parietal lobe (angular gyrus or supramarginal gyrus). Metachromatic leukodystrophy is a disorder caused by a deficiency in the enzyme arylsulfatase A resulting in destruction of myelin sheaths. In the juvenile form, patients initially develop normally but later have significant regression in school, eventually leading to muscle weakness, rigidity, vision loss, seizures, and dementia (*see* Bradley's NiCP, 7th edn, Ch. 90, pp. 1301–1323).

17. D. There is no indication for an MRI of the brain in postural orthostatic tachycardiac syndrome (POTS). This is a syndrome defined by having a heart rate increase of more than 30 beats per minute from supine to standing (5–30 minutes), exaggeration of symptoms when standing, and improvement with recumbence. Further, patients must have symptoms for 6 months or longer, and must have standing plasma norepinephrine levels of 600 pg/mL or more (both standing and supine plasma norepinephrine levels are collected). POTS-associated symptoms may include mental clouding, blurred or tunneled vision, shortness of breath, palpitations, tremors, dizziness, or nausea. There is also a higher incidence of anxiety and chronic fatigue in patients with POTS. Importantly, patients usually do not lose consciousness with this condition, and blood pressure is generally normal. Mimickers of POTS include pheochromocytoma, neutrally neurally-mediated syncope (e.g. vasovagal syncope), or mast cell activation. Diagnosis of POTS is typically made with a tilt-table test. Treatment includes an increase of dietary salt; compression stockings; exercise; or medications such as fludrocortisone, clonidine (which decreases sympathetic tone), propranolol, midodrine, pyridostigmine, or modafinil. A Holter monitor would ensure that only sinus tachycardia is present, because other arrhythmias can mimic POTS (*see* Bradley's NiCP, 7th edn, Ch. 2, pp. 8–16).

18. D. The suprachiasmatic nucleus of the hypothalamus controls circadian rhythm. The supraoptic nucleus synthesizes antidiuretic hormone and oxytocin. The lateral nucleus controls appetite (as opposed to the ventromedial nucleus, which inhibits appetite). The anterior nucleus controls body temperature, preventing overheating through activation of the parasympathetic nervous system when necessary. The arcuate nucleus produces dopamine (*see* Bradley's NiCP, 7th edn, Ch. 52, pp. 696–712).

19. D. The imaging appearance of an avidly and homogeneously enhancing intraparenchymal mass that abuts a cerebrospinal fluid space is classical for CNS lymphoma. Further, restricted diffusion of water, as shown on the ADC map, is common with CNS lymphoma, representing the increased cellularity of the mass. Primary CNS lymphoma, which may include affected sites in the brain, spine, spinal fluid, or vitreous, does not affect other parts of the body and may have normal blood work. Glioblastoma, although an enhancing, intraparenchymal disease, is generally peripherally or heterogeneously enhancing due to central necrosis. Meningiomas, although brightly and solidly enhancing, are extraparenchymal tumors that arise from the meninges. Metastatic lung cancer would often be associated with multiple ring-enhancing lesions, with edema disproportionate to the size of the tumor(s). PML, although generally affecting the white matter, is usually a nonenhancing disease. Additionally, this infection with the John Cunningham (JC) virus tends to be associated with severe immunosuppression, which was not mentioned in this patient (*see* Bradley's NiCP, 7th edn, Ch. 41, pp. 486–503). Figure from Naidich TP, Castillo M, Cha S, Smirniotopoulos JG (eds.) 2013 *Imaging of the Brain* (Expert Radiology Series), Saunders, with permission.

20. E. Upon suspicion or diagnosis of central nervous system (CNS) lymphoma, it is important to first identify the presence of systemic lymphoma involvement (if present), which requires separate treatment by medical oncologists. Second, it is important to identify the extent of disease involvement within the CNS before beginning therapy in order to accurately monitor the efficacy of therapy with subsequent imaging. Generally, extent of disease evaluation for the CNS includes MRI with contrast of the brain and entire spine, ophthalmological examination with a slit lamp, and lumbar puncture with cerebrospinal fluid analysis for glucose, protein, cellularity, bacterial cultures, cytology, and flow cytometry. Ensuring there is no systemic involvement of the cancer is done with either computed tomography, with and without contrast of the chest, abdomen, and pelvis, or with a positron emission tomography scan of the whole body. In older men, a testicular ultrasound may additionally be considered, as this is the most common site of lymphoma in this population. Whereas John Cunningham (JC) virus

DNA levels are usually detectable in cases of progressive multifocal leukoencephalopathy, there is no reason to routinely evaluate for this infection in CNS lymphoma.

21. C. Taking into account the patient's medical and family history, as well as the MRI, the most likely cause of his hearing difficulties is bilateral vestibular schwannomas. These are noted to have bright, fairly homogeneous enhancement, as well as the classical ice cream cone shape on MRI, with the "cone" represented by the enhancing portion of the tumor entering the internal auditory canal. Medulloblastoma is a tumor of the posterior fossa, generally involving the cerebellum, but is not bilateral or homogeneously enhancing. Therefore involvement of the internal auditory canals is not easily explained by this diagnosis. Leptomeningeal metastasis does often affect cranial nerves, such as the acoustic nerves, but would be rare to present so slowly or with such large tumor burden on MRI. Further, there is no leptomeningeal enhancement on MRI. Glioblastoma is exceedingly rare in the posterior fossa, and would not explain the internal auditory canal involvement or the enhancement homogeneity. Meningiomas are a reasonable consideration given the radiographic appearance, but the specific internal auditory canal involvement and lack of dural tail point away from this diagnosis. Also the positive family history suggests only vestibular schwannomas out of the available choices (see Bradley's NiCP, 7th edn, Ch. 100, pp. 1538–1562). Figure from Terry AR, Plotkin SR 2012 Chemotherapy in vestibular schwannoma: evidence-based treatment. *Otolaryngologic Clinics of North America* 45(2): 471–486, with permission.

22. E. Neurofibromatosis type 2 is an autosomal-dominant tumor predisposition syndrome that most classically presents with bilateral vestibular schwannomas, but may also involve juvenile posterior subcapsular cataracts, neurofibromas, meningiomas, or gliomas. The inactive gene leading to this syndrome is *NF2* on chromosome 22q11, which normally encodes a protein called *merlin*. The tumors are unlikely to be sporadic, given their bilateral nature and the positive family history. Neurofibromatosis type 1 is a separate autosomal-dominant tumor predisposition syndrome caused by mutations in the *NF1* gene on chromosome 17 encoding a protein called *neurofibromin*. This disease is more common than neurofibromatosis type 2 and is associated with café-au-lait spots, freckling of the axilla and inguinal regions, Lisch nodules, neurofibromas, optic pathway gliomas, scoliosis, and learning disabilities. Tuberous sclerosis is an autosomal-dominant disorder that affects multiple organ systems, related to the *TSC1* (encoding hamartin) and *TSC2* (encoding tuberin) genes. Affected individuals may demonstrate subependymal giant cell astrocytomas, cortical tubers, subependymal nodules, facial angiofibromas, and Shagreen patches, as well as difficulties with the heart, lungs, and kidneys. Ionizing radiation may increase the risk of gliomas and meningiomas, but without mention of exposure and with positive family history, this is less likely (see Bradley's NiCP, 7th edn, Ch. 100, pp. 1538–1562).

23. B. The MRI shows a small lesion in the pituitary gland, which is likely a pituitary microadenoma (<10 mm). Approximately 60%–70% of pituitary adenomas are hormone secreting, with the remainder being clinically silent. The gonadotrophic adenomas are the most common type of pituitary macroadenoma (>10 mm).

Of those that are silent, it is usually not until there is a bitemporal hemianopsia or headache that the neoplasm is found. Other symptoms can include cerebrospinal fluid rhinorrhea and pituitary apoplexy. Diagnosis is usually made using a combination of history (visual complaints, fatigue, decreased libido, erectile dysfunction, amenorrhea) and MRI imaging, as well as serological studies such as prolactin (lactotrophic adenomas), IGF-1 (somatotrophic adenomas), 24-hour urine-free cortisol (corticotrophic adenomas), and luteinizing hormone or follicle-stimulating hormone, both gonadotrophic adenomas. These adenomas can also cause pituitary hypofunction when nonsecreting adenomas compress the normal pituitary cells. Once diagnosed, one can proceed with therapy such as bromocriptine or transsphenoidal surgery with or without adjuvant radiotherapy (see Bradley's NiCP, 7th edn, Ch. 52, pp. 696–712). Figure from Rennert J, Doerfler A 2007 Imaging of sellar and parasellar lesions. *Clinical Neurology and Neurosurgery* 109(2): 111–124, with permission.

24. C. The patient is suffering from fatal familial insomnia. This is an autosomal-dominant prion disease that can be transmitted to others who come in contact with the prion protein. This disease is marked by dramatic insomnia and disruption of the typical sleep cycles. REM is almost nonexistent. Over time, patients develop ataxia, myoclonus, an abnormal gait, and memory loss. There is also increased sympathetic activation, which can lead to very high levels of serum catecholamines. MRI can show atrophy of the thalamus, particularly the anterior ventral and dorsomedial nuclei. Positron emission tomography scans show hypometabolism of the thalamus and cingulate cortex. The disorder leads to coma and death in a short period. IVIG could be used in cases of an autoimmune encephalitis, but this patient's family history suggests an inherited disorder. The MRI findings are not consistent with limbic encephalitis (see Bradley's NiCP, 7th edn, Ch. 102, pp. 1615–1685).

25. A. A classic amnestic syndrome refers to loss of recent (short-term) episodic memory, which generally relates to bilateral hippocampal damage. Patients with such syndromes generally have impaired recent memory and orientation, but preserved procedural memory, immediate memory, and remote memory (see Bradley's NiCP, 7th edn, Ch. 7, pp. 57–65).

26. E. The pattern demonstrates typical hypsarrhythmia. This involves a chaotic pattern with multifocal spike and waves. The seizure discussed in the question stem is consistent with infantile spasm, which may be either as described in the question or with truncal extension and arm extension. West syndrome involves the triad of infantile spasms, arrest of development, and hypsarrhythmia. Slow spike and wave at 1–2.5 Hz is consistent with Lennox-Gastaut syndrome (LGS). Frequently, children with a hypsarrhythmia pattern will transition into an LGS pattern later in childhood. This brief clip from the EEG does show an area of attenuation in the midportion of the recording, but this is not considered a burst suppression pattern, which would be dominated by suppression with brief bursts of activity arising from the suppressed background. The attenuation shown is when the epileptic spasms occur. This EEG also demonstrates multifocal spikes, not solely left temporal spikes. Finally, quiet sleep is a pattern seen in neonates. It is the precursor to slow wave sleep and is marked by a

pattern of tracé alternans (*see* Bradley's NiCP, 7th edn, Ch. 101, pp. 1563–1614). Figure from Daroff RB, Jankovic J, Mazziotta JC, Pomeroy SL 2016 *Bradley's Neurology in Clinical Practice*, 7th edn, Elsevier, with permission.

27. E. The patient suffered a spinal column fracture at T12–L1 that severed the spinal cord just above the level of the conus medullaris. All of the symptoms listed are commonly seen with severe spinal cord injury, except for hyperreflexia. In the immediate postinjury setting, spinal shock is usually associated with low tone and absent reflexes. Symptoms of cauda equina syndrome and conus medullaris syndrome are also likely in this young man, and are delineated in the table (*see* Bradley's NiCP, 7th edn, Ch. 63, pp. 881–902). Figure from Daroff RB, Jankovic J, Mazziotta JC, Pomeroy SL 2016 *Bradley's Neurology in Clinical Practice*, 7th edn, Elsevier, with permission.

TABLE FOR ANSWER 2.27 Similarities and Differences between Conus Medullaris Syndrome and Cauda Equina Syndrome

Conus medullaris syndrome	Cauda equina syndrome
Upper and lower motor neuron involvement	Lower motor neuron involvement
Symmetrical motor impairment	Asymmetrical motor impairment
Vertebral column injuries between T12 and L2	Vertebral column injuries distal to L2
Absent deep tendon reflexes	Absent deep tendon reflexes
Permanent areflexic bladder	Permanent areflexic bladder
Absent bulbocavernosus reflex	Absent bulbocavernosus reflex

28. B. The patient presented with an oculomotor palsy, an entity that is conceptually divided by whether or not the pupil is involved. Given that the pupillary parasympathetic fibers are located superomedially on the oculomotor nerve, they are particularly at risk of compression by an aneurysm of the adjacent posterior communicating artery. The patient described in the question stem has pupil involvement in her oculomotor neuropathy, and therefore should be evaluated for an enlarging aneurysm as the cause of her symptoms. If her pupil were not involved, one might consider an evaluation for ischemic cause of the neuropathy, especially given her smoking history (*see* Bradley's NiCP, Ch. 104, pp. 1720–1735).

29. A. The patient has been declared brain dead, and therefore is legally dead in most states. This can be a confusing situation for families because the circulatory and respiratory systems can keep working for some time after all cerebral activity has ceased, making the concept of brain death hard to comprehend. In this situation the physician is acting ethically by refusing further procedures and should have a discussion with the family about why these procedures are being withheld. Physicians are not obligated to perform futile procedures. Neither transferring the patient to a different hospital nor complying with family requests is ethical, as the patient is dead and no further interventions will benefit her care. Contacting organ donation services may be reasonable, but can only be performed at the request of the family. Ethics consultation is not necessary, but could be helpful in the discussion with family.

30. A. Although all antipsychotics have a mild risk of weight gain, olanzapine is notorious for causing weight gain, metabolic syndrome, and diabetes. This is an important consideration because patients usually require long-term treatment with antipsychotics. Clozapine can cause agranulocytosis and requires frequent complete blood count monitoring. Haloperidol and ziprasidone can cause QT prolongation, and periodic electrocardiograms are recommended. Aripiprazole is unique in its mechanism of action because it is a partial dopamine agonist at D2 receptors. At low dopaminergic activity, it acts as an agonist, but at higher levels it is an antagonist. The main side effects include akathisia, somnolence, and worsening of extrapyramidal symptoms (*see* Bradley's NiCP, 7th edn, Ch. 10, pp. 92–114).

31. D. Hypercarbia, often causing a respiratory acidosis, may lead to encephalopathy with confusion and altered level of consciousness, especially when acute. Hypercarbia may result from untreated obstructive sleep apnea or obesity-related hypoventilation (both of which may be contributing to the current case), medication side effect as with opiates, or other causes of reduced ventilation. Other causes of encephalopathy and altered level of consciousness, including hyperammonemia and uremia, are generally not related to respiratory dysfunction. Hyperventilation, often caused by panic, dyspnea, or in response to metabolic acidosis (as with ketoacidosis), may lead to respiratory alkalosis and is commonly associated with lightheadedness, paresthesias, and sudden loss of consciousness. Hypoxia is generally associated with intrinsic lung disease rather than obstructive disease, and may cause lightheadedness, confusion, or loss of consciousness in severe cases (*see* Bradley's NiCP, 7th edn, Ch. 58, pp. 814–834).

32. C. The patient presents with illness anxiety disorder, which is a somatic symptom disorder (formerly somatoform disorder) in which patients are preoccupied with the idea that they are ill or that they may acquire an undiagnosed medical condition. Reassurance and negative workups do nothing to alleviate the anxiety, and ultimately the illness becomes part of the patient's identity. Illness anxiety disorder is a new diagnosis in the fifth edition of the *Diagnostic and Statistical Manual of Mental Disorders* and captures a large portion of patients formerly classified as hypochondriacs. Conversion disorder involves a loss or change in motor and/or sensory function without abnormal neurological function to explain the symptoms. One of the more typical manifestations of conversion disorder is a nonepileptic seizure. Acute stressors are not required at the onset for a diagnosis of conversion disorder, and the lack of severe anxiety distinguishes it from illness anxiety disorder. Malingering involves the intentional feigning of disease for personal gain, and there is nothing in the question to suggest this. Factitious disorder involves the intentional production of symptoms without a clear secondary gain. Generalized anxiety disorder is a persistent and excessive feeling of worry or tension about daily activities that makes one easily fatigued, irritable, causes sleep disturbance, impairs concentration, and leads to muscle tension.

33. D. Babbling usually occurs by 6 months, and simple "mama," "dada," and "bye-bye" by 9 months. By 1 year, children generally have about a 10-word vocabulary. A child should be able to use two-word sentences by 2 years of age, and should speak in complete sentences that can be understood by strangers by 3 years of age (*see* Bradley's NiCP, 7th edn, Ch. 8, pp. 66–72).

34. B. The detrusor and urethral sphincter muscles function in opposite tasks, and their working in concert requires input from various levels of the nervous system, including the brain and local spinal reflex. In the storage state, sympathetic outflow and local pudendal control are primarily responsible for urethral contraction, and a lack of parasympathetic input prevents detrusor activity. The pontine micturition center (with input from the hypothalamus, periaqueductal gray matter, and medial prefrontal cortex) is responsible for switching from the storage to voiding state, which is completed with additional parasympathetic input causing the detrusor muscle to contract (see Bradley's NiCP, 7th edn, Ch. 47).

35. B. Innervation of taste and the tongue involves multiple cranial nerves. CN VII through the chorda tympani branch innervates the taste buds on the fungiform papillae, which are located on the anterior tip and lateral portions of the tongue. CN VII also innervates the soft palate. CN IX innervates circumvallate taste buds across the posterior tongue. CN X innervates the taste sensation present in the pharynx. CN V is involved in pain, temperature, and touch sensation on the oral mucosa, but does not innervate taste buds (see Bradley's NiCP, 7th edn, Ch. 19, pp. 190–196).

36. E. The patient has a history of a recent herpes zoster infection in the left T4 dermatome distribution, with severe pain in the same region, which is consistent with postherpetic neuralgia (PHN). Both herpes zoster cutaneous infections and PHN are most common in patients over 60 years old, as well as those who are immunocompromised. It is thought that both central and peripheral pain receptors are involved in the pathophysiology of PHN. The pain is often described as burning, sharp, and stabbing, and can be associated with allodynia (pain evoked by normally nonpainful stimuli). The pain can occur after reactivation of the virus, with or without cutaneous eruption, as it resides in the dorsal root ganglion of the affected dermatome. In fact, even after the initial infection, patients may continue to have flare-ups of PHN without a rash (especially in the immunocompromised). Those who have trigeminal nerve involvement, especially in the V1 distribution, have the highest risk of PHN, whereas those with sacral or lumbar involvement have the lowest risk. Most often, the history makes the diagnosis, but a high index of suspicion is required, as there may not be a preceding rash. Treatment often involves the use of antiepileptics such as gabapentin or pregabalin, tricyclic antidepressants such as nortriptyline, or topical analgesics such as capsaicin as single agents or in combination. Antivirals may shorten the course, and vaccines may prevent the outbreak of herpes zoster (see Bradley's NiCP, 7th edn, Chs. 78, pp. 1121–1146 and 103, pp. 1686–1719).

37. B. Vascular injury is common with penetrating traumas to the brain (25%–36% incidence). Traumatic pseudoaneurysms develop when all layers of the vessel wall are damaged and surrounding brain tissue forms an aneurysmal wall. Patients with penetrating injuries to the brain should undergo early angiogram to screen for pseudoaneurysm, as well as a follow-up angiogram within the first several months. Generally, the risk of surgery for bullet fragment removal outweighs the benefits. Further, the heat associated with a bullet leaves the fragments sterile, so neither antibiotics nor fragment removal are generally required. MRI and transcranial magnetic stimulation should be avoided due to the potential ferromagnetism of remaining bullet fragments (see Bradley's NiCP, 7th edn, Ch. 62, pp. 867–880).

38. B. For women who suffer migraine headaches during menses but not at other times during the month, short-term prophylactic therapy may be efficacious for migraine prevention. Generally, scheduled nonsteroidal antiinflammatory drugs or triptans may be started 2–3 days before menses and continued for up to 2 weeks after menses for migraine prevention. There is no evidence of efficacy with short-term prophylaxis using beta-blockers or antiepileptics. Magnesium oxide and riboflavin both have limited evidence for migraine prevention when taken daily, but not only perimenstrually. Opioids are generally avoided for headache therapy, either abortive or preventive, due to risk of medication overuse headache, as well as rebound headaches (see Bradley's NiCP, 7th edn, Ch. 103, pp. 1686–1719).

39. C. Conceptual apraxia is a disorder in which patients are unable to point out a tool when its function is discussed or they are unable to discuss actions of particular tools. These patients do not have problems with coordinating their movements or following commands, but they demonstrate errors in mechanical knowledge. Ideomotor apraxia results in impaired control of skilled movements, so these patients have incorrect posture when using a tool, but know what it should be used for. For example, a patient knows what a hammer is, but attempts to hammer a nail with the handle instead of the head. Ideational apraxia is the inability to correctly order a series of movements to perform an action, making multistep actions quite confusing. Limb-kinetic apraxia results in a loss of fine motor movements and dexterity not related to weakness, making movements like tying shoes difficult. Dissociation apraxia occurs when a certain stimulus cannot evoke the proper reaction; patients cannot perform an action when verbally asked to do so, but they can mimic the action (see Bradley's NiCP, 7th edn, Ch. 12, pp. 122–127).

40. E. The etiology of her acute stroke is most likely an arterial dissection, as shown in the image. The axial image shows an intramural hematoma along the left internal carotid artery (crescent sign). Usually, dissections present with pain followed by acute neurological deficits (in this case, referable to the left frontal region). Common history clues include chiropractic manipulation, recent trauma (football injury, motor vehicle collision, fall), roller coaster ride, or aggressive coughing. Management for extracranial dissections includes antithrombotics (antiplatelets or anticoagulation) for at least 3–6 months followed by a repeat vessel imaging study such as computed tomography angiogram or magnetic resonance angiogram. Occasionally, pseudoaneurysms can form after dissections. Although venous sinus thrombosis can also present with headaches and lead to strokes in a young person, they often have more global findings and can be associated with strokes of the deep structures. One would expect to find a lack of venous flow on imaging rather than arterial disruption. There is no indication of atrial fibrillation in the question stem, but certainly this should be considered in a stroke where vessel imaging and echocardiogram are

normal. A hypercoagulable state from a neoplasm is another cause of stroke, especially recurring strokes with an otherwise negative workup. This can also predispose patients to venous thrombosis. Oral contraception pills may also increase the risk of stroke, especially in women over 35 years old who smoke (*see* Bradley's NiCP, 7th edn, Ch. 65, pp. 920–967). Figure from Mauro MA, Murphy KPJ, Thomson KR, Venbrux AC, Morgan RA 2014 *Image-Guided Interventions*, 2nd edn, Saunders, with permission.

41. D. Williams syndrome is a rare neurodevelopmental disorder caused by a multigene deletion on 7q. Characteristic findings in Williams syndrome include a facial appearance described as "elfin," as shown in the following image, and developmental delay with mildly decreased IQ, but strong language skills and knack for small talk. Physically, individuals with Williams syndrome may also have difficulty gaining weight (with failure to thrive), hypotonia, widely spaced teeth, and various heart malformations, including supravalvular aortic stenosis. Asperger syndrome is associated with poor social interaction, and is on the autism spectrum. Down syndrome and fragile X syndrome are associated with various levels of intellectual disability, but are not known for particularly good verbal abilities. Angelman syndrome is associated with intellectual disability and a characteristic happy personality, but verbal communication is generally poor (*see* Bradley's NiCP, 7th edn, Chs. 50, pp. 648–675 and 90, pp. 1324–1341).

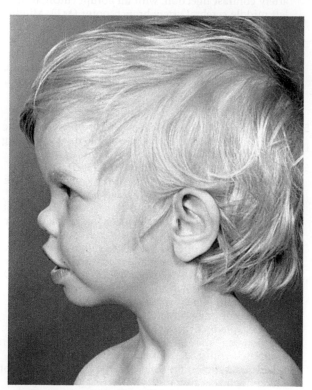

Figure for Answer 2.41 *(from Haldeman-Englert CR, et al. 2012 Specific chromosome disorders in newborns. In: Gleason CA, Juul SE (eds.) Avery's Diseases of the Newborn, 9th edn, Elsevier, with permission.)*

42. B. Medicare is a federally administered insurance program, managed through the Centers for Medicare and Medicaid Services (CMS), which is a component of the federal Department of Health and Human Services.

Medicare is available to individuals over the age of 65 who have paid Medicare tax from earned wages. Additional special populations covered by Medicare include any patient with end-stage renal disease (on dialysis) or any patient with amyotrophic lateral sclerosis. Medicaid is an insurance program administered by each individual state, although it receives a large proportion of its funding from CMS. Medicaid is generally reserved for individuals with low income or limited financial resources. The Affordable Care Act is a multifaceted federal law that, among other things, increased the number of insured Americans by expanding Medicaid coverage, establishing a federal insurance marketplace and providing monetary disincentives for remaining uninsured by choice, increasing the age until which a child may be on their parent's insurance (26 years), and preventing insurance denial for preexisting conditions. Aetna is a private medical insurance provider. Tricare is an insurance program administered by the U.S. Department of Defense to provide civilian health benefits for military personnel, military retirees, and their families.

43. C. The image demonstrates endomysial lymphocyte infiltration indicative of polymyositis. This pattern is in contrast to dermatomyositis, where biopsy shows perifascicular inflammatory infiltrate only. Emery Dreifuss muscular dystrophy is an X-linked disease that tends to affect boys between the ages of 5 and 15, with no inflammatory pathological findings, but with dystrophic features, including wide variation in fiber size and increased fibrous and adipose tissues. Inclusion body myositis is an inflammatory myopathy, with pathology showing vacuoles with basophilic granules (*see* Bradley's NiCP, 7th edn, Ch. 110, pp. 1915–1955). Figure from Uchino M, Yamashita S, Uchino K, et al. 2013 Muscle biopsy findings predictive of malignancy in rare infiltrative dermatomyositis. *Clinical Neurology and Neurosurgery* 115(5): 603–606, with permission.

44. A. Paraneoplastic syndromes are generally immune-mediated constellations of symptoms indirectly related to the presence of a tumor through molecular mimicry. Paraneoplastic cerebellar degeneration is associated with anti-Yo (PCA1) antibodies in many cases (*see* Bradley's NiCP, 7th edn, Table 97.1). Whereas the treatment of underlying cancers most often improves paraneoplastic syndromes, a clinician should be suspicious of cancer recurrence or progression when a treated cancer patient develops a paraneoplastic syndrome. Additional immunosuppressive therapy may be required for the treatment of paraneoplastic disorders, depending on the type, severity, and response to antineoplastic therapy. The severity and broad distribution of symptoms in this patient makes it unlikely that a microscopic brain metastasis could be causative. Paclitaxel causes peripheral neuropathy in many patients, but that would generally not cause speech change. Radiation to areas outside of the brain would not account for the symptoms listed. Although spine metastases may affect sensory function, they would not affect speech (*see* Bradley's NiCP, 7th edn, Ch. 97, pp. 1461–1483).

45. E. Ulnar neuropathy at the wrist is uncommon, but has four main types of entrapment. Type 1 entrapment is the most common and most proximal, where both motor and sensory fibers are affected, resulting in

weakness, numbness, and nerve conduction abnormalities in sensory and motor fibers. In severe cases, abnormal spontaneous activity and neurogenic motor units with reduced recruitment can be seen. The dorsal ulnar cutaneous nerve branches before the wrist, so it is not injured in ulnar neuropathy at the wrist. Froment sign is indicative of adductor pollicis weakness. To test for Froment sign, a patient should hold a piece of paper between the thumb and index finger; if the patient bends the distal portion of the thumb (using the flexor pollicis longus) to hold the paper in place, Froment sign is present (*see* Bradley's NiCP, 7th edn, Ch. 107, pp. 1791–1866).

46. A. Seizure is not a common symptom of sCJD, although a patient's electroencephalogram is often abnormal with periodic sharp wave discharges. Myoclonus, akinetic mutism, and visual and cerebellar disturbance are all common, as well as pyramidal and/or extrapyramidal signs. Additionally, magnetic resonance imaging often shows hyperintensity in the caudate and putamen, and there may be fluid attenuated inversion recovery (FLAIR) or diffusion weighted imaging (DWI) hyperintensity in the temporoparietal cortex. Cerebrospinal fluid 14-3-3 assay is often used for diagnostic confirmation in the absence of a brain biopsy (*see* Bradley's NiCP, 7th edn, Ch. 94, pp. 1365–1379).

47. A. Myasthenia gravis first affects the eyes in about half of the patients, with symptoms of diplopia or ptosis. Patients commonly complain of symptoms worsening with exercise or fatigue or in the evenings. Acetylcholine receptor–directed antibodies block acetylcholine receptors at the neuromuscular junction, leading to motor weakness in the affected muscle. Calcium channel–directed antibodies (P/Q) are associated with Lambert-Eaton myasthenic syndrome (LEMS), a paraneoplastic disorder. Although this patient does have a long history of smoking, this fact is a red herring. LEMS patients commonly complain of proximal muscle weakness and constipation, with improvement in the former after exercise. Further, bulbar symptoms are rare in LEMS. Thyroid-stimulating hormone receptor–directed antibodies are associated with Grave disease. Although this is associated with ophthalmopathy, including exophthalmos, diplopia is fairly rare among patients. Further, one would not expect fluctuation if diplopia were due to thyroid ophthalmopathy, given that the ocular and extraocular muscular changes are static. Aquaporin-4 antibodies are associated with neuromyelitis optica (Devic disease). Although patients commonly present with optic neuritis (frequently bilateral), fluctuating diplopia is not common. Retinal-directed antibodies are found in cancer-associated retinopathy, a paraneoplastic disorder commonly seen with melanoma and other cancers. Patients generally complain of progressive loss of visual acuity, whereas diplopia is not common (*see* Bradley's NiCP, 7th edn, Chs. 44, pp. 528–572 and 109, pp. 1896–1914).

48. B. The most common receptor implicated in schizophrenia is the D_2 receptor. There is increased dopamine receptor density in the limbic regions of schizophrenics and increased D_2 receptor occupancy on positron emission tomography imaging. Most D_2 receptors are located in the striatum, whereas D_1 receptors are located in the cerebral cortex and basal ganglia, D_3 and D_4 are in the limbic system, and D_5 receptors are in the thalamus, hippocampus, and hypothalamus.

49. B. Donepezil, rivastigmine, and galantamine are all reversible acetylcholinesterase inhibitors used in the treatment of Alzheimer disease. Common side effects include nausea, diarrhea, anorexia, headaches, and depression. More serious side effects include atrioventricular block, bradycardia, syncope, seizures, or gastrointestinal hemorrhage. Memantine is a glutamate receptor antagonist used in the treatment of moderate to severe dementia or as an add-on therapy to an acetylcholinesterase inhibitor. Common side effects include dizziness, headaches, confusion, somnolence, and rarely Stevens-Johnson syndrome. Edrophonium is a short-acting, reversible acetylcholinesterase inhibitor that can be injected intravenously to reverse acute symptoms of myasthenia gravis to assist in making the diagnosis. Rasagiline is a monoamine oxidase B inhibitor used in the treatment of Parkinson disease. Vitamin E was studied in Alzheimer disease and has had mixed findings of possibly slowing the progression from moderate to severe disease, but not mild cognitive impairment to mild Alzheimer disease. The role of vitamin E in Alzheimer disease treatment is yet to be determined (*see* Bradley's NiCP, 7th edn, Ch. 95, pp. 1380–1421).

50. D. The angiogram demonstrates a left common carotid artery contrast injection, with an abrupt cutoff at the left middle cerebral artery branch point (M1). Middle cerebral artery strokes generally cause hemiparesis and sensory loss, hemianopsia, and an expressive (or nonfluent) aphasia if in the dominant hemisphere (*see* Bradley's NiCP, 7th edn, Ch. 65, pp. 920–967). Figure from Daroff RB, Jankovic J, Mazziotta JC, Pomeroy SL 2017 *Bradley's Neurology in Clinical Practice*, 7th edn, Elsevier, with permission.

51. E. The patient in this case has Lesch-Nyhan syndrome (LNS), an X-linked recessive metabolic disease causing elevation of uric acid due to hypoxanthine-guanine-phosphoribosyl transferase (HPRT) deficiency. Clinically, LNS is associated with motor and cognitive regression after 3–6 months of age, with early hypotonia, which later becomes spasticity. The patient may also have movement disorders, such as chorea or athetosis, as well as aggressive and self-harming behavior. Serum uric acid levels are often elevated. The diagnosis of LNS can be made by clinical examination and by mutational analysis of the *HPRT* gene on the X chromosome. Allopurinol is a xanthine oxidase inhibitor and benefits patients with LNS due to reduction of uric acid levels. A purine-restricted diet also helps reduce uric acid. Both levodopa and tetrabenazine may be used for the movement disorders associated with LNS. Although patients may have seizures, levetiracetam would not be the best choice of antiepileptic because it may worsen aggression (*see* Bradley's NiCP, 7th edn, Ch. 91, pp. 1324–1341).

52. B. The correct answer is the older Caucasian man who has a history of substance abuse and access to weapons. In general, women attempt suicide more frequently than men, but men complete suicide more frequently than women. Those with an increased risk of suicide include previous suicide attempts, older age, men, Caucasian, socially isolated, substance abuse, and chronic illness. Those with a decreased risk of suicide

include no prior attempts, younger age, lack of impulsivity, women, African-American, married, lack of plan or exposure of weapons, and good health. The woman in choice A has a decreased risk of suicide because of her strong support system, age, and ethnicity. The woman in choice C has a history of borderline personality disorder and performs these attempts in order to attract attention. Although she is at an increased risk of suicide attempt, her risk is slightly lower for actual completion. The man in choice D has both a family at home and hope of a cancer cure, giving him likely reasons to not commit suicide. The woman in choice E also has a lack of impulsivity and a strong family network to lower her risk of suicide.

53. E. CSF is continually produced by the choroid plexus throughout the ventricular system and is reabsorbed by the arachnoid villi. Pericytes surround the endothelial cells of blood vessels in the brain. Ependyma refers to the glial-cell inner lining of the ventricles in the brain and central canal of the spinal cord. Chorionic villi are a part of the placenta (*see* Bradley's NiCP, 7th edn, Ch. 88, pp. 1261–1278).

54. E. The MRI shows the classic "molar tooth sign" often seen in Joubert syndrome. This is a condition associated with hypoplasia of the cerebellar vermis, usually inherited in an autosomal-recessive fashion. It is accompanied by breathing abnormalities, including hyperpnea alternating with periods of apnea, limb and truncal ataxia, oculomotor apraxia with nystagmus, and hypotonia. Many other signs and symptoms may also be associated with Joubert syndrome, including kidney and liver abnormalities, distinct facial features (widely spaced eyes, low-set ears, ptosis, broad forehead), polydactyly, and vision abnormalities including retinal dystrophy. Other cerebellar hypoplastic syndromes include Dandy-Walker syndrome and pontocerebellar hypoplasia (PCH). Dandy-Walker syndrome is characterized by agenesis of the cerebellar vermis, cystic dilatation of the fourth ventricle, and an enlarged posterior fossa with elevation of the tentorium. PCH involves atrophy of the pons and cerebellum that causes breathing abnormalities, intellectual disability, motor neuron degeneration, seizures, and corticospinal abnormalities, all depending on the type of PCH (*see* Bradley's NiCP, 7th edn, Ch. 44, pp. 528–572). Figure from Hoyt CS, Taylor D 2013 *Pediatric Ophthalmology and Strabismus*, Saunders, with permission.

55. B. Glycine is the main inhibitory neurotransmitter of the spinal cord. GABA is a major inhibitory neurotransmitter in the brain. Dopamine, serotonin, and glutamate are excitatory transmitters.

56. B. The mixed-mechanism antidepressants are known for their dual mechanism of action, usually involving the serotonin system, dopaminergic, and/or noradrenergic syndrome. Bupropion works by blocking the reuptake of norepinephrine and dopamine, and is used for smoking cessation and depression. It can increase the risk of seizures at doses above 450 mg/day and is generally thought to be contraindicated in patients with epilepsy. Duloxetine inhibits the reuptake of serotonin and norepinephrine, and is used for depression, fibromyalgia, and neuropathic pain. Venlafaxine also is used for the same indications, but works by blocking the reuptake of serotonin at low doses and norepinephrine and dopamine at higher doses. Mirtazapine increases the release of norepinephrine and serotonin and antagonizes histamine and alpha$_2$-adrenergic receptors. It is mostly used for depression, and has been shown to improve appetite and sleep. Trazodone, which antagonizes serotonin receptors but inhibits synaptic uptake, also helps relieve insomnia and depression. Priapism is a unique side effect of trazodone.

57. E. The presenting symptoms of Klumpke paralysis are weak finger and wrist flexors, weak intrinsic hand muscles, and occasionally weak triceps. Additionally, patients often have numbness in the C8 and/or T1 dermatome, although this may be challenging to test in a newborn. The cause of Klumpke paralysis is dysfunction of the lower trunk, often resulting from stretching injury to either the C8 or T1 nerve root. The fact that this child also has evidence of Horner syndrome suggests that the T1 root is affected. Injury to the C5 or C6 nerve root can affect the upper trunk, and often result from stretch injury of the neck away from the affected side. This injury may lead to Erb–Duchenne paralysis ("waiter's tip" palsy), including internal rotation of the arm with an extended elbow and pronated forearm due to weakness of shoulder abduction and elbow flexion. Isolated C7 injury is fairly rare due to the anatomical location of the root. It generally results in triceps weakness and dermatomal sensory loss (*see* Bradley's NiCP, 7th edn, Ch. 106, pp. 1766–1790).

58. A. The child likely has benign paroxysmal torticollis in infancy. This is an idiopathic condition characterized by periods of cervical dystonia that begin and end suddenly lasting for a few hours to a few days. During this time, the child is usually alert and responsive without other adventitious movements of the arms or legs. Occasionally these movements can be accompanied by vomiting, pallor, irritability, or ataxia. Some consider paroxysmal torticollis in infancy to be a migraine equivalent, and a relationship with the *CACN1A* gene, which is linked to familial hemiplegic migraine, has been discovered in some families. This condition is self-limiting and almost always disappears by 5 years of age. There is no indication that the child is having seizures, and electroencephalograms are almost always normal in this condition. Sandifer syndrome is also a possibility and typically presents with extraneous movements caused by gastroesophageal reflux. However, these are paroxysmal episodes typically induced after feedings and are shorter in duration. Spasmus nutans is associated with cervical dystonia, but should also have nystagmus and head nodding (*see* Bradley's NiCP, 7th edn, Ch. 103, pp. 1686–1719).

59. B. Rasagiline is a monoamine oxidase B inhibitor, which is involved in the breakdown of dopamine and norepinephrine, so it has a potentially serious side effect of malignant hypertension, particularly when combined with some selective serotonin reuptake inhibitors, resulting in serotonin syndrome. Entacapone is a catecholamine methyltransferase inhibitor (catechol-O-methyl transferase) that slows the degradation of dopamine. Serious complications include orthostasis, syncope, hallucinations, and psychosis. Amantadine is an antiviral agent also used in Parkinson disease that has possible side effects of psychosis, seizures, and arrhythmias. L-dopa and ropinirole have similar side effect profiles, including orthostasis, excessive reward-seeking behavior, psychosis, dyskinesias, and arrhythmias (*see* Bradley's NiCP, 7th edn, Ch. 96, pp. 1422–1460).

60. D. Diastematomyelia is a congenital disorder of the spinal cord, which has two different types. In type 1 lesions, the spinal cord splits into two spinal canals separated by a bony septum. In a type 2 lesion, as is shown in the MRI, the spinal cord divides in half and is separated by a fibrous septum in a single spinal canal. Clinically this can present as a myelopathy in childhood. Treatment involves surgery to remove the fibrous septum that tethers the cord in place. Syringomyelia involves an enlarged central canal in the spinal cord. On T2 imaging this would be seen as a hyperintense lesion in the central portion of the spinal cord. Transverse myelitis shows hyperintense lesions in the spinal cord, which may involve part of or the entire spinal cord and generally enhances with gadolinium. Subacute combined degeneration shows T2 hyperintense lesions in the posterior columns and lateral corticospinal tracts. Congenital spinal stenosis demonstrates a small spinal canal. On T2 imaging, cerebrospinal fluid space would be greatly reduced and the spinal cord should appear normal, unless significant compression has occurred (*see* Bradley's NiCP, 7th edn, Ch. 105, pp. 1736–1765). Figure from Fenton D 2011 *Imaging Painful Spine Disorders*, Elsevier, with permission.

61. E. Social media presents new ethical challenges in communication with patients and their families. Each facility has its own policy on the use of social media by physicians and staff. Using social media to start a romantic relationship with a patient or a former patient is considered an inappropriate use of social media. If a physician uses social media, he or she should separate professional and personal accounts to help protect personal information. No personal identifying information about patients should be posted. Reporting unprofessional behavior by colleagues is important if the content violates medical ethics or is below the standard expected of a physician. Social media and e-mail are not preferred to communicate with patients about their medical conditions, but may be used as long as patients are aware that the conversations and e-mails may not be as secure as patient portals, phone conversations, or face-to-face conversations.

62. C. Spongiform changes are consistent with Creutzfeldt-Jakob disease. The pathological hallmark of HSV encephalitis is Cowdry type A inclusions. Dementia with Lewy bodies shows eosinophilic cytoplasmic inclusions. Alzheimer disease shows neurofibrillary tangles. Oligodendroglioma shows multiple cells with a "fried egg" appearance, with a white halo around the nucleus (*see* Bradley's NiCP, 7th edn, Ch. 94, pp. 1365–1379). Figure from Klatt EC 2014 *Robbins and Cotran Atlas of Pathology*, 3rd edn, Saunders, with permission.

63. B. With an underlying diagnosis of AIDS, the patient is at risk for multiple opportunistic infections. The constellation of significantly elevated intracranial pressure with CSF lymphocytosis, low glucose, and high protein is classic for cryptococcal meningitis. Treatment with amphotericin B and flucytosine should be initiated, as well as daily lumbar punctures to reduce intracranial pressure. Although lumbar drain may be used in place of daily lumbar punctures, and chronic obstructive hydrocephalus may be treated with a ventriculoperitoneal (VP) shunt, during the acute course of the infection a VP shunt should be avoided due to risk of fungal seeding into the abdomen. The other treatments mentioned are inappropriate and/or insufficient (in the case of acetazolamide) for this patient (*see* Bradley's NiCP, 7th edn, Chs. 77, pp. 1102–1120 and 79, pp. 1147–1158).

64. B. Confirmation bias results when a diagnostic error is made by seeking out only information that will confirm a diagnosis, not ruling out alternative diagnoses. There are many reasons a patient could have arm weakness that would not be apparent on a brain MRI, so other potential etiologies should be considered. Availability bias involves making a diagnosis because of a recent experience with a similar diagnosis. Anchoring bias involves continuing with a diagnosis despite evidence contrary to that diagnosis. Premature closure bias involves closing the diagnostic process early because of a characteristic presentation leading to a diagnosis. Diagnosis momentum involves accepting a diagnosis passed on from another physician without reconfirming that diagnosis.

65. C. Rods contain the photopigment rhodopsin, which is an achromatic pigment. Rods perceive light and are activated by very low levels of light. These receptors are predominantly in the peripheral portion of the retina, whereas cones are in the fovea. Rods are larger cells than cones and contain more pigment, making them more easily activated. Rods help with night or low-light vision (*see* Bradley's NiCP, 7th edn, Ch. 17, pp. 163–179).

66. B. The EEG demonstrates diffuse rhythmic, high-amplitude slow waves with occasional spikes, which is consistent with nonconvulsive status epilepticus. This condition is more common in the ICU, in critically ill patients, or in patients who have suffered convulsive status epilepticus but have yet to return to normal mentation. This condition is considered equally emergent and critical as convulsive status epilepticus and requires immediate treatment. The EEG in herpes encephalitis shows temporal periodic lateralized epileptiform discharges. The EEG in hepatic encephalopathy classically shows triphasic waves. Medication-induced encephalopathy can have many patterns on EEG, including varying degrees of generalized slowing to a burst suppression pattern. Meningitis can cause seizures, but in this patient his vital signs had stabilized, so it is unlikely that he is suffering from bacterial meningitis (*see* Bradley's NiCP, 7th edn, Ch. 55, pp. 742–758). Figure from Fernández-Torre JL, Rebollo M, Gutiérrez A, López-Espadas F, Hernández-Hernández MA 2012 Nonconvulsive status epilepticus in adults: electroclinical differences between proper and comatose forms. *Clinical Neurophysiology* 123(2): 244–251, with permission.

67. B. PTSD occurs when a person experiences or witnesses an actual or threatened traumatic event that invokes fear, helplessness, or horror. Each time the patient reexperiences a trigger or cue that reminds him or her of the initial event, the patient may have recurrent recollections of the event, dreams, and enhanced physiological reactivity such as startle, tachycardia, or hypervigilance. This ultimately leads to avoidance of activities, places, or people that arouse memories of the inciting event. Symptoms must be present for longer than 1 month to be diagnosed with PTSD (shorter than 1 month is acute stress disorder). Treatment includes antidepressants, benzodiazepines, mood stabilizers, or antipsychotics. Psychotherapy and

desensitization are also very helpful. Although panic disorder (and attacks) can occur with PTSD, the recurring flashbacks sparked by an initial traumatic event are better explained by PTSD. There is no indication that these symptoms occur in sleep, nor that they coexist with another neurodegenerative process, thus making REM sleep behavior disorder unlikely. Although the patient avoids symptom-triggering situations, there is no indication of excessive worry, such as in generalized anxiety disorder.

68. E. The patient presents with myasthenia gravis that started during pregnancy. This is clinically suspected by eye movements that do not follow specific cranial neuropathies, fatigable eye weakness with ptosis, and a nasal voice, which is common in neuromuscular disorders. In addition she recently started magnesium, which can precipitate a myasthenic crisis. Many other medications can precipitate a crisis, including antibiotics and anesthetics. Prednisone is considered first-line treatment, even in pregnancy. IVIG is an option in pregnancy and has been found to be relatively safe, although only studied in a small number of patients. Transient neonatal myasthenia can occur by transplacental transfer of antibodies to the baby. Symptoms can last up to 6 weeks after birth. Breastfeeding does not typically transmit the disease to the child. There is no mendelian pattern of inheritance associated with myasthenia gravis (*see* Bradley's NiCP, Ch. 112, pp. 1973–1991).

69. E. The autonomic nervous system (ANS) uses acetylcholine as its preganglionic neurotransmitter, which binds to nicotinic receptors. Muscarinic receptors are cholinergic receptors involved in sweat glands as well as postganglionic parasympathetic activation. Alpha 2 receptors are adrenergic receptors not involved in the ANS. NMDA receptors are glutamate receptors in the central nervous system that are excitatory. Mu receptors are targets of opioids and result in analgesia (*see* Bradley's NiCP, 7th edn, Ch. 108, pp. 1867–1895).

70. C. The symptoms of headache and blurred vision with a finding of papilledema imply increased intracranial pressure. As such, the woman is most likely suffering from a cerebral venous sinus thrombosis, which was precipitated by intravascular volume depletion from sun exposure. Given her renal insufficiency of unnamed cause and her strong autoimmune family history, lupus anticoagulant antibodies (which are a type of antiphospholipid antibody) are the most likely choice. Asking about prior spontaneous abortions would also help guide the differential diagnosis. von Willebrand deficiency is a genetic cause of impaired coagulation. *JAK2* mutation is associated with polycythemia vera and essential thrombocytosis. Although either of these may increase the risk of thrombosis, neither is specifically implicated by the clinical history given. Elevated vitamin A levels may correlate with classic pseudotumor cerebri, although this has no bearing on venous sinus thrombosis. Vitamin K deficiency may be seen with prolonged antibiotic use (depleting vitamin K–producing gut bacteria) or more commonly with warfarin use, causing prolonged international normalization ratio and therefore increased risk of bleeding (*see* Bradley's NiCP, 7th edn, Ch. 65, pp. 920–967).

71. C. The anterior cingulate gyrus is the anatomical substrate for motivation. Lesions to the anterior cingulate gyrus can result in a lack of motivation and initiation. This is common in frontotemporal dementia, Alzheimer disease, Huntington disease, and even depression. The dorsolateral prefrontal cortex controls executive functions like organization and planning ability. The lateral orbitofrontal cortex controls impulsivity. The Papez circuit involves the hippocampus, mammillary bodies, anterior thalamic nuclei, and the cingulate gyrus. The left parasylvian cortex is involved in generation of speech (*see* Bradley's NiCP, 7th edn, Ch. 43, pp. 511–527).

72. D. The patient likely has fibromyalgia as evidenced by a normal physical and neurological examination; presence of at least 11 of 18 specific areas of point tenderness; and a history of fatigue, musculoskeletal aching, and comorbid psychiatric conditions. The pathophysiology of fibromyalgia is unknown, but new evidence suggests that there are alterations of central pain processing, sleep abnormalities, neurohormonal axis abnormalities, autonomic nervous system changes, and peripheral pain receptor alterations. Patients are diagnosed with fibromyalgia when they fit the clinical picture mentioned earlier along with normal laboratory testing, including complete blood count, erythrocyte sedimentation rate, C-reactive protein, creatine kinase, and thyroid-stimulating hormone. These laboratory tests are often done to exclude other conditions, including inflammatory myopathies, connective tissue diseases, polymyalgia rheumatica, and hypothyroidism. Conditions coexisting with fibromyalgia often include systemic exertion intolerance disease (formally chronic fatigue syndrome), irritable bowel syndrome, migraine, temporomandibular disorder, interstitial cystitis, and vulvodynia. Treatment includes tricyclic antidepressants, serotonin and norepinephrine reuptake inhibitors, exercise programs, physical therapy, and cognitive behavioral therapy (*see* Bradley's NiCP, 7th edn, Ch. 105, pp. 1736–1765).

73. B. Topiramate has significant side effects of acute-angle glaucoma, teratogenicity, metabolic acidosis, and nephrolithiasis. Valproic acid has many significant side effects, including hepatotoxicity, encephalopathy, pancreatitis, and teratogenicity. Amitriptyline has significant side effects of worsening depression, anticholinergic side effects, and cardiac arrhythmias. Propranolol can cause arrhythmias, worsen asthma, and lead to depression. Verapamil can cause arrhythmias, paralytic ileus, and hepatic toxicity (*see* Bradley's NiCP, 7th edn, Ch. 101, pp. 1563–1614).

74. C. This patient presents with typical features seen in acute porphyria. Porphyria is marked by autonomic dysfunction (constipation, abdominal pain, nausea, tachycardia, labile blood pressures, and orthostasis). Later in the course patients can develop an acute motor neuropathy that looks like Guillain-Barré syndrome (GBS). They may also develop encephalopathy, hallucinations, or even seizures. Urine porphobilinogen and δ-aminolevulinic acid are increased in most types of porphyria. Lumbar puncture for cytoalbuminological dissociation would rule out GBS, which is less likely because of her encephalopathic state and hallucinations. Although EMG/NCS would be helpful for determining pure motor involvement, it would not give a specific diagnosis. This patient's history is not typical for botulism because of the significant cognitive symptoms. Niacin deficiency can cause a mild sensorimotor neuropathy, but does not generally cause

significant motor weakness. The triad of niacin deficiency is dermatitis, diarrhea, and dementia (*see* Bradley's NiCP, 7th edn, Ch. 107, pp. 1791–1867).

75. B. After head injury, the pattern of initial loss of consciousness, then brief lucidity, then loss of consciousness again is classic for epidural hematoma. Upon direct impact, the temporal bone is fractured and the underlying middle meningeal artery is torn. As the hematoma expands, the level of consciousness decreases. Imaging reveals a classical convex hyperdensity, which does not cross skull suture lines. Bridging vein tearing tends to occur after rotational or acceleration–deceleration injury, and leads to development of subdural hematoma. Imaging shows a concave hyperdensity that may cross skull suture lines. Axonal shearing is seen in traumatic brain injury with diffuse axonal injury, and magnetic resonance imaging may show microhemorrhages along white matter tracts and in subcortical gray matter. Cerebral contusions result from coup–contrecoup injuries and first appear as multiple microhemorrhages that convalesce and "blossom" into a larger hematoma within the first 24 hours. Concussion refers to traumatic brain injury with associated symptoms (e.g. loss of consciousness, confusion, dizziness, amnesia) but no radiographic abnormalities (*see* Bradley's NiCP, 7th edn, Ch. 62, pp. 867–880).

76. D. The initial segmentation of the neural tube gives rise to the prosencephalon, the mesencephalon, and the rhombencephalon. From there, the prosencephalon divides into the diencephalon (thalamus, hypothalamus, globus pallidus, substantia nigra, subthalamic nucleus) and the telencephalon (cerebral cortex, caudate, putamen). The mesencephalon becomes the midbrain. The rhombencephalon divides into the metencephalon (pons, cerebellum) and the myelencephalon (medulla).

77. D. The case is one of attention-deficit/hyperactivity disorder (ADHD). This is characterized by at least 6 or more months of inattention, difficulty listening, disorganization, avoidance of tasks, losing objects needed to complete tasks, distractibility, and forgetfulness. At least some of the symptoms must occur before the age of 7. Typically, there are hyperactive and inattentive subtypes. In this particular case, the correct treatment of choice is a psychostimulant such as amphetamine or methylphenidate. Alpha-agonists such as clonidine or guanfacine may also be used. Although structure and discipline can help organize behavior in children, it is important to recognize medical and psychological causes of behavioral dysfunction. There is nothing in the history that suggests a learning disability or cognitive decline for which a change in the curriculum is needed. Finally, although psychotherapy is important for comorbidities that can occur with ADHD (i.e. depression), this would not be the first treatment of choice.

78. A. The findings shown on this gradient echo sequence on magnetic resonance imaging (MRI) are consistent with cerebral amyloid angiopathy (CAA). CAA is a condition in which amyloid deposits in the media and adventitia of small and medium vessels. Although microhemorrhages are often seen on MRI, patients are often at increased risk of lobar hemorrhages. The risk of cerebral hemorrhage with either anticoagulation or antiplatelet agents is increased in this population. Caution must also be taken when using statins in this

population, due to a slightly higher risk of bleeding. Chronic hypertension usually leads to bleeding in deep structures of the brain such as the pons, basal ganglia, thalamus, or cerebellum. An AVM can be identified on this sequence on MRI, but usually shows a conglomeration of arteries and veins rather than small microhemorrhages. A subarachnoid hemorrhage usually follows the cortical convexity in the leptomeningeal space. A traumatic brain injury may result in contusion from a coup/contrecoup injury but usually is not associated with microhemorrhages (*see* Bradley's NiCP, 7th edn, Chs. 66, pp. 968–980 and 95, pp. 1380–1421). Figure from, Caldas AC, Silva C, Albuquerque L, Pimentel J, Silva V, Ferro JM 2015 Cerebral amyloid angiopathy associated with inflammation: report of 3 cases and systematic review. *Journal of Stroke and Cerebrovascular Diseases* 24(9): 2039–2048, with permission.

79. A. Psilocybin is a structural analog of serotonin, whose actions resemble lysergic acid diethylamide. It is found in various species of mushroom, although accounts for only one of several mushroom neurotoxins. The puffer fish has been associated with tetrodotoxin, which blocks voltage-gated sodium channels and causes perioral and acral paresthesias, progressive ascending weakness, dysphagia, and hypoventilation. Home-distilled ethanol may contain methanol as a byproduct, which breaks down to formic acid and causes permanent optic nerve damage and blindness. Shellfish are associated with various neurotoxins, most notably saxitoxin and brevetoxin, which affect the voltage-gated sodium channels in different ways (saxitoxin inhibits the channel; brevetoxin activates the channel) and cause perioral and acral paresthesias, ataxia, and paralysis. Peyote is a small cactus that contains mescaline, which has hallucinogenic action similar to psilocybin (*see* Bradley's NiCP, 7th edn, Ch. 86, pp. 1237–1253).

80. C. The treatment of the motor features of Huntington disease (and other hyperkinetic movement disorders) is typically aimed at reducing dopaminergic action. Other treatments are aimed at treating the nonmotor features of Huntington disease. Dopamine depleters, such as tetrabenazine, work by inhibiting the vesicular monoamine transporter (VMAT) protein, thereby decreasing dopamine. Antipsychotics block dopamine's action at the D2 receptor. Both SSRIs and benzodiazepines are aimed at treating the nonmotor manifestations of obsessive-compulsive disorder tendencies, anxiety, and insomnia (*see* Bradley's NiCP, 7th edn, Ch. 96, pp. 1422–1460).

81. D. Syndrome of inappropriate antidiuretic hormone (SIADH) secretion has been reported in Guillain-Barré syndrome (GBS), though the pathophysiology is not known. Among patients with GBS, SIADH is an independent risk factor for increased mortality, as are age >50, requirement of ventilator support, hyponatremia, and bulbar weakness. In SIADH, excess antidiuretic hormone (ADH) prevents water loss in the kidneys, leading to decreased serum osmolality and serum sodium concentration with elevated urine osmolality and urine sodium concentration. Other etiologies of hyponatremia include excessive water intake (psychogenic polydipsia), functional hypovolemia (congestive heart failure [CHF] and cirrhosis), and some cases of dehydration (hypovolemic hyponatremia). It is notable that patients with SIADH generally appear euvolemic, as opposed to

cerebral salt wasting, where patients appear hypovolemic. Cerebral salt wasting is most often seen in brain injuries or central nervous system (CNS) tumors, and is associated with large urinary output due to inability to retain sodium in the body, and therefore high urinary excretion of sodium. Treatment for cerebral salt wasting is replacement of fluid and sodium, whereas treatment for SIADH is fluid restriction. The excess fluid given with IVIG can cause pseudohyponatremia, but this patient has not received any treatment yet (*see* Bradley's NiCP, 7th edn, Chs. 52, pp. 696–712 and 55, pp. 742-757).

82. C. Pulsatile tinnitus is a common complaint of patients with idiopathic intracranial hypertension, which is related to a pressure gradient between the cranial and cervical vascular structures, causing a bruit. Patients generally report a whooshing sound without tone. Conductive hearing loss occurs when vibrations are not appropriately transmitted through the outer or middle ear. This may be related to cerumen, tympanic membrane dysfunction or rupture, fluid in the middle ear, or ossicle dysfunction. Sensorineural hearing loss results from dysfunction of inner ear structures such as hair cells, dysfunction of the vestibulocochlear nerve, or cerebral processing of auditory input. This may be congenital (as in the case of perinatal infections including cytomegalovirus or rubella), traumatic (chronic exposure to loud noises), toxic (aminoglycosides, loop diuretics, salicylates), focal neurological dysfunction (as in cerebellopontine angle masses), or age-related. Persistent tinnitus is a more constant, tonal type of tinnitus. Associated causes vary widely, including ototoxic medications, Meniere disease, hearing loss, head injury, and others. The pathophysiology of persistent tinnitus is not well understood. Palatal myoclonus consists of rhythmic myoclonic activity of the soft palate with associated clicking sound. This may relate to Whipple disease, gluten sensitivity, or structural disruption of the Guillain-Mollaret triangle (dentato-rubro-olivary network; *see* Bradley's NiCP, 7th edn, Ch. 103, pp. 1686–1719).

83. C. Simultagnosia is the inability to visually perceive multiple objects at one time. Patients with this condition may see parts of a picture but miss large portions due to visual inattention (not visual field loss). Visual agnosia is the inability to recognize objects by sight, whereas prosopagnosia is the inability to recognize faces. Phonagnosia is the inability to recognize voices. Amusia is the loss of musical abilities, including both production and appreciation of music (*see* Bradley's NiCP, 7th edn, Ch. 12, pp. 122–127).

84. B. This demonstrates obstructive sleep apnea. In the oronasal channel, flow of air stops four different times (indicated by the flat line). During this same time the thorax and abdominal channels have continued effort. A central apnea occurs when there is no airflow and no thoracic or abdominal effort. A mixed apnea starts initially with no flow and no effort, but near the end effort begins without any airflow. Cheyne-Stokes breathing involves bursts of progressively faster and deeper breaths with a gradual decrease and stop of respiration. This is a type of central apnea. Paradoxical breathing occurs when airflow is positive with positive thoracic effort and negative abdominal effort. This implies inspiration is caused by thoracic muscles rather than diaphragmatic excursion (*see* Bradley's NiCP, 7th edn, Ch. 102, pp. 1615–1685). Figure from Daroff RB,

Jankovic J, Mazziotta JC, Pomeroy SL 2016 *Bradley's Neurology in Clinical Practice*, 7th edn, Elsevier, with permission.

85. A. Thunderclap headaches may result from one of several underlying pathologies, the most threatening of which is subarachnoid hemorrhage. Other less frequently reported causes include pituitary apoplexy, cerebral venous thrombosis, cervical artery dissection, hypertensive crisis, and intracranial hypotension. Although cranial CT is very sensitive for subarachnoid hemorrhage, a lumbar puncture should always be performed if subarachnoid hemorrhage is suspected but not confirmed by CT. Angiography and nimodipine therapy would be important if subarachnoid hemorrhage were identified on CT or lumbar puncture to identify the source of the bleed and to reduce the risk of delayed vasospasm, but would not yet be necessary in this case. Ergotamine therapy should be avoided in suspected cases of subarachnoid hemorrhage, given the risk of symptomatic vasoconstriction. Venography would be helpful to identify cerebral venous thrombosis, although this is lower on the differential and on the acuity scale than subarachnoid hemorrhage (*see* Bradley's NiCP, 7th edn, Ch. 103, pp. 1686–1719).

86. D. Type I muscle fibers are slow-twitch fibers with lower contractile strength, utilize mostly aerobic respiration, and have long endurance. Type II fibers involve fewer mitochondria, are used in quick movements, have higher contractile strength, have lower numbers of mitochondria, and have a mix of aerobic and anaerobic respiration (*see* Bradley's NiCP, 7th edn, Ch. 110, pp. 1915–1956).

87. D. Carotid body injury may affect vagal output and lead to heart rate irregularities. The nerves responsible for the remainder of the listed symptoms would not be present in the neck (*see* Bradley's NiCP, 7th edn, Ch. 104, pp. 1720–1735).

88. D. Somatosensory evoked potentials are used to evaluate the sensory system from the lumbar roots to the somatosensory cortex. Peripheral nerves are stimulated with repeated electric shocks, which move up the dorsal columns of the spinal cord to the somatosensory cortex. Along the path various waveforms can be recorded, which are either positive (P) or negative (N), and a number that corresponds to the typical latency expected. The N13 peak represents a near-field potential recorded over the cervical spine. Erb's point is represented by the N9 peak. The brainstem and medial meniscus are involved in the P14, which is a far-field potential. The N20 is the cortical response and is usually best recorded over the contralateral hemisphere (*see* Bradley's NiCP, 7th edn, Ch. 34, pp. 348–366).

89. C. The MRI is an example of an encephalocele, which results from failure of skull closure and allows cranial contents to herniate outside the skull. Lissencephaly is a disorder of neuronal migration that involves a smooth, poorly organized cerebral cortex. Patients with lissencephaly demonstrate severe developmental delay and seizures. It may also result from mutations in certain genes, including *LIS1*, *DCX*, and *ARX*. Pachygyria can be seen in lissencephaly, and involves a cortex with relatively few gyri. Porencephaly is a cyst or cleft in the brain in which there is a connection between the ependyma and the subarachnoid space, and the cyst is lined by white matter. Schizencephaly is

an abnormality that involves a cleft in the brain that extends from the ependyma to the pia mater and is lined with gray matter (*see* Bradley's NiCP, 7th edn, Ch. 89, pp. 1279–1300). Figure from Winn H 2011 *Youmans Neurological Surgery*, Saunders, with permission.

90. E. Landau-Kleffner syndrome presents between the ages of 2 and 8 years old. It most commonly presents with verbal auditory agnosia (an inability to recognize or differentiate different sounds or words not because of poor hearing) and can progress to involve other areas of speech. The EEG hallmark is continuous spike and slow waves seen during slow wave sleep with a normal EEG when awake. Childhood absence epilepsy has a pattern of generalized 3-Hz spike and wave. Lennox-Gastaut demonstrates an abnormal background with frequent slow spike and wave abnormalities. Juvenile myoclonic epilepsy demonstrates a pattern of polyspike and wave at a rate of 4–6 Hz. Autosomal-dominant nocturnal frontal lobe epilepsy demonstrates frontal spikes during sleep, not generalized discharges as is seen during this segment (*see* Bradley's NiCP, 7th edn, Ch. 101, pp. 1563–1614). Figure from Daroff RB, Jankovic J, Mazziotta JC, Pomeroy SL 2016 *Bradley's Neurology in Clinical Practice*, 7th edn, Elsevier, with permission.

91. A. Immediate memory (sometimes known as *working memory*) is tested by digit span. Asking historical facts tests remote memory. Implicit memory is tested in many ways, including through studies of memory priming wherein subjects are shown a list of words and then asked later if they have seen specific words. Calculation is tested through mathematical problems. Language is tested through many means, including assessment of fluency, naming, repeating, reading, writing, and following commands (*see* Bradley's NiCP, 7th edn, Ch. 4, pp. 23–33).

92. C. *Neisseria meningitides*. A chart with common bacterial causes of meningitis based on age range or comorbidities is shown here.

TABLE FOR ANSWER 2.92

Age or comorbidity	Bacteria
Newborn	Group B streptococci, *E. coli*
Toddler	*S. pneumoniae, N. meningitidis, H. influenzae*
Adolescent through adult	*S. pneumoniae, N. meningitidis*
Elderly	*S. pneumoniae, H. influenzae, E. coli, L. monocytogenes*
Neurosurgical patients	*S. pneumoniae, H. influenzae, S. aureus*
Immunosuppressed	*L. monocytogenes*
Sinusitis or otitis media	*H. influenzae, S. pneumoniae*

93. C. Substance P is closely related to neurokinin A and is an important messenger in pain perception, as well as in the vomiting center of the medulla. Of note, aprepitant is a novel antiemetic that inhibits substance P. Voluntary muscle contraction and sweat production both rely on acetylcholine. Circadian rhythm is regulated, in part, by melatonin. Endocrine function relies, in part, on somatostatin as a peptide neurotransmitter (*see* Bradley's NiCP, 7th edn, Ch. 52, pp. 696–712).

94. C. The image depicts noncommunicating hydrocephalus, identifiable by a small fourth ventricle contrasting with enlarged lateral ventricles. This differs from communicating hydrocephalus, where the entire ventricular system is enlarged. The etiology in this case is cerebral aqueductal stenosis, a common cause of hydrocephalus in children. Other causes of hydrocephalus in infants and children can include posterior fossa abnormalities such as Dandy-Walker syndrome or Chiari malformation, mass lesions such as pilocytic astrocytoma or medulloblastoma, infectious causes such as toxoplasmosis, or vascular causes such as venous sinus thrombosis. The patient's examination reveals restricted vertical gaze, related to midbrain tectal dysfunction in the setting of elevated intracranial pressure (ICP). Sometimes, the eyelids retract and there can be a forced downgaze, often called the *setting-sun sign*. If the pressure continues to increase, Parinaud syndrome can occur, manifested by light-near dissociation, convergence-retraction nystagmus, and eyelid retraction (eyelid retraction is also known as *Collier sign*). Other findings can include unilateral or bilateral papilledema, bilateral cranial nerve VI palsies, or macrocephaly. The treatment of noncommunicating hydrocephalus usually includes placement of a ventriculoperitoneal shunt. Although acetazolamide may be used for increased ICP in the short term, it is almost never indicated for long-term management of hydrocephalus. Because his parents do not have macrocephaly and because of his abnormal imaging of the brain, benign familial macrocephaly is not the correct diagnosis (*see* Bradley's NiCP, 7th edn, Ch. 39, pp. 411–458). Figure from Daroff RB, Jankovic J, Mazziotta JC, Pomeroy SL 2016 *Bradley's Neurology in Clinical Practice*, 7th edn, Elsevier, with permission.

95. D. Older adults, particularly those suffering from dementia, are at great risk of being abused, which should be considered in patients who have unexplained weight loss and unexplained injuries. Local regulations may differ, but in most states, suspected abuse must be reported to local authorities. Confronting the son about possible neglect will erode the patient–physician relationship, would not resolve the issue, and could even result in more injuries to the patient. Ignoring the possible signs of abuse could result in more serious injuries to the patient. Taking immediate action by calling the police to arrest the son is not the best situation because the patient is not in immediate danger of death or serious injury. This will also cause great animosity between the patient's family and the physician, and could result in a disastrous situation for the patient. Although adding donepezil and recommending dietary supplements may be medically helpful, these ignore the concern for abuse and neglect.

96. E. The image demonstrates infarcts in bilateral watershed territories between the anterior cerebral arteries and the middle cerebral arteries. Given that arterial density is least in watershed locations, low perfusion pressure may lead to localized infarcts. Low perfusion pressure may relate to hypotension (as in the case of sepsis) or to reduced arterial luminal diameter (as with severe atherosclerosis or dissection). There are no indications in the image of viral encephalitis, paraneoplastic syndrome, seizure, or neuritic plaque accumulation (*see* Bradley's NiCP, 7th edn, Ch. 65, pp. 920–967). Figure from Yachnis AT 2012 *Neuropathology*, 2nd edn, pp. 40–74, Elsevier, with permission.

97. A. Von Hippel-Lindau (VHL) syndrome is an autosomal-dominant disorder associated with loss of function mutations in the VHL tumor suppressor gene. Patients with this syndrome are predisposed to hemangioblastomas in the brain and spine, renal and pancreatic cysts, renal cell carcinoma, pheochromocytoma, and angiomatosis of the eye. Neurofibromatosis 2 is an autosomal-dominant disorder associated with loss of function mutations in the *NF2* tumor suppressor gene. Affected patients are predisposed to several types of benign tumors, including schwannomas (often bilateral vestibular nerve schwannomas), meningiomas, and ependymomas. Retinoblastoma is a cancer of the retina that is associated with a loss of function mutation in the *Rb1* gene. Although retinoblastoma is the most commonly associated tumor with *Rb1* mutation, nearly half of the cases are sporadic and the mutation is localized to the tumor. In patients who inherit a germline *Rb1* mutation, however, there is an increased risk of other types of tumors, including pinealoma, sarcoma, and melanoma. Neurofibromatosis 1 is an autosomal-dominant cancer predisposition syndrome associated with mutation in the *NF1* tumor suppressor gene. Individuals with neurofibromatosis 1 have multiple associated signs and symptoms, including café-au-lait patches, skinfold freckling, cutaneous neurofibromas, malignant peripheral nerve sheath tumors, optic gliomas, and developmental delay. Cowden syndrome is an autosomal-dominant disorder associated with loss of function of the tumor suppressor gene *PTEN*. Patients with this syndrome have an increased risk of multiple types of tumors, most commonly skin and mucosal surface hamartomas, breast cancer, thyroid cancer, endometrial cancer, and dysplastic gangliocytoma (cerebellar hamartoma). When a dysplastic gangliocytoma is present, the term *Lhermitte-Duclos* is used (*see* Bradley's NiCP, 7th edn, Ch. 100, pp. 1538–1562).

98. C. The patient's symptoms and examination findings are most consistent with idiopathic intracranial hypertension (IIH). Lumbar puncture should demonstrate increased opening pressure (>25 cm). Abducens palsy is commonly associated with increased intracranial pressure from this or other entities (such as trauma). Acetazolamide is first-line therapy for IIH. Although multiple sclerosis may cause abducens palsy with a demyelinating lesion of the pons, this patient's overall picture and lack of demyelination on MRI is more consistent with IIH. Glatiramer would be an appropriate immunomodulatory therapy for multiple sclerosis after resolution of an acute flare, although generally corticosteroids would be used to treat the acute symptoms. Plasma exchange may also be used to treat multiple sclerosis, although is generally reserved for severe, refractory flares that do not improve with corticosteroids. Warfarin would be an appropriate treatment if the cause of intracranial hypertension was cerebral venous sinus thrombosis; however, no such evidence was found on venography. Myasthenia gravis often causes diplopia, including abductor weakness. However, the findings of papilledema argue against myasthenia, as does the absence of fluctuating symptoms. Pyridostigmine would be an appropriate treatment for myasthenia, but not for IIH (*see* Bradley's NiCP, 7th edn, Ch. 103, pp. 1686–1719).

99. A. Phencyclidine (PCP) is a relatively uncommon drug of abuse. Initially it can lead to euphoria, dysphoria, paranoia, or hallucinations, but later in the intoxication it can lead to severe aggression, bizarre behaviors, catatonia, myoglobinuria, fever, hypertension, and nystagmus. Oftentimes patients intoxicated with PCP will be quite difficult to restrain and seemingly feel no pain even with injurious behavior. Treatment is supportive. Cocaine intoxication can cause euphoria, hallucination, paranoia, hypertension, fevers, strokes, and seizures, but is not associated with aggression, myoglobinuria, or nystagmus. Alcohol intoxication usually results in a sense of euphoria or dysphoria, tachycardia, nystagmus, and somnolence. Marijuana intoxication can result in euphoria, dysphoria, hallucinations, somnolence, and rarely strokes or seizures. Opioid intoxication results in euphoria or dysphoria, hallucinations, hypotension, hypothermia, respiratory depression, and coma (*see* Bradley's NiCP, 7th edn, Ch. 87, pp. 1254–1260).

100. C. Among other adverse reactions, including gastrointestinal symptoms and immunosuppression, mitoxantrone may cause an irreversible cardiomyopathy. Therefore regular monitoring with echocardiograms or multigated acquisition scans is recommended, as well as a lifetime maximum dose of mitoxantrone due to cumulative risk. Seizure is a risk with dalfampridine, which is used to improve walking in patients with multiple sclerosis. Headache is a risk of beta-interferon therapy. Allergic reactions, mostly injection site specific, are seen with interferons. Progressive multifocal leukoencephalopathy has been associated with natalizumab, fingolimod, and dimethyl fumarate (*see* Bradley's NiCP, 7th edn, Ch. 80, pp. 1159–1186).

101. A. Seizure is a dose-dependent side effect of dalfampridine, and may occur in up to 4% of patients. If a patient has a seizure while on dalfampridine, the drug should be discontinued. Further, history of seizure is a contraindication to starting dalfampridine. Although patients may have headache as a general side effect to dalfampridine therapy, complicated migraine is not a contraindication for its use. Liver impairment does not preclude a patient from receiving dalfampridine, although renal impairment may increase the likelihood of seizure and should be considered before starting therapy. There is no immune suppression that results from dalfampridine, so history of tuberculosis is not a contraindication. Transverse myelitis is a symptom of multiple sclerosis, and may be an indication for dalfampridine use to improve motor function (*see* Bradley's NiCP, 7th edn, Ch. 80, pp. 1159–1186).

102. A. All of the listed medications can precipitate a myasthenic crisis except for lisinopril. Other medications to be used with caution include any neuromuscular junction–blocking anesthetics, most antibiotics (particularly quinolones, macrolides, and aminoglycosides), lidocaine, cimetidine, phenytoin, carbamazepine, and gabapentin (*see* Bradley's NiCP, 7th edn, Ch. 109, pp. 1895–1914).

103. B. Valproic acid is a strong hepatic enzyme inhibitor, which means it can greatly increase the availability of other medications by slowing their metabolism. This interaction is particularly important when prescribing lamotrigine and valproic acid together because lamotrigine levels can be greatly increased, resulting in

a serious risk of rash, including Stevens-Johnson syndrome. Phenytoin and carbamazepine are hepatic enzyme inducers, so they may increase the metabolism of hepatically cleared medications. Levetiracetam and zonisamide do not affect hepatic enzyme function. Levetiracetam is not affected by inducers or inhibitors because it is primarily excreted in the urine without being metabolized. Zonisamide is hepatically metabolized and affected by both inducers and inhibitors (*see* Bradley's NiCP, 7th edn, Ch. 101, pp. 1563–1614).

104. C. The voltage-gated sodium channel has an activation gate and an inactivation gate. At the resting membrane potential, the activation gate is closed and the inactivation gate is open. With slight depolarization, the activation gate opens, allowing an influx of sodium and further depolarization. As the membrane potential reaches +60 mV, the inactivation gate closes and remains closed until the membrane potential returns to −60 mV. This hyperpolarization closes the activation gate, returning it to its original state. The voltage-gated sodium channels cluster in the nodes of Ranvier to facilitate saltatory conduction in myelinated fibers.

105. D. Conduction aphasia comes from lesions of the superior temporal lobe or the inferior parietal region, and is marked by inability to repeat, with relatively preserved speech production (aside from mild paraphasic errors) and preserved speech comprehension. Due to the surrounding anatomical structures, symptoms that often accompany conduction aphasia include apraxia of the left side, right hemiparesis, right sensory loss, or right-sided hemianopsia. Broca aphasia comes from lesions in the posterior part of the inferior frontal gyrus and results in nonfluent speech, or even mutism at an extreme, and comprehension is intact. Transcortical aphasia has several patterns of speech impairment, all of which share in common preserved repetition. Mixed transcortical aphasia results in nonfluent speech with impaired comprehension, but repetition is intact. Transcortical motor aphasia results in nonfluent speech, intact comprehension, and intact repetition. Transcortical sensory aphasia involves fluent speech, impaired comprehension, and intact repetition. Anomic aphasia involves fluent speech with word-finding pauses, circumlocution, and impaired naming. This can be seen in disorders like Alzheimer disease, but can be caused by lesions to the left angular gyrus. Wernicke aphasia involves impaired comprehension and repetition, but intact fluent speech (*see* Bradley's NiCP, 7th edn, Ch. 13, pp. 128–144).

Test Three

QUESTIONS

1. A 6-year-old obese girl is evaluated for intellectual disability and marked hyperphagia. She requires special education for all classes at school, and her parents have recently put padlocks on the refrigerator and cabinets to keep the patient from unsupervised eating. Which of the following is true of this condition?

   A. Paternally inherited mutation on 15q

   B. Maternally inherited mutation on 15q

   C. Sporadic development of XXY

   D. Sporadic development of trisomy 21

   E. Sporadic development of trisomy 13

2. A 6-year-old boy suffered *Mycoplasma* pneumonia 2 weeks ago, from which he fully recovered. He now presents to the emergency room with headache, confusion, and generalized weakness. A computed tomography (CT) scan is shown here. Based on the most likely diagnosis, which of the following is the best course of therapy?

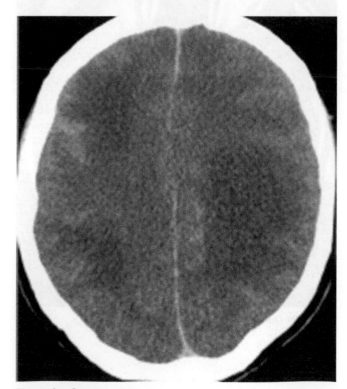

Figure for Question 3.2.

A. Anticoagulation

B. Corticosteroids

C. Antibiotics

D. Observation

E. Hemicraniectomy

3. Which of the following is *not* a hereditary disorder of myelin metabolism?

   A. Alexander disease

   B. Adrenoleukodystrophy

   C. Marchiafava-Bignami syndrome

   D. Canavan disease

   E. Metachromatic leukodystrophy

4. Which of the following is *not* an important component of the blood–brain barrier (BBB)?

   A. Astrocytes

   B. Pericytes

   C. Tight junctions

   D. Oligodendroglia

   E. Basement membrane

5. A 53-year-old man with a history of depression, hypertension, and asthma presents to clinic for tremor that began gradually. His tremor will often worsen with stress or anxiety, and will improve slightly with a glass of wine. His wife also notes an occasional head tremor, mostly at the end of the day. On examination, there is an action tremor bilaterally, occurring mostly in the distal extremities. Further, there is slight imbalance with tandem gait and mild hearing loss. There is no evidence of a resting component to his tremor, nor loss of dexterity or rigidity with activating maneuvers. Which of the following is considered the best first-line agent to treat this patient?

   A. Carbidopa/levodopa

   B. Clonazepam

   C. Propranolol

   D. Primidone

   E. Topiramate

6. A 33-year-old female with a history of prior deep venous thrombosis (DVT), ischemic stroke, and antiphospholipid antibody syndrome presents to the office for an evaluation. She has concerns about her medical history because she would like to become pregnant. Which of the following medications would be the safest for stroke prevention?

A. Warfarin

B. Dabigatran

C. Low molecular weight heparin

D. Aspirin

E. Rivaroxaban

7. The patient whose autopsy photo is shown here most likely died of what?

A. Epidural hemorrhage

B. Subarachnoid hemorrhage

C. Subdural hemorrhage

D. Bacterial meningitis

E. Intraparenchymal hemorrhage

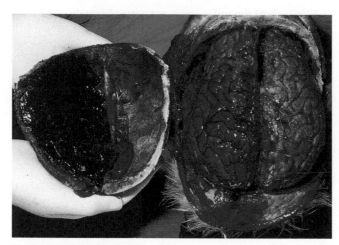

Figure for Question 3.7.

8. Which of the following is *not* a potential source of ototoxicity?

A. Salicylates

B. Gentamycin

C. Cisplatin

D. Levetiracetam

E. Vancomycin

9. Which of the following is the most common treatable cause of neuropathy in the world?

A. Hypothyroidism

B. Diabetes

C. Paraproteinemia

D. Lead toxicity

E. Leprosy

10. Which of the following is *not* commonly seen in fragile X syndrome?

A. Large ears

B. Large testes

C. Dextrocardia

D. Late-onset ataxia

E. Mental retardation

11. A 53-year-old male with no significant medical history presents for evaluation of confusion. In the past month, he developed intermittent jerking movements in his right arm and leg occurring multiple times per day. Additionally, his wife states that he recently lost his keys, couldn't find his car in a parking lot, and even forgot close friends' names. In the emergency department he is afebrile with an elevated white blood cell count. His examination is nonfocal with periodic jerking movements in the right arm. He is noted to have hyponatremia, but otherwise a metabolic panel and hepatic enzymes are normal. Lumbar puncture shows no white blood cells, no red blood cells, protein of 95 mg/dL (normal is <45 mg/dL), and glucose of 63 mg/dL (normal is 45–80 mg/dL). Herpes simplex virus polymerase chain reaction is negative. His magnetic resonance image (MRI) is shown here. Which of the following is the most likely diagnosis?

A. Cerebral autosomal-dominant arteriopathy with subcortical infarcts and leukoencephalopathy (CADASIL)

B. Corticobasal degeneration (CBD)

C. Limbic encephalitis

D. Early-onset Alzheimer's disease

E. Streptococcal meningitis

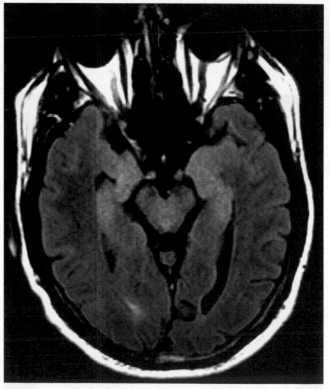

Figure for Question 3.11.

12. In reference to the patient in Question 3.11, which of the following abnormal findings would be expected in this patient?

   A. Anti-voltage-gated calcium channel antibodies
   B. *NOTCH3* gene mutation
   C. Neurofibrillary tangles
   D. Anti-voltage-gated potassium channel antibodies
   E. Cowdry A inclusions

13. Myelin increases the speed of an action potential by doing which of the following?

   A. Reducing membrane capacitance and increasing membrane resistance
   B. Reducing membrane capacitance and reducing membrane resistance
   C. Increasing membrane capacitance and increasing membrane resistance
   D. Increasing membrane capacitance and reducing membrane resistance
   E. No effect on membrane capacitance and reduces membrane resistance

14. A 21-year-old female presented to the emergency department after a new-onset seizure. Before this, she was complaining of a severe headache with blurred vision for the last 2 days. Physical examination demonstrates a somnolent female with normal vitial signs and bilateral papilledema. She has mild weakness of her right face, arm, and leg. Computed tomographic (CT) imaging of the head without contrast and CT angiography of the brain with contrast are shown. Which of the following is the most appropriate treatment?

   A. Intravenous (IV) antihypertensive
   B. IV unfractionated heparin
   C. Oral aspirin
   D. Hematoma evacuation
   E. IV corticosteroids

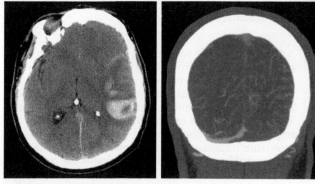

Figure for Question 3.14.

15. Transcranial motor evoked potentials (tcMEPs) and somatosensory evoked potentials (SSEPs) are monitored during a cervical spinal surgery. Halfway through the surgery, the tcMEP responses disappear, but the SSEPs are still present. All of the following can cause this pattern except?

   A. Anterior spinal infarct
   B. Hypotension
   C. Displacement of stimulating electrodes
   D. Posterior spinal infarct
   E. Bolus of rocuronium

16. A 7-year-old boy presents for evaluation of side-to-side head movements and frequent throat clearing in the last 3 months. Each movement is preceded by the urge to move and a sense of relief after. His parents have noted frequent hand washing and the need to flip the light switch multiple times before going to sleep. All of the following could be used to treat this patient except?

   A. Pimozide
   B. Clonidine
   C. Tetrabenazine
   D. Fluoxetine
   E. Methylphenidate

17. A 6-year-old boy who had hypotonia at birth is brought to the neurologist for developmental delay. His mother notes that his eyes move abnormally, his head bobs, and he has weakness and incoordination in his legs. He has never walked like other children, and is not performing well in school. There are two male cousins with similar symptoms, but no affected female family members. On neurological examination, he has nystagmus, truncal titubation, and spasticity in the bilateral lower extremities. His magnetic resonance image is shown. What is the most likely genetic abnormality in this patient?

   A. *GFAP* mutation
   B. Deletion of *PMP22*
   C. *HTT* mutation
   D. *PLP1* mutation
   E. Mutation in *FXN* gene

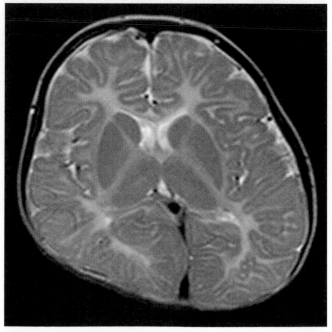

Figure for Question 3.17.

18. After a stroke, a 67-year-old woman is left with Dejerine-Roussy syndrome. Which of the following is the most likely location of her initial infarct?

    A. Ventral posterior lateral nucleus

    B. Pulvinar

    C. Lateral geniculate nucleus

    D. Ventral posterior medial nucleus

    E. Anterior nuclear group

19. A 32-year-old, previously healthy woman presents with left leg weakness and urinary incontinence that developed over the course of 1 day. She has never had this or other neurological symptoms previously. Her thoracic spine magnetic resonance image (MRI) reveals an enhancing lesion at T4, and her brain MRI is shown. Based on this information, which of the following best describes her diagnosis?

    A. Multiple sclerosis

    B. Neuromyelitis optica

    C. Clinically isolated syndrome

    D. Radiographically isolated syndrome

    E. Cerebral autosomal-dominant arteriopathy with subcortical infarcts and leukoencephalopathy (CADASIL)

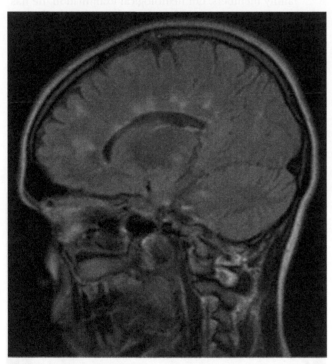

Figure for Question 3.19.

20. For the woman in Question 3.19, after acute treatment for her illness, which of the following is the best choice of therapy thereafter?

    A. Observation

    B. Mitoxantrone

    C. Monthly steroids

    D. Interferon beta-1a

    E. Rituximab

21. A 36-year-old female presents to the emergency department with several falls and a tightness around her upper abdomen over the last 3 days. Her neurological examination demonstrates intact cranial nerves. She has normal strength, sensation, and reflexes in her upper extremities. In her lower extremities she has weakness of hip flexors, knee flexors, and ankle dorsiflexors. Numbness is noted to all modalities below her upper abdomen. Magnetic resonance imaging (MRI) is performed, from which a T2 sagittal image and a T1 sagittal image with contrast are shown here. Which of the following is the most appropriate treatment?

    A. Intravenous immunoglobulin (IVIG) at 0.4 g/kg for 5 days

    B. Intravenous (IV) methylprednisolone at 1000 mg daily for 5 days

    C. Five treatments of plasmapheresis

    D. Oral prednisone at 60 mg followed by a taper over 2 weeks

    E. Anticoagulation with a goal international normalized ratio of 2–3

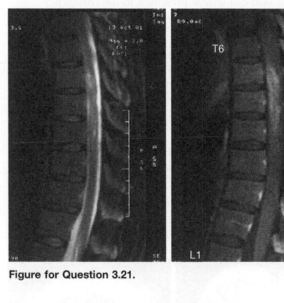

Figure for Question 3.21.

22. A 59-year-old male with a long history of human immunodeficiency virus (HIV) and medical noncompliance presents with a 3-month history of progressive painless gait disturbance and incontinence. His examination demonstrates diffuse weakness in his legs, spasticity, brisk reflexes, and bilateral Babinski responses. No sensory level is present. Magnetic resonance images of his brain and spinal cord are unremarkable. Which of the following is the most likely diagnosis?

    A. Vacuolar myelopathy (VM)

    B. Cytomegalovirus (CMV) myelitis

    C. Varicella zoster virus (VZV) myelitis

    D. Hereditary spastic paraparesis

    E. Cryptococcal meningitis

23. A 54-year-old man is seen in the emergency room for vision changes. For the last month, he has had progressive worsening of vision out of the left and right temporal visual fields, though central and medial vision has been normal bilaterally. His wife states that he has not been himself and that his appearance has even changed. He also complains of mild headaches, which are improved with nonsteroidal antiinflammatory drugs. On examination, he has a bitemporal hemianopsia, as well as coarse facial features, oily skin, and a square jaw. He notes an increase in his glove and shoe size recently. Given the likely diagnosis, which of the following is true of the condition?

    A. Elevated insulinlike growth factor 1 (IGF-1)

    B. Decreased gonadotropin-releasing hormone (GnRH)

    C. Low cortisol

    D. Normal magnetic resonance imaging (MRI) of the brain

    E. Normal x-ray of mandible

24. A 26-year-old male presented to the sleep laboratory for daytime hypersomnolence. His overnight polysomnogram was normal. A multiple sleep latency test (MSLT) was performed the next morning, demonstrating two episodes of sleep-onset rapid eye movement (REM) and an average sleep-onset latency of 5 minutes. All of the following conditions could cause this except?

    A. Behaviorally induced sleep deprivation

    B. Shift-work sleep disorder

    C. Narcolepsy

    D. Recent heavy alcohol use

    E. Somnambulism

25. Which of the following has been shown to benefit nonepileptic attacks?

    A. Obtaining multiple neurological opinions

    B. Continuing anticonvulsant drugs until attacks have stopped

    C. Antidepressant medications

    D. Electroconvulsive therapy

    E. Cognitive behavioral therapy

26. A 15-month-old girl is brought to the emergency room by her mother because of concern for seizures. The patient had been reaching milestones until 3 months ago, when she seemed to have regression. At 6 months old, she had a single seizure associated with a fever. Magnetic resonance imaging and electroencephalography (EEG) at the time were unremarkable. Today, the patient developed recurrent clonic episodes in the absence of a fever. The mother has noted quick jerking movements of both arms over the last several weeks. Neurological examination revealed myoclonic jerks but was otherwise nonfocal. Which of the following is the most likely diagnosis?

    A. Ohtahara syndrome

    B. Benign familial neonatal epilepsy

    C. Dravet syndrome

    D. Panayiotopoulos syndrome

    E. Lennox-Gastaut syndrome

27. A man was seemingly healthy until the age of 25 years, at which point he slowly developed paraparesis, lower extremity neuropathy, hypogonadism, and incontinence. He additionally suffered from dizziness and syncope upon standing. His symptoms were slowly progressive over a couple years, and he ultimately died. An autopsy was performed. Given the most likely diagnosis from the pathological photo shown here, which of the following blood tests would have been abnormal if analyzed premortem?

    A. Very-long-chain fatty acids

    B. Glial fibrillary acid protein (GFAP) genetic testing

    C. Urinary N-acetylaspartate (NAA) level

    D. Sulfatide level

    E. Myelin proteolipid protein (PLP)

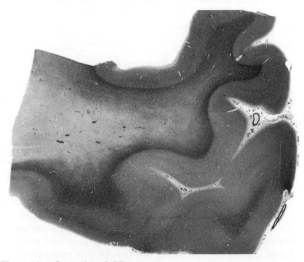

Figure for Question 3.27.

28. A 60-year-old man notes increasingly severe pain on the left side of his midface for about 3 days, followed by the eruption of a vesicular lesion on the side of his nose. Which of the following may he be at increased risk of experiencing?

    A. Ocular complication

    B. Disseminated infection

    C. Cavernous sinus invasion

    D. Infectious meningitis

    E. Trigeminal neuralgia

29. A 72-year-old female presents to the clinic alone for evaluation of abnormal movements. On examination she is demented and has chorea; you suspect Huntington's disease as the cause. Next week you are giving a lecture to medical students and feel this patient would be an excellent example of chorea and you would like to film the patient. Which of the following is the most appropriate response?

    A. Film the patient without asking because she won't remember.

    B. Ask the patient for permission to film her movements.

    C. Ask the nursing facility's medical assistant for permission to film her.

    D. Under no circumstances film the patient.

    E. Film the patient and ask her family for consent before use.

30. A 37-year-old female with multiple sclerosis recently adjusted her treatment. She now presents with new-onset seizures. Which of the following medications was likely added, leading to her seizure?

    A. Glatiramer

    B. Fingolimod

    C. Dalfampridine

    D. Dimethyl fumarate

    E. Natalizumab

31. A 38-year-old man notes that his shoe size has increased from 11 to 13 over the last year, his wedding band no longer fits his finger, and he has a new gap in his lower teeth. After appropriate blood work is performed and demonstrates the direct cause of his symptoms, which of the following is the most rational next test to find the source of the blood abnormality?

    A. Renal ultrasound

    B. Hepatic ultrasound

    C. Magnetic resonance imaging (MRI) of the brain

    D. Computed tomography of the chest

    E. Whole-body positron emission tomography scan

32. A 16-year-old female is brought to her primary care physician's office because of concerns about weight loss. The family has noticed that despite eating large meals on a regular basis, she cannot maintain a normal weight. Her mother says that she even ate four slices of pizza last weekend, yet is still losing weight. The patient feels that she needs to monitor her weight daily to avoid becoming obese. Her physical examination shows a cachectic female, thinning hair, malodorous breath, and scarring on the dorsal aspect of her right hand. All of the following are true of this condition except?

    A. Inability to control self when eating

    B. Binge eating at least once a week for a 3-month period

    C. Eating more than what a normal person would eat in a short period of time

    D. BMI must be <17

    E. Use of laxatives, diuretics, or other agents to lower weight

33. Which of the following is innervated by the anterior interosseous nerve?

    A. Abductor pollicis brevis

    B. Pronator teres

    C. Extensor indicis proprius

    D. Flexor pollicis longus

    E. First dorsal interosseous muscle

34. Which of the following is a parasympathetic activity?

    A. Perspiration

    B. Ejaculation

    C. Urinary storage

    D. Bowel evacuation

    E. Mydriasis

35. Anosmia is common in all of the following conditions except?

    A. Alzheimer disease

    B. Idiopathic Parkinson disease

    C. Dementia with Lewy bodies

    D. Progressive supranuclear palsy

    E. Huntington disease

36. A 63-year-old male smoker presented to the hospital with fever and lower extremity pain. He is found to have elevated inflammatory markers and osteomyelitis of his left foot. He endorses a very long history of poor wound healing and numbness in both feet. He has a hemoglobin A1C of 13.1% (normal is <6%). Despite aggressive intravenous antibiotics, he requires an amputation of the left leg below the knee. The patient wonders how this could occur in the first place and what he should have done to prevent it. What is the best response to the patient?

    A. Increased physical activity could have prevented this complication.

    B. Frequent skin checks and early medical care for wounds or infections is critical in patients with poorly controlled diabetes.

    C. This was likely the result of connective tissue disorder he inherited from his mother.

    D. Even aggressive glucose control could not have prevented this complication.

    E. This likely had to do with smoking rather than poorly controlled diabetes.

37. A 32-year-old man is brought to the emergency room after a bar fight. He complains of severe headache and has a large hematoma over his right temple, but he is otherwise asymptomatic. He is sent home without further evaluation. Then, the next morning he awakes with severe right facial weakness, including the forehead. Given the most likely cause of his new symptom, which of the following should be done?

    A. High-resolution computed tomography (CT) of the temporal bones

    B. Valacyclovir and prednisone

    C. Human immunodeficiency virus serology

    D. Magnetic resonance imaging of the brain

    E. Acetylcholine receptor antibody serology

38. A 34-year-old man with history of migraine develops acute left hemiparesis along with a lateralized, pulsatile headache. The headache resolves within 6 hours, though the weakness persists for the next 24 hours. The patient's sister has suffered similar episodes. Which of the following is true of the underlying diagnosis?

    A. Spike and slow wave on electroencephalogram

    B. Indomethacin sensitive

    C. Associated with cerebrospinal fluid (CSF) pleocytosis

    D. Associated with calcium channel mutation

    E. Autosomal-recessive disorder

39. A 9-year-old boy with short stature is developmentally delayed. He presents to the hospital in the setting of a gastrointestinal illness and has now developed acute blindness. A magnetic resonance image (MRI) of the brain is shown. His strength is normal, and blood work is only notable for an elevated leukocyte count and elevated lactate. Which of the following is the most likely explanation?

    A. Kearns-Sayre syndrome
    B. Leber hereditary optic neuropathy
    C. Myoclonic epilepsy with ragged red fibers (MERRF)
    D. Mitochondrial encephalomyopathy, lactic acidosis, and strokelike episodes (MELAS)
    E. Leigh disease

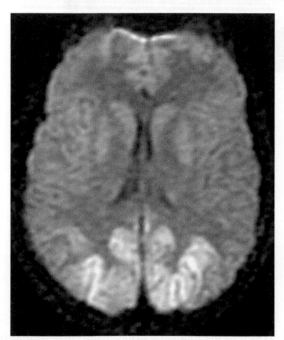

Figure for Question 3.39.

40. A 63-year-old man with a history of diabetes, hypertension, and renal failure on dialysis presents with acute onset of left upper extremity weakness and numbness and left facial droop. His symptoms last only for 1 hour and then resolve, leaving him back to his baseline. His spouse makes him go to the emergency room 5 hours after symptom onset for further evaluation. On examination in the emergency room, his vitals show a pulse of 103, blood pressure (BP) of 153/93, respirations of 12, and oxygen saturation of 98% on room air. He has a normal neurological examination except for numbness and tingling on the plantar aspects of both feet and an irregular pulse. A noncontrast head computed tomography is performed and shows no hemorrhage or blurring of the gray/white margin. He is admitted to the hospital, and further evaluation shows a normal magnetic resonance imaging (MRI) of the brain and magnetic resonance angiography of the head and neck. His transthoracic echo shows only a slightly dilated right atrium, but is otherwise normal. His labs are notable for HbA1C of 7.2 and low-density lipoprotein (LDL) cholesterol of 164. In addition to controlling lipids, blood pressure, and glucose, what is considered the most appropriate regimen for secondary stroke prevention?

    A. Aspirin
    B. Clopidogrel
    C. Warfarin
    D. Rivaroxaban
    E. Aspirin/extended-release dipyridamole combination

41. Which of the following is *not* true of Tay-Sachs disease?

    A. Associated with deficient hexosaminidase A activity
    B. Autosomal-recessive inheritance pattern
    C. Relatively high incidence among individuals from Cajun and French Canadian backgrounds
    D. Classically associated with cherry-red spot on ophthalmoscopy
    E. Reversible with enzyme replacement

42. Which of the following is not considered a component of meaningful use for electronic medical records?

    A. E-prescribing
    B. Automated drug-drug and drug-allergy checks
    C. Maintain active medication and allergy lists
    D. Record smoking status for patients over 13 years old
    E. Copy-forward previous notes

43. A 6-year-old boy has high arches and hammer toes. He begins to trip over his own feet. Examination reveals normal arm strength and sensation, but distal weakness and numbness in his legs, as well as a postural and action tremor in both hands. His nerve conduction and electromyography were abnormal both in his arms and legs, and a sural nerve biopsy was undertaken and is shown below. Which of the following was the most likely abnormality on his nerve conduction testing in his arms?

    A. Decreased motor unit action potential amplitude
    B. Decreased motor unit recruitment
    C. Myotonia
    D. Decreased sensory nerve action potential amplitude
    E. Decreased conduction velocity

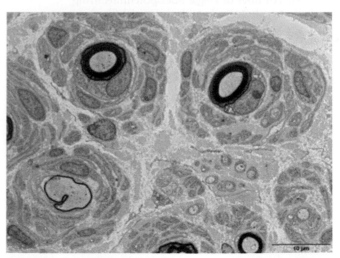

Figure for Question 3.43.

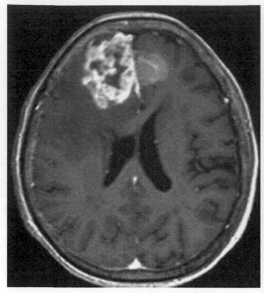 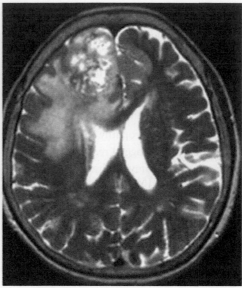

Figure for Question 3.44.

44. A 56-year-old otherwise healthy man presents with 2 weeks of progressive headaches and 2 days of personality change. His primary care physician refers him for a magnetic resonance image (MRI), which is shown here. Which of the following is the next best course of action?

    A. Stereotactic biopsy
    B. Maximal safe resection
    C. Whole-brain radiation
    D. Focal radiation
    E. Chemotherapy

45. Which of the following describes increased jitter seen on single-fiber electromyography (EMG)?

    A. Variability in firing time between two muscle fibers in the same motor unit
    B. Variability in firing time between two motor units in the same muscle
    C. Intermittent transmission failure of one muscle fiber potential
    D. Number of single-fiber potentials firing synchronously with the initial fiber
    E. Measure of quanta of acetylcholine released from the presynaptic terminal

46. In comparing genetic prion disease with sporadic prion disease, which of the following is *not* true of genetic prion disease?

    A. Younger age of onset
    B. Initial parkinsonism or ataxia
    C. Slower disease course
    D. Severe personality changes early on
    E. Longer survival

47. A mass lesion in the pineal gland, compressing the adjacent dorsal midbrain, pretectum, and superior colliculi, is most likely to cause which of the following?

    A. Mobius syndrome
    B. Adie pupil
    C. Parinaud syndrome
    D. Argyll Robertson pupil
    E. Marcus Gunn pupil

48. Which of the following neurotransmitters is thought to play a role in psychosis?

    A. Dopamine
    B. Serotonin
    C. Gamma aminobutyric acid (GABA)
    D. Norepinephrine
    E. All the above

49. Which of the following neurodegenerative conditions caused the pathological findings seen in the figure?

    A. Alzheimer disease
    B. Human immunodeficiency virus dementia
    C. Pick disease
    D. Parkinson disease
    E. Huntington disease

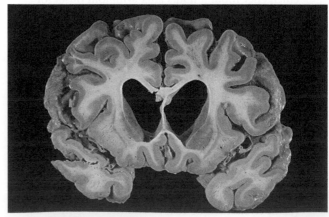

Figure for Question 3.49.

50. A 64-year-old smoker is found comatose. Magnetic resonance imaging reveals well-defined restricted diffusion indicative of a stroke, but no other acute pathological processes or cerebral edema. Laboratory tests and toxicology are relatively unremarkable. What is the most likely artery involved in this stroke?

    A. Left middle cerebral artery
    B. Left posterior cerebral artery
    C. Artery of Percheron
    D. Recurrent artery of Huebner
    E. Artery of Adamkiewicz

51. An 11-year-old boy is admitted to the hospital because of respiratory distress related to respiratory syncytial virus infection. While in the hospital, he develops progressive deterioration of his mental status and seizures. His examination shows obtundation, generalized dystonia, and mild orofacial dyskinesias. On laboratory evaluation, he has ketoacidosis, elevated ammonia, and hypoglycemia. Urine organic acids reveal elevated glutaric acid. A magnetic resonance image of his brain is shown. Which of the following is *not* part of the possible treatment?

    A. Low-protein diet
    B. Riboflavin
    C. L-carnitine
    D. Supplementation of lysine and tryptophan
    E. Intravenous hydration

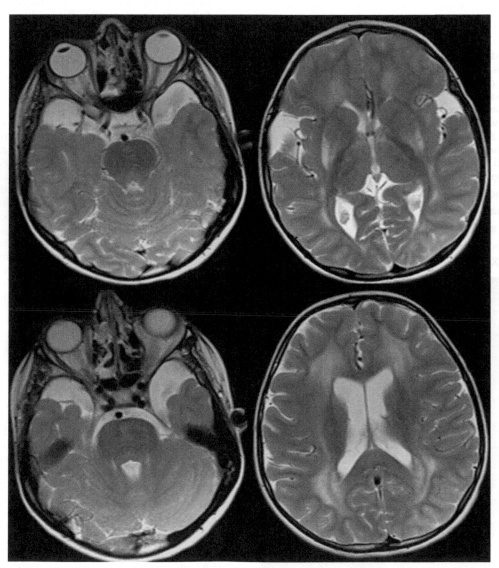

Figure for Question 3.51.

67. A 21-year-old woman presents to the neurologist with a number of complaints that include headache, generalized weakness, and whole-body numbness. Other complaints include pain with intercourse, nausea, and anxiety. She has seen four other providers, and has undergone an exhaustive workup, including neurological imaging, nerve conduction studies, and gastroenterological evaluation, which were all normal. Given her suspected diagnosis, which of the following is most likely to be found upon further questioning?

    A. The patient has a history of physical and sexual abuse, along with comorbid depression.

    B. The patient has a history of flashing lights, photophobia, and nausea that precedes her headaches.

    C. The patient has a history of joint pain across many body parts along with fatigue, poor sleep, and poor concentration.

    D. She is seeking medical disability and needs someone to fill out her paperwork.

    E. She has a history of tick bite followed by targetoid rash.

68. A 24-year-old female who is 36 weeks pregnant comes to the office for evaluation of pain. She describes a burning pain on her right thigh that has been present for 3 weeks. The pain is mostly on the lateral thigh and never goes below the knee. It is worse with standing and is better with sitting or lying down. Her neurological examination is normal. Which of the following is true of this condition?

    A. Electromyography (EMG) and nerve conduction studies are necessary for the diagnosis.

    B. Treatment involves an injection of local steroid and anesthetic around the femoral nerve.

    C. Permanent weakness can occur if left untreated.

    D. Treatment involves avoidance of tight-fitting clothing.

    E. Lumbar puncture is necessary for the diagnosis.

69. Parasympathetic activation leads to which of the following physiological changes?

    A. Pupil dilation

    B. Sweating

    C. Increased cardiac contractility

    D. Increased detrusor activity

    E. Bronchiolar dilatation

70. A 35-year-old Pakistani man presents to the emergency room with 3 days of tremor, weakness, and incoordination in his right arm. Additionally, he developed painful, blurred vision in the left eye about 1 week before. He has a history of recurrent oral ulcers, although he has found no benefit from antiviral medications. On magnetic resonance imaging (MRI) evaluation, an enhancing lesion with no associated edema is identified in the left basal ganglia. Nurses also tell you that he's developed ulcerative lesions at all phlebotomy sites. Which of the following is the most likely diagnosis?

    A. Sarcoidosis

    B. Acute disseminated encephalomyelitis (ADEM)

    C. Lupus cerebritis

    D. Multiple sclerosis

    E. Behçet disease

71. A 78-year-old male presents after having a fluorodeoxyglucose (FDG) positron emission tomography (PET) scan performed in the evaluation of memory loss. This scan shows decreased fluorodeoxyglucose metabolism in the posterior parietotemporal region and posterior cingulate gyrus. Which of the following is the most likely diagnosis?

    A. Dementia with Lewy bodies

    B. Alzheimer disease

    C. Huntington disease

    D. Frontotemporal dementia

    E. Primary progressive aphasia

72. A 73-year-old man presents with shooting pain in his posterior left hip that radiates down his lateral leg and the dorsal aspect of his left foot. The pain began after a fall, and is described as paroxysmal with improvement upon leaning forward. On examination, he has sensory loss in the same distribution of his pain, but normal strength and reflexes. Which of the following would *not* be considered a reasonable first option for treatment of his condition?

    A. Lumbar laminectomy

    B. Physical therapy

    C. Opioids

    D. Nonsteroidal antiinflammatory drug (NSAID)

    E. Temporary activity modification

73. Which of the following is the mechanism of action for rituximab?

    A. Sphingosine-1-phosphatase inhibitor

    B. CD20 monoclonal antibody

    C. Alpha-4-integrin adhesion molecule antibody

    D. CD52 monoclonal antibody

    E. Sodium channel blocker

74. A 53-year-old male presents to clinic with a several-month history of falls. He has a history significant for smoking. His neurological examination reveals normal cranial nerves, normal strength, decreased sensation to all modalities in his extremities, and absent reflexes. He has a positive Romberg and demonstrates sensory ataxia. Pseudoathetosis is present. Which of the following is most commonly associated with this condition?

    A. Anti–N-methyl-D-aspartate (anti-NMDA) receptor antibody

    B. Anti-Jo antibody

    C. Anti-GM1 antibody

    D. Anti-GQ1b antibody

    E. Anti-antineuronal nuclear antibody 1 (anti-ANNA-1)

75. All are true of severe, acute traumatic spinal cord injury *except* which of the following?

    A. Presents with areflexia, weakness, numbness, and incontinence

    B. High-dose steroids may improve ambulation at 3 months

    C. Often associated with significant autonomic instability

    D. Cord contusion may lead to worse arm weakness than leg

    E. Requires immediate magnetic resonance imaging (MRI) in case of reversible compression

76. A 45-year-old man suffers a partial spinal cord transection at T12 on the left. Among the affected Rexed laminae, the substantia gelatinosa appears to be damaged on magnetic resonance imaging. Which of the following leg deficits correlates with this radiographic finding?

    A. Monoplegia

    B. Absent vibratory sensation

    C. Absent noxious stimulus sensation

    D. Ataxia

    E. Absent reflexes

77. A 23-year-old woman was abducted from her home and taken to a basement where she was sexually and physically abused for 1 week. Upon the arrival of authorities, the woman does not remember her name, where she lives, or how she got in the basement. She is also unable to give any details of what happened to her. Which of the following is the most likely diagnosis?

    A. Posttraumatic stress disorder

    B. Concussion

    C. Dissociative identity disorder

    D. Depersonalization

    E. Dissociative amnesia

78. A 23-year-old woman with a history of kidney disease has an acute onset of headache that stopped her midsentence, and was followed immediately by nausea and vomiting. She is rushed to hospital via ambulance. Her head computed tomography (CT) is shown. When is her peak risk of vasospasm?

    A. 1 hour

    B. 1 day

    C. 1 week

    D. 1 month

    E. 1 year

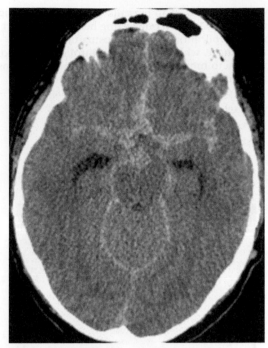

Figure for Question 3.78.

79. All of the following neurotoxins affect voltage-gated sodium channels *except*?

    A. Tetrodotoxin

    B. Saxitoxin

    C. Brevetoxin

    D. α-latrotoxin

    E. Ciguatoxin

80. A 12-year-old boy presents with the inability to sit still. On examination, he has choreiform movements, worse on the left upper extremity than the right. Otherwise, he has a normal neurological examination. His mother states that these movements started gradually about 3 months ago. Further, over the last 2 months he has been increasingly irritable, hyperactive, and obsessed with making sure that his shoelaces are double-knotted. His medical history is generally unremarkable, except for a sore throat approximately 4 months ago. There is no family history of similar neurological or psychological features. Which of the following is indicated?

    A. Penicillin G

    B. Habit reversal therapy

    C. Genetic counseling

    D. Carbidopa/levodopa

    E. Stimulant medication

81. A 34-year-old woman presents with an excruciating headache 3 days after delivering her first baby. Her only complication was mild postpartum vaginal hemorrhage, which was easily controlled. She reports inability to breastfeed since delivery and complains of polydipsia and polyuria. Brain imaging is shown. Which of the following is the correct diagnosis?

    A. Cerebral venous sinus thrombosis

    B. Postpartum angiopathy

    C. Sheehan syndrome

    D. Postepidural spinal headache

    E. Migraine

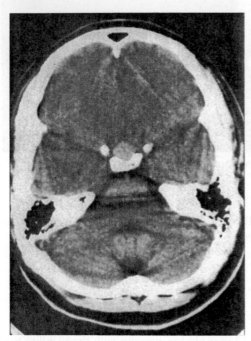

Figure for Question 3.81.

82. If vertigo and a right beating nystagmus are observed 30 seconds after performing a Dix-Hallpike maneuver with the right ear toward the ground, what is the most likely localization of the patient's underlying problem?

    A. Left posterior semicircular canal

    B. Left lateral semicircular canal

    C. Right posterior semicircular canal

    D. Right lateral semicircular canal

    E. Cerebellar vermis

83. A patient who suffered a stroke has intact sensation in his extremities. With his eyes closed, he cannot identify objects placed in his hand affected by the stroke. What is this disorder called?

    A. Astereognosia

    B. Agraphesthesia

    C. Prosopagnosia

    D. Simultagnosia

    E. Visual agnosia

84. All of the following are necessary criteria for the diagnosis of restless legs syndrome (RLS) *except*?

    A. An urge to move the legs caused by uncomfortable sensation in the legs

    B. An urge to move occurring during periods of rest

    C. Discomfort relieved by movement

    D. Diagnosed on overnight polysomnogram with periodic electromyogram (EMG) activity occurring every 20–40 seconds

    E. An urge to move that is worse at night

85. For a woman with recurrent pressurelike headaches, papilledema, and pulsatile tinnitus, which of the following is *not* a therapeutic consideration?

    A. Ventriculoperitoneal shunt

    B. Optic nerve sheath fenestration

    C. Acetazolamide

    D. Isotretinoin

    E. Large-volume lumbar puncture

86. In muscle contraction, which of the following is the mobile part of the sarcomere resulting in a decrease in sarcomere length?

    A. Myosin

    B. Nebulin

    C. Actin

    D. Titin

    E. Troponin

87. Which of the following is highest on the differential diagnosis for an otherwise-healthy 24-year-old woman presenting with new trigeminal neuralgia?

    A. Multiple sclerosis

    B. Conversion disorder

    C. Sjögren syndrome

    D. Facial trauma

    E. Tumor

88. A 27-year-old female presents to the hospital with an episode of suspected thoracic transverse myelitis. Unfortunately the magnetic resonance imaging machine is broken and will not be repaired for days. Somatosensory evoked potentials (SSEPs) are performed to help confirm the diagnosis. Which of the following abnormalities would be expected?

    A. Prolonged N22–P34 interpeak latency

    B. Absent N22

    C. Prolonged N9–N13 interpeak latency

    D. Absent N20

    E. Prolonged P34–P37 interpeak latency

89. Which of the following is demonstrated in the following picture?

    A. Agenesis of the corpus callosum
    B. Pachygyria
    C. Holoprosencephaly
    D. Lissencephaly
    E. Polymicrogyria

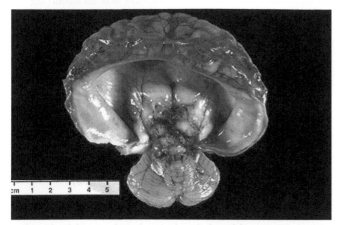

Figure for Question 3.89.

90. A 9-year-old boy presents with episodes of uncontrollable laughing for no reason and at inappropriate times. These outbursts usually last <1 minute, but they have been occurring more frequently over the last few months. Despite his best efforts, he cannot control these episodes. In addition he has complained of headaches, mostly at night. His neurological examination is unremarkable. Which of the following is the most likely cause of his symptoms?

    A. Mesial temporal lobe sclerosis
    B. Autism
    C. Parasagittal meningioma
    D. Hypothalamic hamartoma
    E. Use of levetiracetam

91. Which of the following is not a part of the classic construct of grief?

    A. Denial
    B. Anger
    C. Bargaining
    D. Acceptance
    E. Projection

92. Which of the following is an unlikely cause of meningitis in a 30 year old, but should be considered in an 80 year old?

    A. Group B streptococci
    B. *Listeria monocytogenes*
    C. *Neisseria meningitidis*
    D. *Pseudomonas aeruginosa*
    E. *Staphylococcus aureus*

93. Which of the following is absent in individuals with Zellweger syndrome?

    A. Mitochondria
    B. Peroxisomes
    C. Endosomes
    D. Lysosomes
    E. Chylomicrons

94. Which of the following is true regarding the condition depicted in this image?

    A. This condition frequently leads to low-output cardiac failure in neonates.
    B. The malformation consists of arteries draining into capillaries, leading to defective venous drainage.
    C. Strokes or steal phenomena can occur, leading to progressive hemiparesis.
    D. The malformation is self-limiting and usually does not require treatment.
    E. A common etiology includes dehydration or infection.

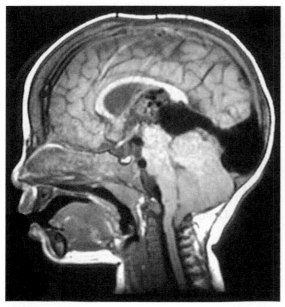
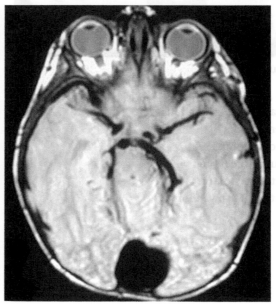

Figure for Question 3.94.

ANSWERS

1. A. Prader-Willi is a genetic syndrome characterized by intellectual disability, cryptorchidism, short stature, hyperphagia, and obesity. This disorder demonstrates the rare genetic principle of parental imprinting, wherein receiving a particular mutation on 15q from the father leads to Prader-Willi syndrome, but maternal inheritance of the same mutation leads to Angelman syndrome. Angelman syndrome is characterized by intellectual disability with seizures, hand flapping, and a characteristic happy demeanor. A karyotype of XXY is found in Klinefelter syndrome, which is associated with decreased muscle mass and body hair, increased breast tissue, and sterility. Trisomy 21 is seen with Down syndrome, with symptoms of intellectual disability, hypotonia, macroglossia, flattened nose, low-set ears, slanting eyes, and a single palmar crease. Trisomy 13 is seen with Patau syndrome, which is associated with microcephaly, craniofacial abnormalities, low-set ears, rocker-bottom feet, genital defects, dextrocardia, and death in infancy (*see* Bradley's NiCP, 7th edn, Ch. 50, pp. 648–675).

2. B. Acute hemorrhagic leukoencephalitis, or acute hemorrhagic encephalopathy, is an acute, monophasic, inflammatory illness associated with demyelination and hemorrhage. This particular variety of acute disseminated encephalomyelitis is almost always associated with a recent respiratory tract infection, most commonly *Mycoplasma*. Immunosuppressive therapy is the best therapy, although with variable success. Cerebral venous sinus thrombosis may have associated infarct and hemorrhage, as one might erroneously suspect from this CT scan. In such a scenario, anticoagulation would be correct. However, without other details to specifically suggest CVST, such as hypercoagulable history or clear imaging evidence of a delta sign, this is a less likely diagnosis. Given the 1-week interval from his *Mycoplasma* infection, central nervous system spread of this infection is less likely than a postinfectious process. Observation would not be an appropriate therapy for any possible diagnosis. There is evidence that hemicraniectomy may improve long-term outcomes and prevent herniation in cases of malignant infarcts, although that is not the underlying diagnosis in this case (*see* Bradley's NiCP, 7th edn, Ch. 80, pp. 1159–1186). Figure from Kao HW, Alexandru D, Kim R, Yanni D, Hasso AN 2012 Value of susceptibility-weighted imaging in acute hemorrhagic leukoencephalitis. *Journal of Clinical Neuroscience* 19(12): 1740–1741, with permission.

3. C. Marchiafava-Bignami syndrome is a toxic/metabolic disease of the myelin that is classically associated with chronic alcoholism and nonspecific nutritional deficiencies. There is no evidence of a hereditary component to this syndrome. All of the other listed disorders of myelin metabolism have a known hereditary basis. Alexander disease is associated with mutations in the *GFAP* gene. Adrenoleukodystrophy is associated with mutations in the *ABCD1* gene, encoding peroxisomal membrane transporter proteins. Canavan disease is associated with mutations in the *ASPA* gene, encoding the protein aspartoacylase. Metachromatic leukodystrophy is associated with mutations in the *ARSA* gene, encoding arylsulfatase A (*see* Bradley's NiCP, 7th edn, Chs. 85, pp. 1226–1236 and 91, pp. 1324–1341).

4. D. The BBB is a highly selective filter that keeps many circulating blood substances away from the brain. The components of the BBB include astrocytic end feet, pericytes, tight junctions, and basement membrane. Oligodendroglia are not involved in the BBB, but instead myelinate neurons in the brain (*see* Bradley's NiCP, 7th edn, Ch. 88, pp. 1261–1278).

5. D. The patient most likely has essential tremor. Most often, this is a familial tremor characterized by a distal action tremor, mild sensorineural hearing loss, and loss of balance. Although there is generally no bradykinesia, rigidity, or postural instability, cogwheeling may still be seen in this disorder. The tremor will occasionally start asymmetrically, but quickly spreads to the other side and may even affect the voice, head, or legs. Commonly, tremors worsen with stress, anxiety, fatigue, or caffeine, and will occasionally improve with alcohol. First-line medical treatment for essential tremor includes primidone or propranolol. Propranolol would not be the most appropriate choice in this patient, as it may worsen both his depression and asthma. Other medications that can be tried include topiramate, clonazepam, and gabapentin. For medically refractory tremors, botulinum toxin or deep brain stimulation of the thalamus (ventral intermediate nucleus) can be considered. Unless the physical examination suggests features of parkinsonism, carbidopa/levodopa is not usually used (*see* Bradley's NiCP, 7th edn, Ch. 96, pp. 1422–1460).

6. C. Decisions on anticoagulation during pregnancy can be difficult. This patient has antiphospholipid antibody syndrome and a history of DVT and ischemic stroke. She is at a high risk of recurrent stroke, especially during pregnancy. Aspirin would reduce the risk of stroke, but not as much as unfractionated heparin, and aspirin is pregnancy class D. Dabigatran and rivaroxaban could be considered if the patient did not desire pregnancy, although there is limited information on the safety of these medications during pregnancy, so they are not recommended. Warfarin is known to be teratogenic and is pregnancy category X. Unfractionated heparin or low-molecular-weight heparin are the recommended anticoagulants to use during pregnancy (*see* Bradley's NiCP, Ch. 112, pp. 1973–1991).

7. C. The image demonstrates a subdural hemorrhage, most easily differentiated from other hemorrhage types because the falx cerebri remains visible and intact within the skull convexity in the examiner's hands (*see* Bradley's NiCP, 7th edn, Ch. 66, pp. 968–980). Figure from Ellison D, Love S, Chimelli L, et al. 2013 *Neuropathology*, 3rd edn, Elsevier, with permission.

8. D. Ototoxicity is a common concern with medications used in neurology, and is often dependent on dose, duration of therapy, metabolic clearance, and concurrent administration with other ototoxic medications. At high doses, salicylates may cause tinnitus or temporary hearing loss. Among aminoglycosides, gentamycin tends to affect both balance and hearing, whereas amikacin tends to only affect the hearing (with profound, permanent hearing loss) and streptomycin tends to only affect balance. Cisplatin can cause tinnitus and profound sensorineural hearing loss. Vancomycin may cause hearing loss, especially in the setting of renal insufficiency. Although some antiepileptic drugs may be associated with temporary vertigo (including

phenytoin, lamotrigine, carbamazepine, and lacosamide), levetiracetam is not associated with vertigo or ototoxicity (*see* Bradley's NiCP, 7th edn, Ch. 46, pp. 583–604).

9. E. Leprosy is the most common treatable cause of neuropathy in the world, particularly in Southeast Asia, Africa, and South America. In the United States diabetes is the most common treatable cause of neuropathy (*see* Bradley's NiCP, 7th edn, Ch. 107, pp. 1791–1867).

10. C. Fragile X syndrome is an autosomal-dominant disease of cytosine-guanine-guanine (CGG) repeats in the coding region of the *FMR-1* gene on chromosome X. Women are carriers of this syndrome, given the presence of a normal X chromosome. Symptoms of fragile X syndrome include mental retardation, large ears, and large testes. Further, patients with fragile X syndrome are at increased risk of a disorder known as *fragile X tremor ataxia syndrome*, which begins in the fifth or sixth decade with tremor and ataxia. Dextrocardia is not seen at an increased rate with relation to fragile X syndrome (*see* Bradley's NiCP, 7th edn, Ch. 90, pp. 1301–1323).

11. C. The patient presents with subacute memory loss and myoclonus with a lumbar puncture showing inflammation without infection. The MRI demonstrates hyperintensities in the bilateral mesial temporal lobes, which is common in limbic encephalitis. CADASIL usually involves headaches, strokelike episodes, and dementia later in the course, and the MRI shows subcortical white matter lesions, particularly in the anterotemporal lobes. CBD involves myoclonus, rigidity, dementia, and alien limb syndrome. There are no diagnostic MRI findings for CBD, although atrophy of the parietal lobe can be present. There are no diagnostic MRI findings for Alzheimer disease, although global atrophy and atrophy of the temporoparietal junction are common. Streptococcal meningitis would present more acutely with high fevers, encephalopathy, seizures, and elevated white blood cells and protein in the spinal fluid. In meningitis, enhancement of the meninges can be seen, but hyperintensities within the parenchyma signify encephalitis, not meningitis (*see* Bradley's NiCP, 7th edn, Ch. 82, pp. 1196–1200). Figure from Mayans D, personal collection, with permission.

12. D. Anti-voltage-gated potassium channel antibodies are auto-antibodies, which may be either paraneoplastic or sporadic, and are associated with limbic encephalitis and neuromyotonia (Isaac syndrome). Anti-voltage-gated calcium channel antibodies are seen in Lambert-Eaton myasthenic syndrome. *NOTCH3* gene mutation is seen in CADASIL. Neurofibrillary tangles are a prominent pathological feature seen in Alzheimer disease. Cowdry A inclusions are the main pathological feature seen in herpes encephalitis (*see* Bradley's NiCP, 7th edn, Ch. 82, pp. 1196–1200).

13. A. Myelin develops an insulating layer around the axons with nodes of Ranvier every 1 to 2 mm. Conduction of an action potential occurs at the node of Ranvier. By decreasing the area where conduction can occur (compared with unmyelinated fibers), the total resistance of the membrane is increased. Capacitance is reduced by the high concentration of sodium channels in the nodes, which allows for more-than-adequate depolarization to occur so that the signal is transmitted to the next node of Ranvier without fail (*see* Bradley's NiCP, 7th edn, Ch. 34–35, pp. 349–391).

14. B. The patient's CT scan demonstrates a left-sided intracerebral hemorrhage, and the CT angiography shows a filling defect in the left transverse sinus. Cerebral venous sinus thrombosis is a neurological emergency for which the primary treatment remains anticoagulation even in the setting of a hemorrhagic stroke. This patient's blood pressure is normal, so no antihypertensives are indicated. Further, while the intracerebral hemorrhage is associated with swelling, hyperosmotic therapy is superior to corticosteroids in such an emergent scenario. Aspirin has no role in acute treatment of a venous thrombosis (*see* Bradley's NiCP, 7th edn, Ch. 66, pp. 968–980). Figure from Mirvis SE, Kubal WS, et al. *Problem Solving in Emergency Radiology*, pp. 53–101, Figure 4-13, Elsevier, with permission.

15. D. tcMEPs and SSEPs are frequently used during intraoperative spinal surgery monitoring. Transcranial motor evoked potentials roughly measure function of the anterior portion of the cord through stimulation of the upper motor neurons through transcranial stimulation, measuring connectivity by electromyography activity in various muscles. Loss of these signals can be due to technical failure (displacement of either recording or stimulating electrodes), hypotension, or anesthetics (particularly neuromuscular blocking agents like rocuronium), or can also indicate a pathological state such as anterior spinal infarct or injury from the surgical procedure. SSEPs are transmitted through the dorsal column and detect injury in that pathway. These are also susceptible to technical failure, anesthetics, and hypotension (*see* Bradley's NiCP, 7th edn, Ch. 36, 391–400 and Ch. 38, pp. 407–410).

16. E. Tourette syndrome is marked by both motor and phonic tics and can be associated with obsessive-compulsive disorder (OCD) and/or attention-deficit/hyperactivity disorder (ADHD). In this question, the patient has motor and vocal tics along with OCD behaviors. Tics can be treated with a variety of medications that block or deplete dopamine, including antipsychotics (risperidone, pimozide, haloperidol, fluphenazine) or tetrabenazine. Other agents used to treat the comorbidities of Tourette syndrome include centrally acting alpha$_2$-antagonists (clonidine, guanfacine) or selective serotonin reuptake inhibitors. Methylphenidate would not be used in this patient because of the lack of ADHD symptoms (*see* Bradley's NiCP, 7th edn, Ch. 96, pp. 1422–1460).

17. D. This case is an example of Pelizaeus-Merzbacher disease, which is caused by a deleterious event (most often duplication) of the *PLP1* gene. Clinically, Pelizaeus-Merzbacher presents with nystagmus, spasticity, athetosis, tremor, and ataxia. Typically symptoms begin in the first 2–4 months of life. Given the X-linked pattern of heredity, this is a disease of males. Motor milestones are often delayed, and children frequently develop spastic quadriparesis. Cognition is also frequently impaired. Brain MRI commonly reveals diffuse leukodystrophy, with increased signal intensity in bilateral hemispheres, cerebellum, and brainstem, which spares the U-fibers. On pathology, there can also be islands of white matter, giving the sample a "tigroid" appearance.

Management for Pelizaeus-Merzbacher is largely supportive. A *GFAP* mutation leads to Alexander disease and presents in an autosomal-recessive fashion. The question stem suggests involvement in a male cousin, with normal females in the family suggesting an X-linked inheritance, typical of Pelizaeus-Merzbacher disease. In addition, Alexander disease of the infant/juvenile type usually has a frontal predominance of white matter change rather than the confluent nature of Pelizaeus-Merzbacher disease. A deletion in the *PMP22* gene leads to hereditary neuropathy with liability for pressure palsies. A trinucleotide expansion of *HTT* leads to Huntington disease. A mutation in the *FXN* gene leads to Friedreich's ataxia (*see* Bradley's NiCP, 7th edn, Ch. 50, pp. 648–675). Figure from Shimojima K, Mano T, Kashiwagi M, et al. 2012 Pelizaeus-Merzbacher disease caused by a duplication-inverted triplication-duplication in chromosomal segments including the PLP1 region. *European Journal of Medical Genetics* 55(6-7): 400–403, with permission.

18. A. The ventral posterior lateral (VPL) nucleus relays sensory information from the limbs to the postcentral gyrus. Whereas an acute lesion in the VPL may cause sensory loss, chronically patients may be left with a thalamic pain syndrome (Dejerine-Roussy syndrome) in the same distribution. The pulvinar is the largest thalamic nucleus and is associated with visual attention and saccade initiation. Also worth noting is the frequent presence of MRI fluid attenuation inversion recovery (FLAIR) sequence hyperintensity in the bilateral pulvinar associated with Creutzfeldt-Jakob disease (pulvinar sign). The lateral geniculate nucleus is a relay of visual input from the optic tract to the primary visual cortex. The ventral posterior medial nucleus is a sensory relay for pain and temperature from the face, as well as taste from all portions of the tongue and epiglottis. The medial geniculate nucleus relays auditory information from the inferior colliculi to the primary auditory nucleus (*see* Bradley's NiCP, 7th edn, Ch. 30, pp. 314–323).

19. A. Based on the 2010 revisions of the McDonald Diagnostic Criteria for Multiple Sclerosis (MS), this patient meets the diagnostic criteria for MS based on one clinical attack and objective clinical evidence of ≥2 lesions. See the table for more information. Neuromyelitis optica is a demyelinating disorder, previously known as *Devic disease*, associated with recurrent demyelinating events of the optic nerves and longitudinally extensive transverse myelitis. This disorder is associated with antibodies against aquaporin-4. Clinically isolated syndrome is diagnosed in an individual with only one attack of demyelination with no radiographic evidence of prior attacks. Radiographically isolated syndrome is diagnosed based on MRI evidence of prior demyelinating episodes (e.g. ovoid, well-circumscribed foci in commonly affected areas) with no clinical history suggestive of demyelinating attacks. CADASIL is a hereditary syndrome associated with recurrent small-vessel strokes, vascular dementia, and migraines. CADASIL is associated with defects in the *NOTCH3* gene (*see* Bradley's NiCP, 7th edn, Ch. 80, pp. 1159–1186). Figure from Calabresi P 2016 Multiple sclerosis and demyelinating conditions of the central nervous system. In: Goldman L, Schafer AI *Goldman-Cecil Medicine*, Elsevier, with permission.

TABLE FOR ANSWER 3.19, 2010 McDonald Diagnostic Criteria for Multiple Sclerosis

Clinical presentation	Additional data needed for diagnosis of multiple sclerosis
Two or more attacks; objective clinical evidence of two or more lesions; or one lesion with a prior attack	None
Two or more attacks; objective clinical evidence of one lesion	Dissemination in space, demonstrated by ≥1 T2 lesion in at least two of four typical regions for MS (periventricular, juxtacortical, infratentorial, spinal cord); or await another attack in a different region
One attack; objective clinical evidence of ≥2 lesions	Dissemination in time, demonstrated by simultaneous presence of asymptomatic enhancing and nonenhancing lesions at any time; or a new lesion developed on follow-up scan; or await a second clinical attack
One attack; objective clinical evidence of 1 lesion (clinically isolated syndrome)	Dissemination in space and time, demonstrated by measures detailed above

20. D. First-line immunomodulatory therapy for relapsing remitting multiple sclerosis (RRMS) may include an interferon (interferon beta-1a or interferon beta-1b), glatiramer, dimethyl fumarate, or fingolimod. Mitoxantrone is approved for progressive forms of MS, but is generally used only for refractory disease due to the risk of cardiac toxicity. Rituximab is an anti-CD20 monoclonal antibody that reduces many immune-mediated diseases and symptoms. Although initial studies are hopeful for rituximab in the use of RRMS, there are no definitive data for this choice. Monthly steroids are generally avoided as a monotherapy due to undue side effects and lack of efficacy in disease modulation. Observation is not the best choice given the definitive diagnosis of MS reached in Question 3.19 (*see* Bradley's NiCP, 7th edn, Ch. 80, pp. 1159–1186).

21. B. This patient presents with an acute transverse myelitis. Symptoms of transverse myelitis depend on the section of the spinal cord involved. Patients with this condition commonly present with a bandlike sensation across the chest or abdomen, a sensory level, and weakness. The MRI scan of her spine demonstrates T2 hyperintense lesions within the cord that enhance with contrast. This is the typical appearance of acute transverse myelitis. Initial treatment begins with IV methylprednisolone given over the course of 5 days. Oral steroids are not an appropriate treatment, but an oral steroid taper could be used after the initial IV steroids are completed. IVIG has no role in transverse myelitis. Plasmapheresis can be considered if there is no response to initial steroids; however, this is not used first line because of risks of hypotension, sepsis, metabolic disturbances, and bleeding. This patient's examination is most consistent with a complete spinal lesion and not an anterior spinal artery syndrome, so anticoagulation is not indicated (*see* Bradley's NiCP, 7th edn, Ch. 80, pp. 1159–1186). Figure from Waldman SD, Campbell RSD 2010 *Imaging of Pain*, Saunders, with permission.

22. A. The patient presents with a painless, progressive, lower extremity myelopathy in the setting of HIV. This is most consistent with a VM or possibly human T-cell lymphotropic virus 1 (HTLV1; which is not an answer choice). VM occurs in up to 50% of HIV patients at autopsy, and pathological samples show vacuolar changes within the myelin sheaths in the thoracic cord. Once the disorder develops, it does not improve with highly active antiretroviral therapy, unlike other complications of HIV. Pain, sensory level, or upper extremity symptoms would point toward CMV myelitis, VZV myelitis, other focal lesions, or inflammation. Hereditary spastic paraparesis can present similarly; however, there is nothing in the question stem to suggest a family history, and the history of HIV should be a red flag for VM. Cryptococcal meningitis does not typically cause a myelopathy, but rather a severe headache with increased intracranial pressure and seizures (*see* Bradley's NiCP, 7th edn, Ch. 77, pp. 1102–1120).

23. A. The patient has a bitemporal hemianopsia, headache, coarsening of facial features, and abnormal growth of the hands and feet (acromegaly). This most likely relates to excessive growth hormone (GH) production. Clinically, patients may also develop gigantism (tall stature, macrocephaly, visual changes, coarse facial features). Most often, the excessive GH is caused from a secreting pituitary adenoma, which is apparent on a contrast-enhanced MRI of the sella. Enlarging masses may result in a bitemporal hemianopsia due to compression of the optic chiasm. X-rays of bones such as the mandible also are abnormal. The diagnosis is made through a combination of history, examination, imaging, and laboratory evidence of elevated IGF-1 and GH level after an oral glucose tolerance test. Administration of 100 grams of glucose would suppress GH secretion normally, but would not suppress excess GH in acromegaly. Treatment often involves a transsphenoidal resection of the tumor, as well as pharmacological therapy with somatostatin analogs (octreotide), or GH-receptor antagonists (pegvisomant), or dopamine agonists (bromocriptine). Decreased GnRH would lead to diminished follicle-stimulating hormone or luteinizing hormone, which would result in infertility or hypogonadism. Low cortisol is seen in adrenal insufficiency (*see* Bradley's NiCP, 7th edn, Ch. 52, pp. 696–712).

24. E. This patient has a positive MSLT. This test is positive if the average sleep-onset latency is <8 minutes and if two out of four (or five) naps have sleep-onset REM. Disorders that reduce REM sleep times can result in a positive MSLT. This can include sleep apnea, shift-work disorder, intentional sleep deprivation (like 30-hour calls), and narcolepsy. Because sleep apnea can cause an MSLT to be positive, a normal overnight polysomnogram is necessary the evening before an MSLT is performed in order to rule this out. Various substances, like alcohol, can suppress REM. Sleep walking does not cause sleep deprivation or suppress REM (*see* Bradley's NiCP, 7th edn, Ch. 102, pp. 1615–1685).

25. E. Cognitive behavioral therapy has the most supportive data for nonepileptic attacks, as well as a wider range of functional symptoms. Generally, it is recommended that additional referrals are not made once a diagnosis of nonepileptic attacks is made and that anticonvulsant drugs be discontinued. Although antidepressant medications (especially tricyclic antidepressants) have been shown to help a variety of functional neurological illnesses, there is no good evidence for their use with nonepileptic attacks specifically. There are also no data for electroconvulsive therapy for nonepileptic attacks (*see* Bradley's NiCP, 7th edn, Ch. 113, p. 1992).

26. C. Of the various options, this patient most likely has Dravet syndrome, also known as *severe myoclonic epilepsy of infancy*. This comes from a mutation affecting the *SCN1A* gene. Initially, children develop normally until they present with a febrile seizure under the age of 1. Over the course of months they continue to have milestone regression and develop multiple seizure types, including myoclonic seizures, atonic seizures, absence seizures, and complex partial seizures. Seizures may be exacerbated by carbamazepine or lamotrigine. An initially normal EEG can change to hypsarrhythmia or even multifocal slow spike and wave. Ohtahara syndrome is also known as *early myoclonic encephalopathy* and involves focal myoclonus that shifts from one region to the next in the first 3 months of life with spasms developing later in the disorder. The neurological examination is abnormal at birth with hypotonia, possible seizures, and a very abnormal EEG. Benign familial neonatal epilepsy is a dominantly inherited disorder with a mutation in voltage-gated potassium channels. This leads to seizures on the second or third day of life, but remits by 6 months of age. The child develops normally despite these seizures. Panayiotopoulos syndrome is a disorder that usually develops at the age of 5. These seizures have prominent autonomic involvement, including ictal vomiting, along with occipital spikes. Lennox-Gastaut typically develops between the ages of 3 and 5 and involves multiple seizure types along with cognitive dysfunction (*see* Bradley's NiCP, 7th edn, Ch. 101, pp. 1563–1614).

27. A. Adrenoleukodystrophy is the most common inherited leukodystrophy. It is an X-linked disorder in the *ABCD1* gene, leading to impaired breakdown of very-long-chain fatty acids in peroxisomes and ultimately severe myelin loss, as is shown in the image. Males commonly present as in the case noted here, whereas heterozygous female carriers may be asymptomatic or develop mild myelopathy or myeloneuropathy later in life. Alexander disease is associated with *GFAP* mutations and generally causes delayed milestones, seizures, macrocephaly, and progressive quadriparesis. Brain biopsy is generally noted to have abnormal accumulation of Rosenthal fibers. Canavan disease is caused by deficiency of the enzyme aspartoacylase, leading to accumulation of NAA in the urine and central nervous system. Clinically, the most severe type of Canavan disease begins in the first months of life and is associated with macrocephaly, seizures, hypotonia, poor visual fixation and tracking, and poor sucking and feeding. Pathologically, Canavan disease causes cerebral vacuolization, which can often be seen as multiple cysts on magnetic resonance imaging, in addition to myelin loss. Metachromatic leukodystrophy is an autosomal-recessive lysosomal storage disorder with distinct phenotypes, depending on age of onset. The presenting symptoms of late infantile cases are ataxia, dysarthria, dysphagia, and cognitive decline, ultimately leading to death. The presenting symptoms of adult

cases, on the other hand, usually are cognitive and psychiatric changes. The disease is caused by impairment of the lysosomal enzyme arylsulfatase A, leading to increased levels of sulfatide. Pelizaeus–Merzbacher disease is an X-linked disorder of myelin with broad phenotypic variation, depending on the underlying genetic change in the *PLP1* gene (and its protein, PLP). Whereas the most severe form of Pelizaeus-Merzbacher disease associated with *PLP1* duplication events occurs in infancy with abnormal eye movements and nystagmus, motor developmental delay, dystonia, and ataxia, there is a milder form associated with *PLP1* missense mutations that causes only spastic paraplegia. Notably, only three inherited leukodystrophies classically involve myelin loss in the subcortical U-fibers (which is a good radiographic or pathological clue for differential diagnosis): Canavan disease, Pelizaeus-Merzbacher disease, and vanishing white matter disease (*see* Bradley's NiCP, 7th edn, Ch. 91, pp. 1324–1341). Figure from Kleinschmidt-DeMasters BK, Simon JH 2012 Dysmyelinating and demyelinating disorders. In: Prayson RA (ed.) *Neuropathology*, pp. 183–239, Elsevier, with permission.

28. A. The patient likely has herpes zoster after a recrudescence of the virus at the trigeminal ganglion. The presence of vesicles on the nose corresponds to the nasociliary branch of the ophthalmic division of the trigeminal nerve, known as *Hutchinson sign*, and strongly predicts subsequent ocular complications (*see* Bradley's NiCP, 7th edn, Ch. 104, pp. 1720–1735).

29. E. Patients can be filmed for educational purposes as long as informed consent is obtained from the patient or his or her caregiver in cases of dementia or when filming children. The film should be considered part of the medical record and as private patient information, which can be shown to others in the medical community who follow similar privacy-related policies. The film should be kept as secure as other medical records and destroyed appropriately so as to not compromise patient information. Filming the patient without telling her is unethical. Asking the demented patient or impaired patient for permission is also unethical because he or she cannot give proper informed consent. The nursing facility staff is not appropriate to give consent because they are not the medical decision maker for the patient. If family or the decision maker is not present, the film could be made but only shown in an educational setting if consent is obtained from the healthcare decision maker before the presentation.

30. C. Dalfampridine is a potassium channel inhibitor used in multiple sclerosis to help improve speed of walking, but it does not affect disease activity. One of the main side effects is that it can precipitate seizures. The rest of the listed medications do not commonly cause seizures as a side effect of the medicines themselves (*see* Bradley's NiCP, 7th edn, Ch. 80, pp. 1159–1186).

31. C. Increasing ring and shoe size and growth of the jaw are classic signs of acromegaly in adults. This disorder relates to increased secretion of growth hormone (GH), which is most commonly from pituitary adenomas. Although other, much rarer, types of tumors may secrete GH, the best test after finding elevated GH levels in the blood would be an MRI of the brain to assess for a pituitary tumor (*see* Bradley's NiCP, 7th edn, Ch. 52, pp. 696–712).

32. D. Bulimia nervosa is an eating disorder that is marked by discrete episodes of recurrent binge eating in which patients eat more than is typical in a short period and/or describe an inability to control what they eat. This is followed by behaviors to prevent weight gain, like mechanically or medically inducing vomiting or diarrhea, or taking diuretics. Binge eating and purging must occur at least once a week for a 3-month period. There are no BMI criteria for a diagnosis of bulimia nervosa, unlike anorexia nervosa in which the patient must have a BMI less than 18.

33. D. The flexor pollicis longus is innervated by the anterior interosseous nerve, which also innervates the pronator quadratus and the first two flexor digitorum profundus muscles. The abductor pollicis brevis and pronator teres are innervated by the median nerve. The extensor indicis proprius is innervated by the posterior interosseus nerve. The first dorsal interosseous nerve is innervated by the ulnar nerve (*see* Bradley's NiCP, 7th edn, Ch. 25, pp. 262–272).

34. D. The sympathetic and parasympathetic autonomic nervous systems are complementary. Colloquially, the sympathetic system may be thought of as "fight or flight" and the parasympathetic system as "rest and digest." Sympathetic input originates in the spine, and is associated with tachycardia, mydriasis, perspiration, urinary and bowel storage, and ejaculation. The parasympathetic system is associated with bradycardia, miosis, urinary and bowel evacuation, and erections (*see* Bradley's NiCP, 7th edn, Ch. 108, pp. 1867–1895).

35. D. Anosmia is now recognized as an early symptom in several neurodegenerative conditions. Idiopathic Parkinson disease. Alzheimer disease, dementia with Lewy bodies, Huntington disease, and idiopathic rapid-eye-movement sleep behavior disorder are frequently associated with a significant loss of smell. Vascular parkinsonism, progressive supranuclear palsy, idiopathic dystonia, essential tremor, and major affective disorder are not associated with loss of smell. Multiple system atrophy, corticobasal degeneration, and frontotemporal dementia may have mild levels of smell loss (*see* Bradley's NiCP, 7th edn, Ch. 19, pp. 190–196).

36. B. This case underscores the importance of glucose control and frequent evaluations by healthcare providers in those who have diabetes. As peripheral nerves are damaged with excessive blood glucose, patients lose their vibratory sensation and may not feel an active infection or laceration to their foot. If an infection persists without intervention, it may cause cellulitis or spread to the bone or bloodstream. Patients should be educated that these complications are preventable and that frequent, proactive care should be taken. Although exercise is important for reducing the incidence of diabetes mellitus type 2, it is not the sole preventer (*see* Bradley's NiCP, 7th edn, Ch. 58, pp. 814–834).

37. A. The patient likely suffered a temporal bone fracture the night before. Only 5%–10% of temporal bone fractures result in facial weakness, and those that develop facial weakness late tend to have better prognosis for facial strength recovery. A CT of the temporal bone should be performed to ensure that surgery is not required (as it would not necessarily be for facial weakness alone). The remainder of the

options listed are reasonable considerations for new facial weakness if there were not preceding trauma and temporal hematoma (*see* Bradley's NiCP, 7th edn, Ch. 62, pp. 867–880).

38. D. Familial hemiplegic migraine is an autosomal-dominant disorder associated with mutations in various voltage-gated calcium channel genes. Often the associated paralysis may outlast the headache in these cases. Although no CSF pleocytosis is described for this condition, it may be seen with the syndrome of transient headache and neurological deficits with cerebrospinal fluid lymphocytosis. While various headache pathologies are particularly sensitive to indomethacin abortive therapy, most notably paroxysmal hemicrania, such efficacy is not reported for hemiplegic migraine. Although epileptiform activity has not been reported with hemiplegic migraine, unilateral or bilateral delta activity has been reported during an attack of hemiplegic migraine (*see* Bradley's NiCP, 7th edn, Ch. 103).

39. D. All of these diseases are mitochondrial in origin. MELAS is specifically implicated by the question stem due to elevated lactic acid and restricted diffusion on MRI. Kearns-Sayre syndrome is a mitochondrial myopathy that nearly always occurs sporadically (thought to be related to somatic mutation in utero). Phenotypically, Kearns-Sayre syndrome results in progressive external ophthalmoplegia and pigmentary retinopathy, with additional risk of cardiac abnormalities, sensorineural deafness, or cerebellar degeneration. Leber hereditary optic neuropathy results from a point mutation in mitochondrial DNA and causes progressive optic neuropathy and blindness. Patients may additionally have cardiac arrhythmias. MERRF causes myoclonic epilepsy, cerebellar dysfunction, myoclonus, short stature, and occasionally lactic acidosis. It is caused by a mutation in mitochondrial DNA encoding the lysine tRNA. Leigh disease (subacute necrotizing encephalomyelopathy) is a mitochondrial syndrome that presents before 2 years of age with developmental delay, ataxia, failure to thrive, weakness, and ophthalmoplegia, which results from pyruvate dehydrogenase and cytochrome oxidase deficiency (*see* Bradley's NiCP, 7th edn, Ch. 93, pp. 1349–1364). Figure from Carmody R 2013 Vascular injury and parenchymal changes. In: Naidich T, Castillo M, Cha S, Smirniotopoulos J (eds.) *Imaging of the Brain*, Elsevier, with permission.

40. C. The patient presented with acute onset of symptoms referable to the right hemisphere with resolution of symptoms in 1 hour, leaving him with a negative MRI (no restricted diffusion on diffusion weighted imaging sequence). The correct diagnosis is a transient ischemic attack (TIA). TIAs warrant admission and further evaluation, given that the stroke risk in the first 48 hours after TIA is approximately 5%. The ABCD2 scale helps predict stroke risk in those with symptoms suggestive of a TIA. The scale uses age, BP, clinical features, duration of symptoms, and the presence or absence of diabetes mellitus to predict the 2-day, 7-day, and 90-day stroke risk. This patient would not have been a candidate for intravenous thrombolysis given that he was outside of the 4.5-hour window and had rapidly resolving symptoms. Once admitted, the evaluation should include an MRI and assessment of anterior circulation vessels to ensure there is not a symptomatic carotid stenosis. Evaluation should also include a transthoracic echo to rule out vegetations, patent foramen ovale, or atrial clots. In this case the examination showed a rhythm likely consistent with atrial fibrillation and a dilated right atrium, which is often seen with atrial fibrillation. His hemoglobin A1c, LDL cholesterol, and BP were also elevated and warrant further intervention to reduce his risk of stroke. This patient should have his atrial fibrillation verified on a 12-lead electrocardiogram or, if paroxysmal, on a loop recorder or Holter monitor. Once verified, anticoagulation, rather than an antiplatelet agent, should be started to reduce his overall stroke risk. Because this patient also has renal failure and is on hemodialysis, novel direct thrombin inhibitors or factor 10a inhibitors such as the one listed in choice D should be avoided. Risk of stroke in those with atrial fibrillation can be further assessed by using the CHA2DS2-VASc score, which in this case, would be calculated at 4 (4% stroke risk per year) because of his diabetes, hypertension, TIA, male sex, and age <65 years old (*see* Bradley's NiCP, 7th edn, Ch. 65).

41. E. Tay-Sachs is an autosomal-recessive gangliosidosis associated with deficient hexosaminidase A activity. The incidence of Tay-Sachs is particularly high among individuals with Ashkenazi Jewish, Cajun, or French Canadian backgrounds. Signs of Tay-Sachs include normal postnatal development until around 6 months of age, when children begin to demonstrate progressive mental and physical regression, including blindness (with associated cherry-red spot), deafness, inability to swallow, and progressive paralysis. To date, no therapy has been developed that reliably stabilizes or reverses the devastation of Tay-Sachs disease (*see* Bradley's NiCP, 7th edn, Ch. 91, pp. 1324–1341).

42. E. Meaningful use of electronic health records (EHRs) is a stipulation of receiving monetary incentives (and ultimately avoiding penalties) from the Medicare and Medicaid Electronic Health Record Incentive Program. Since the creation of this incentive plan in 2014, meaningful-use requirements have been adopted in a stepwise fashion. There are many components to meaningful use, including the use of EHR e-prescribing capabilities, drug-drug and drug-allergy checkers, maintenance of (and reconciliation of) medication and allergy lists, and recording smoking status for patients over 13 years old. Copying previous notes as a template for subsequent patient encounters, however, is not considered meaningful use. Instead, this is a contentious use of EHR because it increases the risk of poor documentation and even fraudulent billing.

43. E. The case and the image are demonstrative of Charcot-Marie-Tooth type 1 (CMT1), a hereditary sensorimotor demyelinating neuropathy. Most cases are autosomal dominant, related to duplication of the *PMP22* gene. Symptoms vary widely, but include distal weakness and numbness that spreads over time, as well as tremor in a large minority of patients. The electron microscopy image demonstrates several myelinated nerve axons with surrounding concentric Schwann cell proliferation (onion bulbs), as well as one abnormally thin myelin sheath in the bottom left. The most common nerve conduction abnormality in CMT1 is slowed conduction velocity due to demyelination. Although symptomatic regions with muscle weakness and numbness may also show decreased compound muscle action potential and sensory nerve action potential amplitudes, as well as decreased motor unit

recruitment, this would be less likely in the patient's asymptomatic arms (see Bradley's NiCP, 7th edn, Ch. 107, pp. 1791–1866). Figure from Tazir M, Mahadouche T, Houioua S, Mathis S, Vallat J-M 2014 Hereditary motor and sensory neuropathies or Charcot-Marie-Tooth diseases: an update. *Journal of the Neurological Sciences* 347(1): 14–22, with permission.

44. B. The history and MRI are both compatible with glioblastoma, the most common primary brain tumor in adults. Maximal surgical resection is not only important for pathological diagnosis and molecular characterization of the tumor, but also plays an important role in a patient's overall survival (survival increases as percent resection increases). Stereotactic biopsy is reserved for tumors in otherwise inoperable locations or in patients too ill to undergo major surgery. Whole-brain radiation is rarely ever used for glioblastoma due to the toxicity of the therapy and to the fact that usual whole-brain radiation doses are below therapeutic levels for glioblastoma. Focal radiation and chemotherapy (temozolomide and/or bevacizumab) are standard therapy for glioblastoma, but almost always postoperatively (see Bradley's NiCP, 7th edn, Ch. 74, pp. 1049–1064). Figure from Khan SN, Linetsky M, Ellingson BM, Pope WB 2013 Magnetic resonance imaging of glioma in the era of antiangiogenic therapy. *PET Clinics* 8(2): 163–182, with permission.

45. A. Jitter is the variability in firing time between two muscle fibers in the same motor unit. With single-fiber EMG (SFEMG), individual muscle fibers are recorded, as opposed to an entire motor unit (which is composed of many muscle fibers) on a regular EMG. These individual fibers are stimulated by the same axon and should fire within a relatively close time of each other. Classically, disorders that affect neuromuscular transmission can increase the variability of firing times and therefore increase jitter. However, myopathies, chronic neuropathies, and motor neuron disease can all cause similar changes. There is no clinical measure of the increased variability in firing time between two motor units in the same muscle. Blocking is the failure of neuromuscular transmission of one of the muscle fibers on SFEMG. Fiber density, also measured on SFEMG, estimates the number of single-fiber potentials firing synchronously. There is no clinical measure of the number of quanta released from the presynaptic terminal (see Bradley's NiCP, 7th edn, Ch. 35, pp. 366–390).

46. D. Genetic forms of prion disease (which are divided into familial Creutzfeldt-Jakob disease, Gerstmann-Straussler-Scheinker disease, and fatal familial insomnia) are all associated with autosomal-dominant mutations in the *PRNP* gene with nearly 100% penetrance. Genetic forms of prion disease generally present at an earlier age (fifth to seventh decade), with early movement symptoms and late personality and cognitive symptoms. Additionally, genetic prion disease usually has a slower course and a longer survival than sporadic prion diseases (see Bradley's NiCP, 7th edn, Ch. 94, pp. 1365–1379).

47. C. Parinaud syndrome is composed of light-near dissociation of pupillary response, eyelid retraction (Collier sign), paralysis of upgaze and accommodation, and convergence-retraction nystagmus on attempted upgaze. This syndrome localizes to the dorsal midbrain region, as described in the question stem, and is commonly seen with pineal tumors. Mobius syndrome is a congenital syndrome of underdeveloped abducens and facial nerves. Patients are noted from infancy to have bilateral lower motor neuron facial weakness and bilateral weakness with abduction of the eyes. Adie's pupil results from a defect in parasympathetic innervation to the iris sphincter. Affected pupils tend to remain large compared with the contralateral pupil and are slow to respond to direct light reflex, but generally respond better to accommodation. Argyll Robertson pupil results in bilateral, abnormally small pupils that respond to accommodation but not light. This syndrome is classically associated with tertiary syphilis. Marcus Gunn pupil is another name for a relative afferent pupillary defect, in which the affected pupil reacts consensually, but not directly, to light. The most common localization for this syndrome is the optic nerve, as in the case of optic neuritis (see Bradley's NiCP, 7th edn, Chs. 18, pp. 179–189 and 21, pp. 205–216).

48. E. All of the neurotransmitters listed play a role in psychosis. Dopamine (D_2 receptor mostly) leads to increased psychosis as evidenced by disease exacerbation under the influence of amphetamines, dopamine agonists, and levodopa. In addition, psychosis improves when dopamine is blocked. Serotonin is also increased (especially 5-HT2a) in psychosis. For example, psychosis increases when lysergic acid diethylamide (LSD), a serotonin agonist, is given. There may also be increased norepinephrine levels as psychosis increases when amphetamines and cocaine are given (which also stimulate dopamine release). Finally, there appears to be a loss of GABA neurons in the hippocampus, which leads to less inhibition of excitatory pathways implicated in psychosis.

49. E. The image demonstrates atrophy of the caudate, with so-called *boxcar ventricles*, which is characteristic of Huntington disease. Alzheimer disease may show atrophy of the mesial temporal lobe and temporoparietal junction. Pick disease would show frontal atrophy. Parkinson disease would show loss of pigmented neurons in the substantia nigra. Human immunodeficiency virus dementia has no identifying gross pathological findings (see Bradley's NiCP, 7th edn, Ch. 95, pp. 1380–1421). Figure from Klatt EC 2014 *Robbins and Cotran Atlas of Pathology*, 3rd edn, Saunders, with permission.

50. C. Whereas the paramedian thalamic blood supply is generally supplied by the paramedian arteries, arising from the posterior cerebral arteries, about one third of humans have variant anatomy in this region. The artery of Percheron is a common pedicle from one posterior cerebral artery, which branches to supply both paramedian arteries. Given the paramedian thalamus's importance in maintenance of consciousness, occlusion of the artery of Percheron may lead to coma. Occlusion of the basilar artery may also lead to coma, due to ischemia in the reticular activating system, although generally concurrent cranial neuropathies and/or long track signs are present. Unilateral occlusion of the middle or posterior cerebral arteries would not lead to coma. The recurrent artery of Huebner is the largest perforating branch arising from the proximal anterior cerebral artery. It delivers blood to the head of the caudate, the anterior limb of the internal capsule, and the anterior lentiform nuclei. A stroke in this artery

may lead to contralateral arm and face weakness, as well as contralateral hemichorea. The artery of Adamkiewicz is the largest radicular artery in the spine, arising from the caudal portion of the anterior spinal artery and supplying the bulk of blood supply to the lumbar cord and cauda equina. Infarction here usually leads to an anterior spinal artery-type syndrome, with paraplegia and urinary and fecal incontinence but preserved dorsal column sensation (*see* Bradley's NiCP, 7th edn, Ch. 44, pp. 528–572).

51. D. The patient presented with a respiratory illness accompanied by acute deterioration of his mental status. The diagnosis is consistent with organic acidemia, specifically glutaric acidemia type 1 (GA1). This is caused by deficiency of the riboflavin-dependent glutaryl-CoA dehydrogenase (GCDH), which is a mitochondrial enzyme that converts glutaryl-CoA to crotonyl-CoA in the breakdown of lysine, hydroxylysine, and tryptophan. Clinically, patients typically present during an episode of illness with an acute metabolic decompensation, characterized by ketoacidosis, elevated ammonia, hypoglycemia, and encephalopathy. Extraneous movements such as dystonia and dyskinesia of the mouth and face are seen. Some patients may have seizures or subdural hemorrhages, which may be confused with evidence of child abuse. Imaging shows enlargement of the sylvian fissures and the cerebrospinal fluid spaces anterior to the temporal lobes, as well as increased signal intensity in the bilateral basal ganglia. The diagnosis is confirmed by identification of elevated urinary concentrations of glutaric acid and 3-hydroxyglutaric acid. Treatment consists of withholding protein from the diet; intravenous hydration; and correction of metabolic derangements such as acidosis, hyperammonemia, hypoglycemia, and electrolyte abnormalities. Riboflavin and L-carnitine are also indicated. L-carnitine and a low-protein diet, coupled with an early diagnosis, help to promote normal development in children with GA1. In this case the supplementation of lysine and tryptophan would worsen the condition, making this the incorrect answer choice (*see* Bradley's NiCP, 7th edn, Ch. 91, pp. 1324–1341). Figure from Kurtcan S, Aksu B, Alkan A, Guler S, Iscan A 2015 MRS features during encephalopathic crisis period in 11-year-old case with GA-1. *Brain and Development* 37(5): 546–551, with permission.

52. E. Dysthymic disorder must be present for at least 22 months in a 2-year period and include at least two of the following: appetite change, sleep disturbance, low energy, low self-esteem, poor concentration, and hopelessness. Most are never without a depressed mood and are often resistant to therapy. There is no psychosis to suggest schizoaffective disorder. Major depressive disorder or episode would not be the correct answer choice, as both of these typically have severe consequences, rendering the patients unable to hold or carry on daily function (such as a job). There is no suggestion for mania, making bipolar disorder less likely.

53. B. Normal cerebrospinal fluid pressure is between 6 and 25 cm H_2O in adults in the lateral decubitus position with legs extended. Pressures below this range indicate a spinal fluid leak, whereas pressures above this range can arise from a wide variety of causes, including idiopathic intracranial hypertension, central nervous system infection, mass lesion, or slow drainage of the arachnoid villi, as with leptomeningeal metastatic disease (*see* Bradley's NiCP, 7th edn, Ch. 88, pp. 1261–1278).

54. C. The case describes a girl with a history of infantile spasms, generalized convulsions, mental retardation, and blindness from chorioretinal lacunae. The MRI demonstrates agenesis of the corpus callosum. This constellation of findings is consistent with Aicardi syndrome, an X-linked dominant condition that occurs in females only (lethal to males). Patients often present in infancy with infantile spasms and progress to have a number of other neurological deficits, as noted earlier. Angelman syndrome, caused by a maternally inherited deletion on the long arm of chromosome 15, causes a very happy/pleasant demeanor with associated mental retardation (MR), hand flapping, ataxia, and seizures. Notably, if the same chromosome 15 mutation is inherited from the father, the child develops Prader-Willi syndrome, causing MR, hypogonadism, and hyperphagia. Rett syndrome occurs mostly in girls and is caused by a mutation in the *MECP2* gene that leads to developmental delay, regression, seizures, hand wringing, and gastrointestinal abnormalities. Autism includes a broad spectrum of neurodevelopmental disorders, characterized by poor verbal and nonverbal communication skills, poor social interaction, and repetitive behaviors. Fragile X syndrome is caused by a mutation in the *FMR1* gene and occurs mostly in boys. It includes global developmental delay, autistic features, seizures, and typical physical characteristics including long face, large ears, and enlarged testicles (*see* Bradley's NiCP, 7th edn, Ch. 89, pp. 1279–1300). Figure from Özkale M, Erol I, Gümüş A, Özkale Y, Alehan F 2012 Vici syndrome associated with sensorineural hearing loss and laryngomalacia *Pediatric Neurology* 47(5): 375–378, with permission.

55. A. Cholinergic neurons in the pedunculopontine tegmentum show the highest firing rates during REM sleep and are considered REM-generating neurons. Norepinephrine (in the locus ceruleus), hypocretin (from the lateral hypothalamus), serotonin (from the dorsal raphe nucleus), and dopamine (in the ventral tegmental area and periaqueductal gray) are all involved in promoting wakefulness. The locus ceruleus shows the highest firing rate during wakefulness (*see* Bradley's NiCP, 7th edn, Ch. 102, pp. 1615–1685).

56. B. Benzodiazepines are usually given to treat anxiety, phobias, sleep disorders, seizures, and alcohol withdrawal and to induce anesthesia. This class of medication works on the $GABA_A$ receptors that are ligand-gated ion channels and allow for the conductance of chloride (ionotropic). The different formulations of benzodiazepines have different half-lives that distinguish one from another. For example, chlordiazepoxide, valium, and clonazepam have longer half-lives; lorazepam and temazepam have a medium half-life; and alprazolam has a short half-life. Notably, whereas most benzodiazepines are hepatically metabolized, lorazepam is uniquely considered safe to give to those with liver dysfunction. The $GABA_B$ receptors are coupled to an inhibitory G protein (metabotropic) that inhibits adenylyl cyclase. Baclofen works on $GABA_B$ receptors. All of these medications can cause dependence if taken consistently and should not be abruptly withdrawn. If toxicity

disease may show day-to-day fluctuations in cognitive abilities, but there are not discrete episodes of amnesia followed by recovery of normal cognitive function (*see* Bradley's NiCP, 7th edn, Ch. 65, pp. 920–967).

63. C. This patient is most likely suffering from aseptic meningitis in the setting of acute human immunodeficiency virus (HIV) infection or seroconversion. Patients may have cranial neuropathies in this setting as well. At the time of presentation, HIV testing (enzyme-linked immunosorbent assay or Western blot) may be negative, but after seroconversion it will be positive. Although a patient may begin empiric therapy until cultures and PCR testing returns, treatment should be deescalated with negative results. The acute aseptic meningitis and associated symptoms generally resolve within 1 to 2 weeks (*see* Bradley's NiCP, 7th edn, Ch. 77, pp. 1102–1120).

64. C. Type I errors are a statistical measure used to describe an incorrect rejection of the null hypothesis. This occurs when a test is positive showing a patient has a disease but they do not actually have that disease. A type I error is essentially a false-positive test. Accepting a prior diagnosis without confirming it is a type of cognitive bias called *diagnosis momentum*. Accepting a diagnosis despite contrary evidence is a cognitive bias called *anchoring bias*. Type II errors are the opposite of a type I error, in which the null hypothesis is false but is not rejected. Seeking out confirmatory evidence without ordering tests to rule out a diagnosis is a cognitive bias called *confirmation bias*.

65. D. The Trail tests evaluate executive function. Trails A involves numbers scattered on a page, and the patient must correctly draw a line from 1 to the last number in sequential order. This assesses processing speed. Trails B involves drawing a line from alternating letters and numbers in sequential order until completed, which assesses attention, concentration, and executive function. The Boston Naming Test is a test of language and aphasia in which patients are to identify pictures of objects. The Wechsler Adult Intelligence Scale is an intelligence quotient (IQ) test. The Clock Draw Test evaluates visuospatial abilities and parietal lobe function. The Wechsler Memory Scale evaluates several types of memory to further define specific deficits patients might have (*see* Bradley's NiCP, 7th edn, Ch. 43, pp. 511–527).

66. E. The main treatments for a myasthenic exacerbation are either IV immunoglobulins or plasmapheresis, both of which are quite effective. The decision depends on comorbid conditions and availability of each treatment. Prednisone immunosuppression is the mainstay of long-term treatment for myasthenia, but prednisone in the short term can precipitate or worsen an exacerbation. She has a very low vital capacity and low NIF, which put her at a high risk of requiring intubation. A NIF of <30 cm H_2O or forced vital capacity of <20 mL/kg (1.4 L for a 70-kg patient) is indicative of impending respiratory failure. Starting prednisone could tip the balance and lead to her requiring mechanical ventilation. IV methylprednisolone has no role in acute myasthenic crises because it can worsen exacerbations. Azathioprine is used in long-term management of myasthenia to help reduce chronic steroid use. Although the patient may need antibiotics, her vital

capacity and NIF are on the edge of requiring ventilation, so acute treatment of her myasthenia should be a priority. Further, fluoroquinolones, especially ciprofloxacin, can worsen myasthenic exacerbations (*see* Bradley's NiCP, 7th edn, Ch. 55, pp. 742–758 and Ch. 109, pp. 1896–1915).

67. A. This patient most likely has somatization disorder, in which there is usually a history of physical and/or emotional abuse. In these patients, there are multiple recurrent somatic complaints of pain in at least four different sites or functions along with at least one sexual complaint, two gastrointestinal symptoms, and at least one neurological symptom. Somatization disorders typically lead to excessive and unnecessary medical workup, and have comorbid psychological disturbances of mood and anxiety. It is important to note that these symptoms are not intentional, nor do they imply the patient is "faking." Treatment involves cognitive behavioral therapy along with treatment of comorbid psychological dysfunction. Although this patient does endorse headaches, one must be careful not to blame other physical symptoms on migraines. Further, the question stem does not provide sufficient detail to meet diagnostic criteria for migraines. There is no indication here that the patient is suffering from fibromyalgia. Unless there is an obvious reason to believe the patient is malingering with hopes of secondary gain, one should reserve this as a diagnosis of exclusion. Finally, although Lyme disease can cause a number of symptoms and signs (fever, myalgia, arthralgia, headache, and cranial neuropathies to name a few), there is nothing on workup or physical examination that suggests Lyme disease.

68. D. This patient presents with meralgia paresthetica. This is a common condition in pregnancy. As the pregnancy progresses, the enlarging abdomen places pressure on the ilioinguinal ligament, which then entraps the lateral femoral cutaneous nerve. EMG and nerve conduction studies are not necessary for the diagnosis. They can be performed to rule out other causes like radiculopathy. The lateral femoral cutaneous nerve can be evaluated by nerve conduction; however, it is technically challenging to perform, and bilateral studies have to be performed for comparison. Furthermore, the condition can be present in the presence of normal electrodiagnostic studies. Diagnosis is primarily clinical. Local injections to the nerve can be helpful. A block of the femoral nerve would not capture the lateral femoral cutaneous nerve as it branches from the femoral nerve proximal to the ilioinguinal ligament. In the case of pregnancy, the main treatment is delivery; however, this is not a condition that should force an early delivery. Loose-fitting clothing around the waist can also be beneficial. The lateral femoral cutaneous nerve is a purely sensory nerve, so no weakness is involved in this condition. Lumbar puncture would not be helpful in the diagnosis (*see* Bradley's NiCP, Ch. 112, pp. 1973–1991).

69. D. The parasympathetic nervous system (PNS) will increase detrusor contraction leading to micturition if the bladder is full. The PNS is involved with slowing of cardiac conduction, decreased cardiac contractility, constriction of bronchioles, constriction of pupils, and lacrimation. The sympathetic nervous system is involved with pupillary dilation, sweating, increasing cardiac conduction and contractility, and dilation of

the bronchioles (*see* Bradley's NiCP, 7th edn, Ch. 108, pp. 1867–1895).

70. E. Behçet disease is an immune-mediated small vessel vasculitis associated with mucosal ulcers, uveitis, and pathergy reaction, leading to papules at sites of minor cutaneous trauma due to robust inflammatory response. It is most common in individuals from the Middle East and Asia. When Behçet's affects the central nervous system, it generally causes enhancing inflammatory lesions as described. Although sarcoidosis is a consideration in the differential diagnosis, mucosal ulcers and pathergy more strongly indicate Behçet's. ADEM generally has associated enhancement on MRI, preceding infection or vaccination, and is not associated with mucosal ulcers. Neurological complications of lupus are present in 25%–50% of patients. However, the concurrent symptoms in this patient are more suggestive of Behçet's than lupus. Multiple sclerosis would have enhancing lesions and vision problems (optic neuritis rather than uveitis), but would not have associated ulcers or pathergy (*see* Bradley's NiCP, 7th edn, Ch. 58, pp. 814–834).

71. B. Fluorodeoxyglucose PET scans are increasingly used to assist in the diagnosis of undifferentiated memory complaints. Fluorodeoxyglucose (FDG) is metabolized by the active brain, and areas of hypometabolism suggest decreased functional activity. In Alzheimer disease, the posterior parietotemporal region and posterior cingulate are often affected first. In dementia with Lewy bodies there is significant hypometabolism in the occipital lobes. Huntington disease causes hypometabolism in the frontal lobes and striatum. In frontotemporal dementia and primary progressive aphasia, there may be significant hypometabolism in the frontal lobes and anterior temporal lobes (*see* Bradley's NiCP, 7th edn, Ch. 41, pp. 486–503).

72. A. The patient has an L5 radiculopathy, which is likely traumatic in origin. On examination, he has radicular pain in the L5 distribution with corresponding sensory loss but no weakness. In this setting, conservative management is recommended initially, including activity modification, nonnarcotic pain medication with NSAIDs, and physical therapy. Opioid pain medication may also be used in the short term, but should be avoided long term. Systemic or epidural steroids may be used in those who have persistent severe radicular pain that is refractory to other agents, although the evidence is more limited for these. Only if the pain is refractory or the patient has progressive neurological decline with weakness is surgical discectomy an option (*see* Bradley's NiCP, 7th edn, Ch. 106, pp. 1766–1790).

73. B. Rituximab is a CD20 monoclonal antibody that is used in a variety of autoimmune conditions such as neuromyelitis optica and refractory myasthenia gravis. Fingolimod is a sphingosine-1-phosphatase inhibitor used in the treatment of multiple sclerosis. Natalizumab is an alpha-4-integrin adhesion molecule antibody used in the treatment of multiple sclerosis. Alemtuzumab is a CD52 monoclonal antibody used in the treatment of multiple sclerosis. Multiple antiepileptics (phenytoin, carbamazepine, lamotrigine, and valproic acid) are voltage-gated sodium channel blockers (*see* Bradley's NiCP, 7th edn, Ch. 51, pp. 676–690).

74. E. This patient presents with signs and symptoms of a purely peripheral sensory disorder consistent with a sensory ganglionopathy (also known as *sensory neuronopathy* or *sensory polyganglioneuropathy*). This is commonly associated with small cell lung cancer, Sjögren syndrome, thiamine toxicity, or human immunodeficiency virus. Paraneoplasia is the most common cause, typically from the ANNA-1 antibody (anti-Hu antibody). Anti-Jo antibody is seen in inflammatory myopathies associated with interstitial lung disease. Anti-GM1 antibody is commonly seen in multifocal motor neuropathy. Anti-GQ1b antibody is seen in the Miller-Fisher variant of Guillian-Barré syndrome. Anti-NMDA receptor antibody is seen in NMDA receptor encephalitis, which involves chorea, personality changes, and refractory seizures and is not associated with neuropathy (*see* Bradley's NiCP, 7th edn, Ch. 107, pp. 1791–1867).

75. B. Although the effect of high-dose methylprednisolone remains incompletely understood, studies have shown small gains in sensory and motor outcomes at 1 year. However, none have reported that patients regain the ability to ambulate. Traumatic spinal cord injury often presents with "spinal shock" with plegia, numbness, areflexia, and decreased sphincter tone. Within weeks, however, tone increases and patients develop spasticity. Upon presentation, any acute spinal cord injury should have an immediate MRI in case a surgically reversible compression is present. Patients may have severe autonomic instability with severe spinal cord injury, including swinging blood pressures or cardiac arrhythmias, especially with patient manipulation or with bowel movements. Cord contusions often result in venous congestion of the central cord, and may therefore affect the upper limbs more than the lower limbs, but still have a sensory level and sphincter tone loss (*see* Bradley's NiCP, 7th edn, Ch. 63, pp. 881–902).

76. C. The substantia gelatinosa is mostly a column of interneurons, transmitting noxious stimuli afferently. There is an additional contribution from this spinal column of producing natural opiates, which reduce the production of substance P from nociceptive neurons. Monoplegia and absent reflexes would be a result of injury to the ventral horn motor fibers. Vibratory sensation travels in the nucleus proprius, along with fine touch, stereognosis, and proprioception. Ataxia from spinal cord injury often relates to injury of Clarke's column, through which joint position sensation is transmitted to the cerebellum. Corresponding spinal anatomy is shown (*see* Bradley's NiCP, 7th edn, Ch. 26, pp. 273–278).

Nuclear cell columns   **Laminae of Rexed**

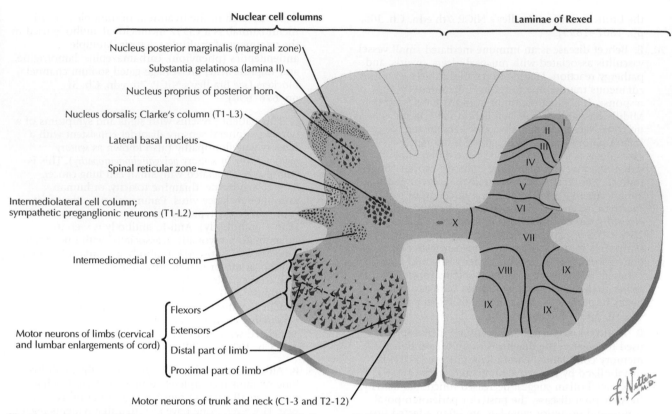

Nucleus posterior marginalis (marginal zone)

Substantia gelatinosa (lamina II)

Nucleus proprius of posterior horn

Nucleus dorsalis; Clarke's column (T1-L3)

Lateral basal nucleus

Spinal reticular zone

Intermediolateral cell column;
sympathetic preganglionic neurons (T1-L2)

Intermediomedial cell column

Motor neurons of limbs (cervical
and lumbar enlargements of cord)
- Flexors
- Extensors
- Distal part of limb
- Proximal part of limb

Motor neurons of trunk and neck (C1-3 and T2-12)

Figure for Answer 3.76 *(from Jones HR, Burns E, Aminoff MJ, Pomeroy S 2013* The Netter Collection of Medical Illustrations: Nervous System, *Vol. 7, Pt. 2, Spinal Cord and Peripheral Motor and Sensory Systems, pp. 49–78, Saunders, with permission.)*

77. E. Dissociative amnesia is a dissociative disorder characterized by the inability to recall personal or situational information, typically associated with a traumatic event. Gaps of memory often exist for long periods and go beyond that of typical amnesia. Memories are still present but repressed as part of a defense mechanism. Some will eventually recall details of the event, but others will remain amnestic to the event forever. Other dissociative disorders listed include dissociative identity disorder (previously called *multiple personality disorder*). This exists when a person has two or more distinct identities, with each identity unaware of the others. There may be differences in speech, attitudes, thoughts, gender orientation, and even right/ left-handedness or eyeglass prescriptions. Depersonalization is the feeling of detachment from one's own body or self. Often, patients with depersonalization will feel as if they are in a dream and unable to control their own actions or movements. The current case does not mention external trauma to the head that would make concussion high on the differential. Although there is memory impairment, there are no other features of concussion mentioned, such as headache, nausea, vomiting, photophobia, or phonophobia. Finally, the patient may later develop posttraumatic stress disorder from her experience, but the initial diagnosis is better explained by dissociative amnesia

78. C. The CT scan and history suggest a subarachnoid hemorrhage (SAH), which typically presents with a thunderclap headache, nausea, vomiting, photophobia, and meningismus. It is often seen on CT scan or by xanthochromia on lumbar puncture if >12 hours after onset. Causes of SAH include trauma, drugs, or ruptured aneurysm. Given her history of kidney disease, one should consider the possibility of a ruptured aneurysm in association with adult polycystic kidney disease. Complications of SAH include hydrocephalus, seizures, rebleeding, hyponatremia, and vasospasm. Vasospasm typically presents 3–15 days (peaks at 1 week) from the onset of bleeding, and is associated with worsening of neurological examination such as headache, nausea, vomiting, or new focal deficits. Nimodipine is used to reduce the risk of vasospasm and is often taken for at least 14–21 days. Treatment of ruptured aneurysms includes clipping or coiling of the aneurysm, along with management of the complications of SAH. Typically, SAH is graded using the Hunt and Hess scale, which is a scale of 1–5 that takes the patient's clinical appearance and helps predict prognosis and outcome. The Fisher grade is a scale that classifies the radiological appearance of SAH (*see* Bradley's NiCP, 7th edn, Chs. 55, pp. 742–757 and 67, pp. 981–995). Figure from Verma RK, Kottke R, Andereggen L, et al. 2013 Detecting subarachnoid hemorrhage: comparison of combined FLAIR/SWI versus CT. *European Journal of Radiology* 82(9): 1539–1545, with permission.

79. D. α-latrotoxin is the neurotoxin produced by black widow spiders, which causes release and blocks

reuptake of neurotransmitters at noradrenergic, cholinergic, and aminergic nerve endings. Symptoms often begin with a target lesion around the bite, then pain and involuntary muscle contractions in the abdomen that later spread to the limbs; this is known as *latrodectism*. Respiratory failure may occur due to diaphragm involvement, and diffuse dysautonomia is common. Tetrodotoxin is found in puffer fish and selectively blocks voltage-gated sodium channels, inhibiting action potential formation in somatic and autonomic nerve fibers. Symptoms include perioral and acral paresthesias, followed by ascending weakness, dysarthria, dysphagia, and respiratory depression. Both saxitoxin and brevetoxin are found in shellfish. Saxitoxin works similar to tetrodotoxin, by blocking activation of voltage-gated sodium channels, whereas brevetoxin activates these channels, leading to membrane depolarization and action potential firing. Both cause perioral and acral paresthesias, headaches, ataxia, and occasionally paralysis. Ciguatoxin is found in the ciguatera fish and modulates the voltage-gated sodium channels by allowing increased sodium permeability at rest, and therefore increased membrane depolarization. Neurological symptoms often include paresthesias that begin around the mouth and spread to the limbs and perineum. Cold allodynia and paradoxical temperature reversal (sensing cold as unbearably hot) are common. Headache, fatigue, and mild diffuse weakness are also common. Symptoms may last for up to 1 week (*see* Bradley's NiCP, 7th edn, Ch. 86, pp. 1237–1253).

80. A. Sydenham disease typically presents up to 6 months after a streptococcal throat infection in children. The chorea is usually asymmetrical and can be associated with other behavioral issues such as irritability, obsessive-compulsive disorder, and hyperactivity. It typically resolves spontaneously within 3 months, but can persist for longer. Evaluation typically includes antistreptolysin-O and anti-DNase B titers. Treatment is secondary prevention with penicillin G until the age of 21, or for at least 10 years after the disease, to reduce the risk of rheumatic carditis. Treatment of the chorea could include prednisone, tetrabenazine, or other antidopaminergic drugs. Habit reversal therapy is typically used for the treatment of Tourette syndrome and would not be indicated here. Although chorea can be mistaken for tics, tics are usually accompanied by a premonitory urge followed by a sense of relief after the action is performed. Genetic counseling would be indicated if Huntington disease was high on the differential. A trial of carbidopa/levodopa would be appropriate for dopamine-responsive dystonia. Stimulant medications are typically used for treating attention-deficit/hyperactivity disorder, which would not be associated with choreiform movements (*see* Bradley's NiCP, 7th edn, Ch. 96, pp. 1422–1460).

81. C. The computed tomography (CT) image shows hyperdensity in the area of the pituitary gland, which likely represents hemorrhage. This, paired with the clinical syndrome described, is consistent with Sheehan syndrome, which is caused by pituitary necrosis after postpartum hemorrhage and associated hypovolemia. The hemorrhage is thought to result from ischemia in the anterior pituitary gland. Symptoms vary widely, and range from mild weakness to failure to lactate, amenorrhea, adrenal insufficiency, and hypothyroidism. Hemorrhages may occasionally

involve the posterior pituitary as well and lead to diabetes insipidus. Commonly, patients have a preexisting pituitary adenoma or lymphocytic hypophysitis. The other answer choices are causes of postpartum headaches, but are not likely, given the other information regarding endocrinological dysfunction in the patient (*see* Bradley's NiCP, 7th edn, Ch. 52, pp. 696–712). Figure from Ferri F 2009 *Ferri's Color Atlas and Text of Clinical Medicine*, Saunders, with permission.

82. C. Benign paroxysmal positional vertigo is a condition caused by otolith malposition in the semicircular canals, causing symptoms of sudden, severe paroxysms of vertigo with oscillopsia and frequent nausea. The most common semicircular canal location of otolithic crystal malpositioning is the posterior canal due to gravitational settling. The Dix-Hallpike maneuver is performed by rotating the head 45 degrees and then rapidly moving from a seated position with head upright to a prone position with neck extended. The Dix-Hallpike is best suited to detect posterior canal dysfunction, which leads to lateral beating nystagmus toward the affected ear when that ear is toward the ground. The lateral canal otolith position more likely produces down-beat nystagmus with Dix-Hallpike or possibly no nystagmus with this maneuver at all. Cerebellar vermis lesions tend to cause gait and trunk ataxia, whereas nystagmus is more commonly associated with cerebellar hemispheric lesions. Further, delayed nystagmus with the Dix-Hallpike maneuver is more commonly associated with semicircular canal localization than cerebellar (*see* Bradley's NiCP, 7th edn, Ch. 46, pp. 583–604).

83. A. Astereognosia is the inability to identify objects by touch despite having intact sensation, and relates to parietal dysfunction. Agraphesthesia is the inability to identify numbers or letters written on the hand. Prosopagnosia is the inability to recognize faces, whereas visual agnosia is the broader inability to recognize objects visually. Simultagnosia is the loss of ability to see multiple objects or an inability to see an entire picture or scene (*see* Bradley's NiCP, 7th edn, Ch. 12, pp. 122–127).

84. D. Restless legs syndrome has five diagnostic criteria. It is (1) an often uncomfortable urge to move the legs (2) at times of inactivity (3) or in the evening (4) that is usually relieved by movement (5) and is not accounted for by another medical or behavioral condition. RLS is thought to be due to the low accumulation of brain iron and is usually treated with dopaminergic agents or agents such as calcium channel alpha$_2$-delta ligands. The diagnosis of RLS is made clinically and does not require diagnostic testing such as a polysomnogram. Periodic limb movements of sleep (PLMS) are characterized by EMG activity seen regularly every 20–40 seconds, with each movement lasting 0.5–10 seconds on polysomnogram. PLMS is highly associated with RLS but not required for the diagnosis. RLS may also be secondary and associated with iron deficiency, neuropathy, radiculopathy, diabetes, uremia, hypothyroidism, caffeine, lithium, calcium channel blockers, and selective serotonin reuptake inhibitors (*see* Bradley's NiCP, 7th edn, Ch. 102, pp. 1615–1685).

85. D. Isotretinoin is associated with the development of idiopathic intracranial hypertension (IIH, also known as *pseudotumor cerebri*) and should be discontinued

upon diagnosis. Similarly, tetracycline, amiodarone, and quinolone antibiotics have been described in association with IIH development. Large-volume lumbar puncture may be helpful in the diagnosis of IIH, and is rarely used as therapy for exacerbations. Acetazolamide is the mainstay of therapy for mild cases of IIH, improving both headaches and vision symptoms. Ventriculoperitoneal shunting is reserved for intractable headaches associated with high pressure, even after treatment with acetazolamide. Optic nerve sheath fenestration is a last-resort therapy to preserve vision when intracranial pressure remains high despite maximal therapy (*see* Bradley's NiCP, 7th edn, Ch. 103, pp. 1686–1719).

86. C. The sarcomere is a repeating unit within muscle fibers leading to muscle contraction. The sarcomere is bordered by a Z-line on each side, which is made up of multiple proteins, including nebulin. From this frame, long chains of myosin are attached and make up the structure of the thick filament. The thin filament is made up of actin polymers. Troponin sits on the actin polymers and blocks the binding of actin to myosin. When a muscle is activated, calcium released from the sarcoplasmic reticulum binds to troponin, releasing troponin from actin and allowing actin to bind to myosin-heavy chains. When this occurs, the motion of actin binding to myosin-heavy chains will shorten the sarcomere and therefore shorten the muscle (*see* Bradley's NiCP, 7th edn, Ch. 110, pp. 1915–1956).

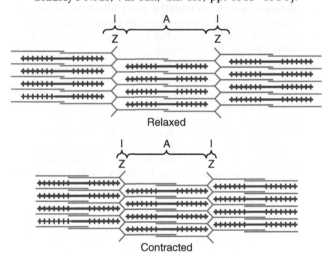

Relaxed

Contracted

Figure for Answer 3.86 *(from Hall JE 2015* Guyton and Hall Textbook of Medical Physiology, *13th edn, Elsevier, with permission.)*

87. A. Approximately 5% of patients with trigeminal neuralgia have multiple sclerosis, and about 2% of patients with multiple sclerosis will have trigeminal neuralgia. Although the most common cause of trigeminal neuralgia is a blood vessel pressing on the trigeminal nerve as it exits the brainstem, compressing and damaging the nerve sheath over time, this is not an answer choice. Less common causes include nerve compression by tumor, arteriovenous malformation, infection, trauma, or inflammatory diseases such as Sjögren syndrome (*see* Bradley's NiCP, 7th edn, Chs. 80, pp. 1159–1186 and 103, pp. 1686–1719).

88. A. The N22–P34 interpeak latency corresponds with conduction between the lumbar roots and the brainstem. This patient has a presumed thoracic

transverse myelitis, which would prolong this latency. The P37 would also likely be prolonged, but P34–P37 interpeak latency (brainstem to cortical response) would be normal, indicating a lesion in the dorsal columns of the spinal cord. An absent N22 would suggest a problem with either peripheral nerve conduction or the spinal roots. N9–N13 peaks are involved in upper extremity SSEPs and would be prolonged with a cervical cord lesion, not a thoracic lesion. N20 is the cortical peak in upper extremity SSEPs and would not be affected (*see* Bradley's NiCP, 7th edn, Ch. 34, pp. 348–366).

89. C. The specimen demonstrates alobar holoprosencephaly in which the brain does not separate into different hemispheres, causing a large central ventricle. This is usually associated with midline facial defects like cyclopia, cleft lip, and cleft palate. Pachygyria involves few smooth gyri along the brain, but both hemispheres are present. Although there is no corpus callosum in this sample, the entire brain is abnormal with a single ventricle, making holoprosencephaly the best answer. Lissencephaly is a genetic disorder that results in pachygyria, mental retardation, and seizures. Polymicrogyria involves many very small gyri on the surface of the brain (*see* Bradley's NiCP, 7th edn, Ch. 89, pp. 1279–1300). Figure from Klatt EC 2014 *Robbins and Cotran Atlas of Pathology*, 3rd edn, Saunders, with permission.

90. D. This patient presents with gelastic seizures. These present with episodes of either uncontrollable laughter or crying, lasting for <1 minute. Many times it can take years for the right diagnosis because the seizures are confused with behavioral episodes. Gelastic seizures are most commonly associated with hypothalamic hamartomas. Nocturnal headaches suggest increased intracranial pressure, and therefore the possibility of a tumor. Levetiracetam can cause behavioral changes, usually increased agitation or aggression, but there is nothing in the question stem to suggest this patient is on levetiracetam. Autistic children can have odd behaviors with inappropriate emotions, but nocturnal headaches should point toward the possibility of an intracranial mass. Mesial temporal lobe sclerosis does not cause primarily laughing seizures. A parasagittal meningioma may cause nocturnal headaches, but does not cause gelastic seizures (*see* Bradley's NiCP, 7th edn, Ch. 101, pp. 1563–1614).

91. E. The five phases of grief are denial, anger, bargaining, depression, and acceptance. Projection is an immature defense mechanism.

92. B. A chart with common bacterial causes of meningitis based on age range or comorbidities is shown here.

TABLE FOR ANSWER 3.92

Age or comorbidity	Bacteria
Newborn	Group B streptococci, *E. coli*
Toddler	*S. pneumoniae, N. meningitidis, H. influenzae*
Adolescent through adult	*S. pneumoniae, N. meningitidis*
Elderly	*S. pneumoniae, H. influenzae, E. coli, L. monocytogenes*
Neurosurgical patients	*S. pneumoniae, H. influenzae, S. aureus*
Immunosuppressed	*L. monocytogenes*
Sinusitis or otitis media	*H. influenzae, S. pneumoniae*

93. B. Zellweger syndrome is an autosomal recessive disorder associated with mutations in several *PEX* genes that encode the proteins required for peroxisomes. As such, individuals with Zellweger syndrome have no peroxisomes, resulting in many developmental abnormalities. This includes impaired neuronal migration and abnormal brain development. Patients frequently have symptoms of hypotonia, seizures, apnea, impaired feeding, craniofacial abnormalities, and organomegaly. Zellweger syndrome may be diagnosed through measurement of very-long-chain fatty acids (especially C26:0 and C26:1) in cultured fibroblasts, which may indicate impaired peroxisomal fatty acid metabolism (*see* Bradley's NiCP, 7th edn, Ch. 91, pp. 1324–1341).

94. C. The images depict a vein of Galen malformation. These malformations form at approximately 6–11 weeks during fetal development and are often identified in the early neonatal period. These malformations often lead to arteriovenous shunting, causing a variety of symptoms, including high-output cardiac failure (manifested by tachypnea, cyanosis, and respiratory distress), strokes from steal phenomena or mass effect, hemorrhages (rarely), cognitive delay, headaches, seizures, or hydrocephalus. Treatment is usually required and may consist of ventriculoperitoneal shunt if hydrocephalus is present and/or vasoocclusive treatment of the malformation. Secondary treatment of the high-output heart failure may also be required. Although dehydration and infection may lead to venous sinus thrombosis, these two factors do not directly relate to the formation of vein of Galen malformations, as these form prenatally. Figure from Swaiman K 2011 *Swaiman's Pediatric Neurology: Principles and Practice*, 5th edn, Saunders, with permission.

95. C. The most appropriate response is to leave the order as originally intended. Changing the order when contrast was not felt to be necessary is performing excessive testing, placing the patient at risk of an adverse event, and increasing medical expenses unnecessarily. No fraudulent billing has occurred, so Medicare or the insurer does not need to be contacted. Without an injury to the patient, malpractice has not occurred, although the patient should be informed of the mistake. Although the radiology technician made a mistake, it is up to the facility to determine whether the error was severe enough to result in termination.

96. D. Prolonged carbon monoxide exposure may lead to necrosis of the globus pallidus, as seen in the photograph. Tobacco does not cause any specific brain injury, but increases the risk of stroke and microvascular disease substantially. Alcohol is associated with brain atrophy, especially the cerebellum, and may indirectly lead to mammillary body hemorrhage through thiamine deficiency. Methanol ingestion is associated with bilateral putamen necrosis. Manganese is most often inhaled by welders and accumulates in the globus pallidus, causing parkinsonism. Although it does deposit in the same area, the patient described would be less likely to have manganism than carbon monoxide poisoning (*see* Bradley's NiCP, 7th edn, Ch. 39, pp. 411–458). Figure from Yachnis AT 2012 *Neuropathology*, 2nd edn, pp. 40–74, Elsevier, with permission.

97. D. Metastatic tumors from systemic cancers are the most common intracranial tumors. Among primary intracranial tumors, meningiomas are the most common, accounting for about one third of tumors. Glioblastomas are the second most common intracranial tumor, occurring at about half the incidence of meningiomas. Pituitary adenomas are slightly less common than glioblastomas. Nerve sheath tumors, a category that includes vestibular schwannomas, occur about half as often as glioblastomas.

98. B. The visual field shown demonstrates a "pie in the sky" field loss, which correlates with a contralateral temporal lobe lesion. The following figure summarizes lesion localizations related to various visual field deficits (*see* Bradley's NiCP, 7th edn, Ch. 16, pp. 158–162). Figure accompanying question text from Liu GT, Volpe NJ, Galetta SL 2010 *Neuro-Ophthalmology: Diagnosis and Management*, 2nd edn, Saunders, with permission.

99. C. Hexacarbon solvents like n-hexane are commonly found in paints, lacquers, and glue. Inhalation leads to a sense of euphoria and hallucinations, and long-term use leads to peripheral neuropathy and dysautonomia. Acrylamide can have similar symptoms, although the exposure comes from manufacturing molded plastics or cardboard, not paints and lacquer. Organophosphates are predominantly used in the agricultural industry in pesticides and herbicides. Organophosphates are acetylcholinesterase inhibitors that cause nausea, salivation, headaches, weakness, bradycardia, diarrhea, seizures, and coma. Pralidoxime is the antidote used in organophosphate poisoning, which binds the organophosphates, releasing them from acetylcholinesterase. Carbon monoxide poisoning typically occurs in gas workers, miners, or garage employees, although home exposure from a malfunctioning furnace or wood-burning stove can occur. Headache is the initial symptom, which can progress to extrapyramidal deficits, seizures, coma, and death. Aluminum toxicity can result in cognitive decline, seizures, and myoclonus. This is seen in chronic dialysis patients in which aluminum exposure is not limited, but may be seen in welders exposed to aluminum dust (*see* Bradley's NiCP, 7th edn, Ch. 87, pp. 1254–1260).

100. E. Rapid increases in steroid doses are known to exacerbate myasthenia symptoms, and may actually send a patient into myasthenic crisis. Although each of the other drugs may be used in the treatment of myasthenia gravis, timing and size of dosage increases have not been associated with symptom exacerbation (*see* Bradley's NiCP, 7th edn, Ch. 109, pp. 1896–1914).

101. A. Factors associated with favorable prognosis with multiple sclerosis include younger age at disease onset, female gender, sensory onset (rather than motor), complete remission after first attack, long remission between first and second attacks, and few lesions on initial magnetic resonance imaging of the brain. Although certain MHC class II alleles (such as HLA-DR2) are associated with increased risk of multiple sclerosis, and possibly worse phenotype, there is no such association with MHC class I. Living in a northern latitude may increase one's overall risk of multiple sclerosis, but is not specifically correlated with prognosis (*see* Bradley's NiCP, 7th edn, Ch. 80, pp. 1159–1186).

102. E. The patient clinically has Lambert-Eaton myasthenia syndrome (LEMS). LEMS presents in the 40s through 60s with progressive proximal weakness. It is frequently

normal. Which of the following would be the most reasonable next step?

A. Restart valproic acid

B. Recommend daily ibuprofen

C. Start propranolol for migraine prevention

D. Recommend no preventative medications

E. Start acetazolamide

7. The photomicrograph of a biopsied thigh muscle is most likely taken from a patient with which disease?

A. Steroid myopathy

B. Normal muscle

C. Duchenne muscular dystrophy

D. Inclusion body myositis

E. Polymyositis

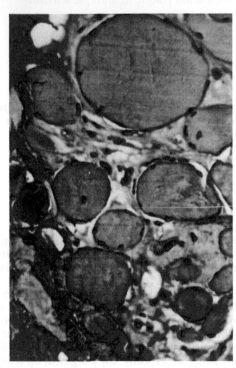

Figure for Question 4.7.

8. Correction of which of the following is most classically deleterious to cerebral myelin?

A. Hyponatremia

B. Hypokalemia

C. Hypernatremia

D. Hypocalcemia

E. Hypoglycemia

9. A 62-year-old male presents with a 6-month history of painless weakness in his right arm. Initially this began with weakness of grip strength, but now involves a wrist drop. He denies any numbness. His examination demonstrates weakness in muscles innervated by the ulnar and radial nerves along with fasciculations. His triceps reflex is absent. Nerve conduction studies in the right arm demonstrate normal sensory responses and abnormal motor responses with conduction blocks present. These conduction blocks are outside of typical sites of compression. Electromyography shows fasciculations and decreased recruitment in ulnar and

radial innervated muscles. Which of the following is true about this condition?

A. Anti-GM1 antibodies are frequently found in this condition.

B. Riluzole is the recommended treatment for this condition.

C. Diagnosis can be confirmed by lumbar puncture demonstrating cytoalbuminological dissociation.

D. This condition responds dramatically to plasmapheresis.

E. This condition is caused by a virus in the Picornaviridae family.

10. A 27-year-old woman presents with subacute paraparesis over the past 2 days. She first noted decreased sensation in her toes, which ascended up her legs, then difficulty with urinary continence, and finally an inability to walk due to weakness. She has never had any similar episodes of weakness or numbness before, although last year she had a 2-week episode of severe vision loss and pain in her right eye that resolved without treatment. Which of the following is the best test to diagnose her underlying condition?

A. Anti-GQ1b antibody

B. Pathergy test

C. Anti–aquaporin-4 antibody

D. Anti–HTLV-1 antibody

E. Anti-GM1 antibody

11. A 63-year-old female presents to the office for evaluation of left arm weakness, which was present upon awakening 2 weeks ago, along with pain in her left shoulder. Her examination is notable for 0/5 strength in the left brachioradialis, extensor digitorum, and extensor indicis muscles, with 5/5 strength elsewhere in the arm. She has a normal biceps reflex and triceps reflex, but the brachioradialis reflex is not present on the left. She has numbness on the dorsal portion of the left thumb. Which of the following is the most likely diagnosis?

A. Lower trunk brachial plexopathy

B. Posterior interosseous neuropathy

C. Posterior cord brachial plexopathy

D. Radial neuropathy at the spiral groove

E. C8 radiculopathy

12. A 15-year-old boy is evaluated for developmental delay. His parents are intellectually normal, and he was the product of an uncomplicated birth. He was never on schedule with motor or cognitive milestones as a small child, and currently requires special education at school. On general examination, he is noted to have an elongated face, large ears, and macroorchidism. Neurologically, he does not make eye contact with the examiner, is moderately delayed in verbal output, and has decreased tone but normal strength. He demonstrates stereotypies with his hands. Which of the following is true of the underlying cause for his symptoms?

A. Caused by CGG triplet repeat

B. Increased risk of leukemia

C. Always associated with autism spectrum disorder

D. Only present if mutation received from father

E. X-linked recessive

13. Which statement about myelinated axons is *true*?

    A. Myelinated axons conduct axon potentials with statutory conduction.

    B. Sodium and potassium channels are distributed equally along the axon.

    C. Voltage-gated potassium channels allow depolarization to occur, propagating the action potential.

    D. Sodium channels are clustered in the nodes of Ranvier, whereas potassium channels reside under myelin sheath.

    E. Normal conduction speeds in myelinated axons are 20 m/s.

14. An 18-year-old male is brought into the emergency department after a motor vehicle accident. On examination he will open his eyes to painful stimulation, makes incomprehensible sounds, and withdraws his extremities to painful stimulation. What is the patient's Glasgow Coma Scale score?

    A. 5

    B. 6

    C. 7

    D. 8

    E. 9

15. In an electroencephalogram (EEG), increasing the high-pass filter will result in which of the following?

    A. Reduce electromyography (EMG) artifact

    B. Reduce sweat artifact

    C. Reduce amplitude of all waveforms

    D. Increase amplitude of all waveforms

    E. Increase electrode impedance

16. All of the following are features of schizotypal personality disorder except?

    A. Acceptance of magical thinking

    B. Eccentric clothing

    C. Talking to one's self in public

    D. Pervasive discomfort with close relationships

    E. Assuming others will exploit one's self

17. A 1-year-old Ashkenazi Jewish girl who was born at full term presents with developmental delay. She has a long history of seizures, blindness, and impaired motor skills. At birth, she had hypotonia, poor head control, and poor feeding. On examination, she has macrocephaly, pale optic discs, and spasticity in the bilateral lower extremities. There is hyperreflexia and positive Babinski signs bilaterally. A magnetic resonance image (MRI) demonstrates diffuse symmetric hyperintensities of bilateral white matter regions with involvement of the U-fibers. A magnetic resonance (MR) spectroscopy shows an increase peak of N-acetylaspartic acid (NAA). Which of the following is the correct diagnosis?

    A. Pelizaeus-Merzbacher disease

    B. Alexander disease

    C. Rett syndrome

    D. Canavan disease

    E. Cerebral palsy

18. Through which of the following does the mandibular nerve exit the skull base?

    A. Superior orbital fissure

    B. Foramen rotundum

    C. Foramen ovale

    D. Jugular foramen

    E. Foramen lacerum

19. After a severe motor vehicle accident, a 50-year-old man arrives at the emergency room unconscious and intubated. A computed tomography scan of his brain is shown here. After the assurance of proper respiratory and circulatory support, as well as spine imaging, which of the following is the next most appropriate evaluation?

    A. Cerebral angiogram

    B. Intracranial pressure monitoring

    C. Transcranial Doppler evaluation

    D. T-tube trial

    E. Electroencephalogram

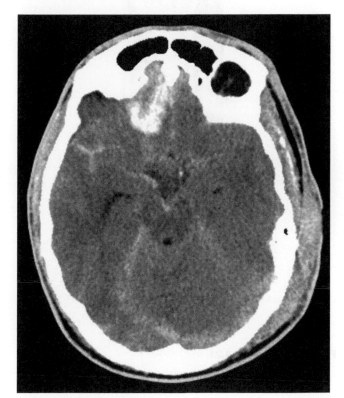

Figure for Question 4.19.

20. The aforementioned patient remains critically ill and intubated. On day 7, transcranial Doppler demonstrates increasing velocities, suggestive of cerebral vasospasm. The next day, his motor response to noxious stimulus weakens significantly. Which of the following would *not* be effective in this scenario?

    A. Hypervolemia

    B. Hypertension

    C. Balloon angioplasty

    D. Hemodilution

    E. Intraarterial beta-blockers

21. A 23-year-old African American female presents to the emergency department with leg weakness, falls, and numbness, which have progressively worsened over the last week. She has been unable to control her bladder and had several episodes of incontinence. Her neurological examination reveals nearly flaccid paralysis of her legs and loss of sensation in her legs to all modalities. She has sensation loss to vibration and pin prick in her hands, and strength is mildly reduced. Her magnetic resonance image (MRI) is shown. Which of the following tests would uncover the diagnosis?

    A. Elevated oligoclonal bands
    B. Cervical spinal angiogram
    C. MRI of the thoracic spine with and without contrast
    D. MRI of the brain with and without contrast
    E. Aquaporin-4 antibody

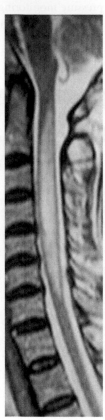

Figure for Question 4.21.

22. A 47-year-old male with a recent history of endocarditis presents with progressive weakness in his legs. He has severe pain in his lower back and is tender to the touch over his vertebral processes. He denies any trauma. On examination, he has a fever of 102.6, weakness in his legs, sensory loss to all modalities in his legs, reduced reflexes, and loss of sphincter tone. White blood cell count is 14 and erythrocyte sedimentation rate (ESR) is 75 mm/h. Which of the following is the most likely diagnosis?

    A. Anterior spinal infarct
    B. Guillan-Barré syndrome
    C. Spinal epidural abscess
    D. Transverse myelitis
    E. Vertebral fracture

23. A 45-year-old man presents to the emergency room with altered mental status. He has a history of myasthenia gravis, but his immunosuppressant regimen is unknown. His wife states that he has poor compliance with his medications. He has not been sick with infectious symptoms recently. On examination, he is hypotensive and encephalopathic. He has central obesity with multiple bruises, round facies, and striae on his abdomen, but the remainder of his neurological examination is normal. Laboratory tests reveal hyponatremia, hyperkalemia, and metabolic acidosis. What is the most appropriate next best step to stabilize the patient?

    A. Plasmaphoresis
    B. Intravenous immunoglobulins (IVIG)
    C. Lower potassium
    D. Administer hydrocortisone
    E. Elevate sodium

24. Which of the following is characteristic of stage 2 sleep?

    A. K complexes and spindles
    B. Slow rolling eye movements
    C. Delta waves comprising 20%–50% of epoch
    D. Delta waves comprising >50% of epoch
    E. Vertex sharp waves

25. Which of the following is an example of a mature coping mechanism?

    A. Sublimation
    B. Denial
    C. Projection
    D. Rationalization
    E. Intellectualization

26. An 8-year-old male presents to the office for evaluation of seizures. His parents state that he has reached all developmental milestones and does well in school. In the last 2 months he has had several nocturnal episodes with twitching of one side of his face and retained consciousness. A sample from his electroencephalogram (EEG) is shown. Which of the following is the most likely diagnosis?

    A. Benign epilepsy with centrotemporal spikes
    B. Autosomal-dominant nocturnal frontal lobe epilepsy
    C. Juvenile absence epilepsy
    D. Juvenile myoclonic epilepsy
    E. Landau-Kleffner syndrome

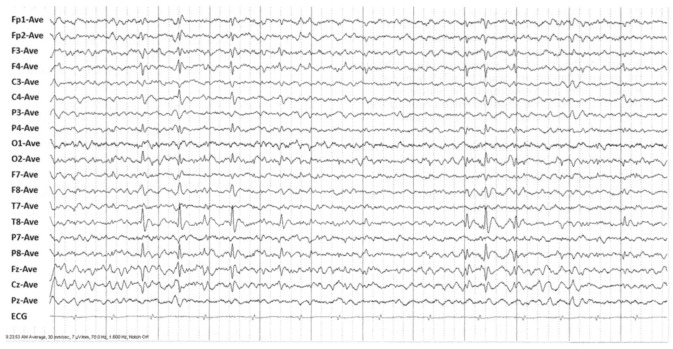

Figure for Question 4.26.

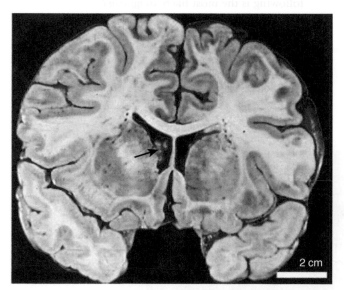

Figure for Question 4.27.

27. The abnormality indicated by the black arrow in the figure is most likely related to an abnormality in which of the following?
    A. Glucose metabolism
    B. Cell growth pathways
    C. Myelin production
    D. Cerebrospinal fluid drainage
    E. Neuronal migration

28. The woman in the figure has which cranial nerve palsy?
    A. Right oculomotor nerve palsy
    B. Left trochlear nerve palsy
    C. Right abducens nerve palsy
    D. Left abducens nerve palsy
    E. Left oculomotor nerve palsy

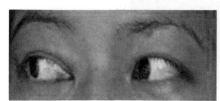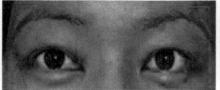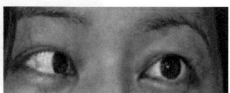

Figure for Question 4.28.

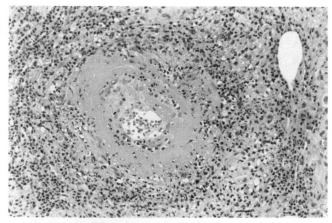

Figure for Question 4.43.

44. A 43-year-old woman received surgery and high-dose focal radiation 2 years ago for the treatment of a left nasopharyngeal carcinoma. She now presents with neurocognitive deficits and imbalance. Examination reveals no local recurrence of cancer in her nasopharynx. Her magnetic resonance imaging (MRI) of the brain with contrast is shown. Based on the most likely diagnosis, which of the following is true about this condition?

A. The patient should be observed.

B. Antifungal therapy should begin immediately.

C. Radiation therapy should begin immediately.

D. Evaluation for paraneoplastic antibodies should be undertaken.

E. Treatment with steroid or antiangiogenic therapy may be necessary.

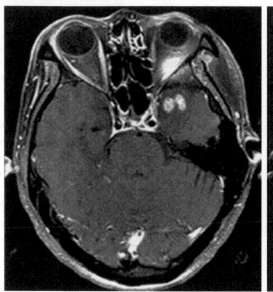

Figure for Question 4.44.

45. Which of the following conditions could cause the pattern seen in this blink reflex?

A. Left Bell palsy

B. Left trigeminal neuralgia

C. Right lateral pontine stroke

D. Right trigeminal neuropathy

E. Right internal capsule stroke

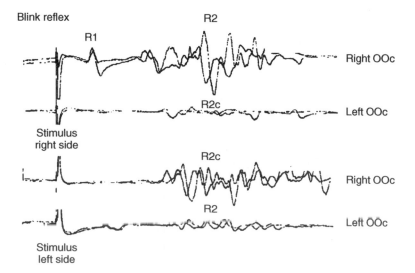

Figure for Question 4.45.

46. Aside from insomnia, which is the most prominent early symptom of fatal familial insomnia?

    A. Dysautonomia
    B. Parkinsonism
    C. Cognitive decline
    D. Ataxia
    E. Myoclonus

47. A 65-year-old man with a long smoking history presents with sudden, profound, painless, monocular vision loss. He reports two recent episodes of transient vision loss in the same eye. Dilated fundoscopy was performed in the emergency room, a picture from which is shown here. Which of the following is the most likely cause of his symptoms?

    A. Paraneoplastic retinopathy
    B. Central retinal vein occlusion
    C. Central retinal artery occlusion
    D. Optic neuritis
    E. Anterior ischemic optic neuropathy

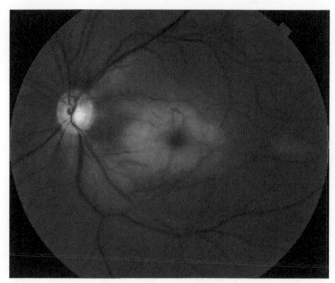

Figure for Question 4.47.

48. A 32-year-old woman with no prior psychiatric history is brought to the emergency room by her family because of a change in behavior. Three days prior, she witnessed a car hit a child while crossing the street. Upon attempting to help the child, she realized he had succumbed to his injuries and passed away. Since the accident, she has seen the child walking throughout her house and even talks to him in front of her family. On examination, she is unkempt and disheveled, frequently crying when the incident is mentioned. At this point in time, what is most likely her diagnosis?

    A. Schizophrenia
    B. Schizophreniform disorder
    C. Schizoaffective disorder
    D. Brief psychotic disorder
    E. Bereavement

49. A 67-year-old male dies after having dementia for the past 5 years, and an autopsy is performed. Which of the following is shown in his pathological specimen?

    A. Neurofibrillary tangles
    B. Spongiform changes
    C. Lewy body
    D. Negri body
    E. Cowdry A inclusions

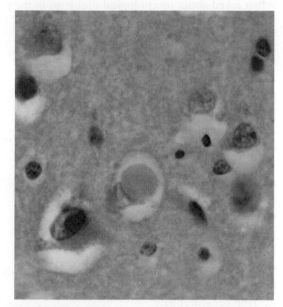

Figure for Question 4.49.

50. The anterior choroidal artery is a branch of which of the following?

    A. Middle cerebral artery
    B. Anterior cerebral artery
    C. Internal carotid artery
    D. Common carotid artery
    E. Ophthalmic artery

51. Which of the following is *not* characteristic of a simple febrile seizure?

    A. History of mild motor milestone delay
    B. Seizure duration more than 15 minutes
    C. Normal neurological examination
    D. Only one seizure per 24 hours
    E. Negative family history for seizures

52. A 31-year-old man presents to the emergency room after being unable to sleep for 1 week. His wife states that he has been rearranging his garage, has had an increased libido, and has even thought of experimenting with drugs, which is uncharacteristic of him. She also recently found out that he has been gambling away their savings with online poker. On examination, he appears tired but has a difficult time sitting still. His speech is sensible but tends to be fast and jumps from one topic to the next. There is no evidence of illegal substances on his urine drug screen. When asked about psychological problems in the past, his wife thinks he had a prior hospitalization for suicide attempt with depression when he was a teenager. What is the most likely diagnosis?

    A. Schizophrenia
    B. Major depressive disorder
    C. Bipolar 1 disorder
    D. Bipolar 2 disorder
    E. Cyclothymic disorder

53. Which of the following is *not* a likely effect of low vitamin B12 (cobalamin)?

    A. Hypercoagulability
    B. Macrocytic anemia
    C. Cognitive decline
    D. Demyelinating myeloneuropathy
    E. Mania

54. Which of the following conditions is depicted in the magnetic resonance image (MRI) shown?

    A. Holoprosencephaly
    B. Schizencephaly
    C. Polymicrogyria
    D. Periventricular nodular heterotopia
    E. Porencephaly

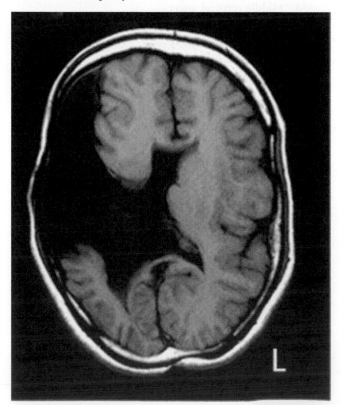

Figure for Question 4.54.

55. Which of the following cell types provides the primary output of the cerebellum?

    A. Granular cells
    B. Mossy fibers
    C. Stellate cells
    D. Purkinje cells
    E. Basket cells

56. A 27-year-old man with a history of poorly controlled schizophrenia comes to the emergency room (ER) in a fit of psychosis. He believes there are cops trying to kill him, and he is talking to the devil to help him out of this situation. He is throwing chairs in the room, placing the healthcare workers in danger. The ER physician administers haloperidol in combination with lorazepam. Which of the following is true regarding haloperidol?

    A. It is not available in an injectable form.
    B. It is an atypical antipsychotic.
    C. It has low potency action on the D_2 receptor.
    D. There is low potential for acute extrapyramidal side effects.
    E. It is useful for the positive, but not the negative, symptoms of schizophrenia.

57. Which of the following cerebellar nuclei send efferent information via the superior cerebellar peduncle?

    A. Dentate
    B. Emboliform
    C. Globose
    D. Fastigial
    E. All of the above

58. A newborn becomes increasingly somnolent over the first 2 days of life, and requires intubation for respiratory alkalosis. Clinically, he is hypothermic, hypotonic, and has significant vomiting. Although he was initially placed on broad-spectrum antibiotics, sepsis is ruled out and antibiotics are discontinued. His ammonia is elevated, although liver function is normal, and there is no evidence of acidemia. A urea cycle defect is suspected. Which of the following is *not* true regarding urea cycle defects?

    A. All have an X-linked inheritance except ornithine transcarbamylase (OTC) deficiency, which is autosomal recessive.
    B. Cerebral edema is a common cause of coma.
    C. Women with OTC deficiency can be normal or have headaches, vomiting, and ophthalmoplegia.
    D. Arginine supplementation is needed for arginosuccinic acid synthetase deficiency.
    E. Sodium benzoate, sodium phenylacetate, and arginine hydrochloride are all treatments for OTC deficiency.

59. Which of the following antiepileptic medications does not enhance the activity of gamma aminobutyric acid (GABA) in the central nervous system?

    A. Clonazepam
    B. Phenobarbital
    C. Tiagabine
    D. Pregabalin
    E. Vigabatrin

60. A 36-year-old female with a history of multiple sclerosis presents to the emergency department with weakness. On neurological examination she is noted to have new weakness of the left finger flexors and extensors, moderate weakness of the left leg, and normal strength on the right. She has loss of vibration and position sense in the left leg, whereas she has loss of temperature and pin prick sense in the right leg. Which is the most likely localization of her symptomatic lesion?

    A. Left side of the cervical cord
    B. Central portion of the cervical cord
    C. Posterior columns in the thoracic cord
    D. Left lateral pontine lesion
    E. Right side of cervical cord

61. A 32-year-old female tragically lost her husband in a motorcycle accident 3 weeks ago. When family members talk to her about her loss, she ignores their questions and talks about her husband as if he is still alive. They are concerned about her being depressed. After a brief evaluation, it is felt that she is going through the normal grieving process. Which stage of grief is she likely experiencing?

    A. Anger
    B. Denial
    C. Bargaining
    D. Depression
    E. Acceptance

62. A 48-year-old male with a history of alcohol abuse presents to your clinic with his family for evaluation of memory loss. His family has noticed short-term memory loss, disorientation, and apathy over the last few weeks. He has suffered three falls in that time. His examination demonstrates an ataxic gait and bilateral partial abducens nerve palsies. All of the following are true of this condition *except*?

    A. If left untreated, this can lead to progressive encephalopathy and death.
    B. This disorder is more common in patients with the APOE4 allele.
    C. Administration of thiamine before glucose can prevent development of the disorder.
    D. Magnetic resonance imaging may show fluid attenuated inversion recovery (FLAIR) abnormalities in the periaqueductal gray matter and mammillary bodies.
    E. Despite adequate treatment, memory may not fully recover.

63. A 31-year-old man in Texas who is current in his routine medical care presents to the hospital in July with symptoms of fever, headache, neck stiffness, and confusion. He has been spending long days in the garden this summer. A magnetic resonance image (MRI) of the brain is unrevealing. After admission, he develops flaccid weakness in his arms and legs, but

with retained bulbar strength and normally reactive pupils. Which of the following is the most likely cause of his symptoms?

    A. West Nile virus
    B. Poliovirus
    C. Guillain-Barré syndrome
    D. Acute disseminated encephalomyelitis (ADEM)
    E. Botulinum toxin

64. On morning rounds, a nurse expresses concerns about the blood pressure medications ordered for a patient due to episodes of hypotension. She refuses to give medications until her concerns are addressed. Which of the following is the best response?

    A. Tell the nurse to give the medications because the physician has ordered them.
    B. Report the nurse to her charge nurse.
    C. Contact the hospital risk management team.
    D. Educate the nurse on why the medications are necessary.
    E. Change the orders to appease nursing concerns.

65. A young girl first developed generalized tonic-clonic seizures with fever during her first year of life. These increased in frequency, and later absence seizures developed as well. She became quite refractory to antiepileptic medications. Along with this, her cognitive development began to slow at about the age of 18 months, falling well behind her peers by the time she was 30 months of age. Which of the following genetic syndromes should be considered?

    A. Rett syndrome
    B. West syndrome
    C. Landau-Kleffner syndrome
    D. Dravet syndrome
    E. Generalized epilepsy with febrile seizures plus (GEFS+)

66. A 37-year-old female is intubated due to hypoxic respiratory failure. Her husband states she had diarrhea for 1 week before her admission and spent several days in bed. Today she complained of shortness of breath and could not get out of bed. Her examination shows diffuse weakness in her extremities, bifacial weakness, double vision, and loss of reflexes. Nerve conduction studies were normal in the arms and legs, except for absent F waves. She was unable to activate any muscles on electromyography (EMG), and no spontaneous activity was seen. Which of the following is the most likely diagnosis?

    A. Polymyositis
    B. Guillain-Barré syndrome
    C. Myasthenia gravis
    D. Critical illness neuropathy
    E. Acid maltase deficiency

79. All of the following are true of Emery-Dreifuss myopathy *except*?
    A. Autosomal-dominant, autosomal-recessive, and X-linked varieties exist
    B. Involve frequent cardiac arrhythmias
    C. Most die in adolescence
    D. Contracture is a common early symptom
    E. Mutated genes encode nuclear envelope proteins

80. An 11-year-old boy is referred to neurology by his otolaryngologist for frequent sniffing despite a lack of congestion or seasonal allergies. For the last year, he frequently sniffed for no reason and began to flick his finger throughout the day. On examination, you appreciate the noted mannerisms, and also note frequent throat clearing. The patient reports that he feels anxious unless he performs the action and has a sense of relief after performing the action. They are also suppressible. Which of the following is a comorbidity of this condition?
    A. Attention-deficit/hyperactivity disorder (ADHD)
    B. Poor impulse control
    C. Obsessive-compulsive disorder (OCD)
    D. Self-injurious behavior
    E. All of the above

81. A 12-year-old boy is brought to the neurologist for pressure-like headaches that worsen when he lies down and improve when he stands up. He denies weakness or gait difficulty, but does endorse frequent urination. His mother states that he "just can't stop drinking fluids." A magnetic resonance imaging of the brain is obtained, and the patient is diagnosed with a Rathke cleft cyst. Which of the following is *not* true about his current condition?
    A. Urine osmolality is typically high.
    B. Serum sodium is typically high.
    C. Treatment involves desmopressin.
    D. Incidence is high after surgical manipulations of the pituitary gland.
    E. Trauma, hemorrhages, and autoimmune conditions are other possible etiologies.

82. A 75-year-old man with 100-pack-year smoking history comes to the emergency room with a chief complaint of vertigo. He reports a few passing moments of vertigo over the last 3 days, at which point he stopped smoking. Then today he developed acute vertigo described as a spinning sensation with associated imbalance and nausea, which has been ongoing for 3 hours. He denies hearing loss or ear pain, and has not had any recent infections. On examination, he has no cranial nerve deficits, weakness, or numbness. He easily maintains fixation on a target with bilateral head thrust testing. Which is the most likely cause of his symptoms?
    A. Labyrinthitis
    B. Vestibular neuritis
    C. Benign paroxysmal positional vertigo (BPPV)
    D. Posterior circulation stroke
    E. Nicotine withdrawal

83. Which of the following is a tauopathy?
    A. Progressive supranuclear palsy
    B. Parkinson disease
    C. Dementia with Lewy bodies
    D. Multiple system atrophy
    E. Amyotrophic lateral sclerosis

84. A 23-year-old female presents to the office with complaints of difficulty falling asleep. Each night when lying down to sleep, she develops cramps in her legs, forcing her to stand up and walk around to relieve the pain. Her husband complains that she kicks him during the middle of the night. She has no significant past health problems except for heavy menstrual cycles. Recent complete blood count, basic metabolic panel, and liver function tests were normal. Which of the following would be the best course of action?
    A. Arterial Doppler of the lower extremities
    B. Overnight polysomnogram
    C. Trial of ropinirole
    D. Nerve conduction study
    E. Serum ferritin level

85. Which of the following is *uncommon* of classic migraine auras?
    A. Duration <30 minutes
    B. Visual disturbance usually monocular
    C. Generally similar symptoms with repeating attacks
    D. May be preceded by prodrome of changes in mood or eating
    E. May include visual, sensory, cognitive, speech, or gait symptoms

86. Stimulation of which types of fibers produces poorly localized, dull, aching pain?
    A. A-delta fibers
    B. C fibers
    C. A-alpha fibers
    D. A-gamma fibers
    E. B fibers

87. A 62-year-old patient with poorly controlled diabetes presents with midface pain and horizontal diplopia, left facial numbness, and left facial weakness. Which of the following is the most likely cause of the symptoms?
    A. Multiple embolic events
    B. Hyperglycemia
    C. Idiopathic inflammatory condition
    D. Fungal infection
    E. Viral infection

88. Which of the following would correlate with this full-field visual evoked potential?
    A. Prechiasmal right optic nerve lesion
    B. Right occipital lobe lesion
    C. Chiasmal lesion
    D. Left occipital lobe lesion
    E. Prechiasmal left optic nerve lesion

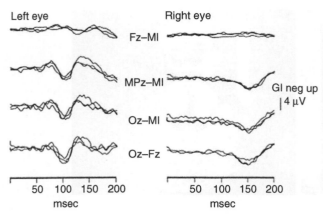

Left eye   Right eye

Fz–MI

MPz–MI
GI neg up
|4 µV

Oz–MI

Oz–Fz

50 100 150 200   50 100 150 200
msec   msec

Figure for Question 4.88.

89. At what age should a child be able to say sentences with two to four words, build a tower of four blocks, stand on tiptoes, and demonstrate parallel play?

    A. 1 year
    B. 18 months
    C. 2 years
    D. 3 years
    E. 4 years

90. A 12-year-old boy presents to clinic for evaluation of recurrent abnormal episodes that occur at night while he's asleep. The episodes start with a noise, and by the time his parents arrive in the room, they witness bicycling of his legs and unresponsiveness for 30 seconds before it stops; afterward he is confused. These have occurred several times per week over the last 3 months. He has even fallen out of bed with these episodes, resulting in bruises and scrapes. With the last episode, his parents noted his right arm was stiff. Which of the following is the most likely diagnosis?

    A. Night terrors
    B. Autosomal-dominant nocturnal frontal lobe epilepsy
    C. Mesial temporal lobe sclerosis
    D. Juvenile myoclonic epilepsy
    E. Nightmares

91. At what age does a child first sense the finality of death?

    A. 18–24 months
    B. 2–4 years
    C. 4–6 years
    D. 6–9 years
    E. 9–12 years

92. A 56-year-old homeless Indian immigrant man presents to the hospital with weeks of cough, malaise, and headache, followed by new-onset diplopia. On examination, he is afebrile. He is noted to have bilateral abducens palsies, as well as dysarthria, dysphagia, and tongue deviation to the left. Otherwise, his strength and sensation are normal. A head computed tomography (CT) is unremarkable, and a chest x-ray reveals a right upper lobe consolidation. Cerebrospinal fluid (CSF) analysis reveals a glucose level of 4 mg/dL (normal is 45–80 mg/dL), protein of

140 mg/dL (normal is 15–45 mg/dL), white blood cells of 223 cells/mL (lymphocytic predominance), and red blood cells of 0 cells/mL. Gram stain and India ink are negative. Based on your greatest suspicion of the underlying cause of this patient's illness, which is the best next step?

A. Whole body position emission tomography-computed tomography (PET-CT) and radiation oncology consult
B. Begin oral antifungal therapy and plan daily lumbar punctures
C. Begin antitreponemal therapy and identify sexual contacts
D. Begin intravenous immunoglobulin and monitor respiratory function
E. Airborne isolation and directed antimicrobial therapy

93. Which of the following is *not* true of porphyria?

A. Acute attacks may be triggered by certain anticonvulsants
B. Associated with decreased production of heme
C. Associated neuropathy may be triggered by cold weather
D. Classically presents with psychosis
E. Classically presents with strokes

94. A 12-year-old boy presents to the neurology clinic due to a history of seizures. As an infant, he was noted to have infantile spasms, and more recently has developed complex partial seizures with staring, lip smacking, and automatisms. A thorough neurological examination demonstrates features of motor stereotypies and poor eye contact. He has minimally delayed language. His skin examination is shown. What is the most likely diagnosis based on history and examination?

A. Hypomelanosis of Ito
B. Sturge-Weber syndrome
C. Ataxia-telangiectasia
D. Von Hippel-Lindau disease
E. Tuberous sclerosis

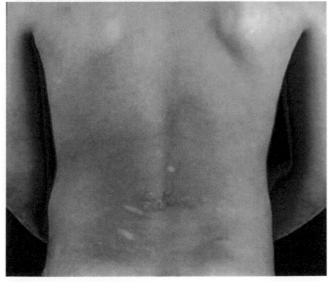

Figure for Question 4.94.

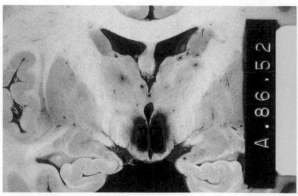
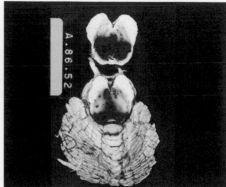

Figure for Question 4.96.

95. A medical student has been showing romantic interest toward one of his neurology attendings. They have been seen on two dates. As chairperson of the department, what is the most appropriate response?

    A. Ask the couple to be discrete until he graduates.

    B. Fire the attending.

    C. Remove the attending from a supervisory role.

    D. Expel the student.

    E. Ignore the relationship.

96. Which of the following was likely deficient in the patient for whom an autopsy photo is shown?

    A. Vitamin B12

    B. Vitamin B6

    C. Vitamin B1

    D. Vitamin D

    E. Vitamin B3

97. A 66-year-old female presents for evaluation of extremity pain. She was recently diagnosed with diabetes after laboratory work showed a hemoglobin A1C of 11%. She started on metformin and insulin and then developed painful burning paresthesias in her fingers and toes. Electromyography (EMG) and nerve conduction studies in the arms and legs are normal. Which of the following is the most likely cause of her symptoms?

    A. Adverse effect of metformin

    B. Diabetic distal sensory polyneuropathy

    C. Diabetic cachexia

    D. Insulin neuritis

    E. Diabetic amyotrophy

98. A 35-year-old healthy man presents with a first-time neurological symptom of diplopia on right lateral gaze. Notable findings from extraocular examination are demonstrated in the figure and include horizontal nystagmus of the right eye in panel B. Which of the following lesion localizations most corresponds with these findings?

    A. Left medial longitudinal fasciculus

    B. Right parapontine reticular formation (PPRF)

    C. Nucleus of Edinger-Westphal

    D. Left oculomotor nucleus

    E. Left abducens nucleus

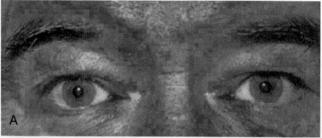
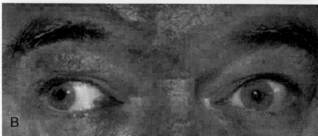
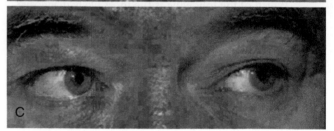

Figure for Question 4.98.

99. A 62-year-old female presents for stroke evaluation due to acute right hemiparesis for the last several hours. On examination, she has a right facial droop with right arm weakness and mild sensory changes in the right arm. She is noted to have effortful and fragmented speech, and is unable to name several objects. Her comprehension is intact, but she has difficulty with repetition. Which of the following arteries is the most likely cause of her stroke?

    A. Inferior division of the middle cerebral artery

    B. Anterior cerebral artery

    C. Lenticulostriate arteries

    D. Artery of Heubner

    E. Superior division of middle cerebral artery

100. In using cyclophosphamide for the treatment of paraneoplastic disorders, which of the following is *not* a clinical risk to be addressed or monitored?

    A. Osteopenia
    B. Infertility
    C. Hemorrhagic cystitis
    D. Immunosuppression
    E. Developing new malignancy

101. Which of the following is the most likely underlying diagnosis for the images shown from a 45-year-old woman?

    A. Metastatic lung cancer
    B. Acute disseminated encephalomyelitis (ADEM)
    C. Balo's concentric sclerosis
    D. Tumefactive multiple sclerosis
    E. Multiple abscesses

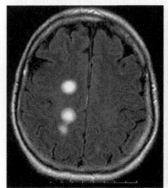 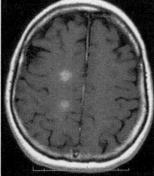

Figure for Question 4.101.

102. An 8-month-old girl presents to the emergency room with poor feeding and weakness over the last 3 days. Examination demonstrates a well-developed child with few movements, decreased tone, ptosis, and dilated pupils. The parents deny any recent illnesses. She spent the last few days with her grandparents where she had tried new foods. Which of the following is true of this condition?

    A. This patient has progressive motor neuron weakness from a mutation in the *SMN1* gene.
    B. Soluble NSF attachment protein receptor (SNARE) proteins are cleaved, leading to an inability of synaptic vesicles to release acetylcholine.
    C. This patient should have increased cerebrospinal fluid (CSF) protein and conduction blocks seen on nerve conduction studies.
    D. Muscle biopsy would reveal necrotic muscle fibers and ragged red fibers.
    E. This is inherited in an autosomal-dominant manner with anticipation.

103. Which of the following is the mechanism of action for pyridostigmine?

    A. Voltage-gated calcium channel agonist
    B. Reversible acetylcholinesterase inhibitor
    C. Muscarinic receptor agonist
    D. Nicotinic receptor antagonist
    E. Irreversible acetylcholinesterase inhibitor

104. Which of the following cerebral blood flow levels correlate with impaired but reversible neuronal function?

    A. 65 mL/100 g/min
    B. 45 mL/100 g/min
    C. 35 mL/100 g/min
    D. 15 mL/100 g/min
    E. 5 mL/100 g/min

105. A 55-year-old male presents with an acute stroke in the right fusiform gyrus. Although he has intact visual fields, he is unable to recognize faces. Interestingly, he is able to identify and name people by their voices. Which of the following best describes his condition?

    A. Optic aphasia
    B. Prosopagnosia
    C. Anomic aphasia
    D. Cortical blindness
    E. Aphemia

ANSWERS

1. **A.** The case and image are consistent with cerebral amyloid angiopathy (CAA). Although the most common form is sporadic, it is important to identify hereditary cases when present. Hereditary CAA is autosomal dominant and is most commonly associated with mutations in the amyloid precursor protein (*APP*) gene. Figure from Ma JM 2010 Biopsy pathology of neurodegenerative disorders in adults. In: *Practical Surgical Neuropathology: A Diagnostic Approach*, Churchill Livingstone, pp. 551–572, with permission.

2. **D.** Natalizumab is a monoclonal antibody against α4-integrin, a cell adhesion molecule necessary for leukocytes to exit blood vessels into the central nervous system (CNS). Studies demonstrated reduced relapses and slower progression of disability for natalizumab compared with placebo. This drug is known to increase the risk of JC virus infection, causing progressive multifocal leukoencephalopathy, with the highest risk in previously immunosuppressed patients, patients with positive JC virus antibodies, or people taking natalizumab for more than 2 years. Glatiramer is a synthetic protein whose exact mechanism of action is unknown. The four amino acids composing the drug are similar to the myelin basic protein, which may cause an immunological diversion. Alternatively, glatiramer has been noted to induce a population switch from proinflammatory Th1 cells to regulatory Th2 cells through an unknown mechanism. Rituximab is a monoclonal antibody against CD-20, a surface protein expressed on B-cells. By targeting CD-20, the B-cell population is reduced, as is autoimmunity. The exact mechanism of action of dimethyl fumarate is not known, although its use is associated with decreased granulocyte invasion into the CNS, potentially through mediation on the HCA2 receptor. Additionally, there is speculation of an antioxidant role of dimethyl fumarate. Fingolimod is a structural analog of a sphingosine, which is thought to sequester lymphocytes in lymph nodes, thereby reducing the number of active, circulating lymphocytes and overall autoimmunity (*see* Bradley's NiCP, 7th edn, Ch. 80, pp. 1159–1186).

3. **D.** Oligodendroglia, the cells responsible for axonal myelination in the brain, are reduced proportionate to myelin loss in the center of a demyelinated plaque, although they are preserved or even increased at the periphery of a plaque. Generally, neuronal axons are preserved within a demyelinated plaque. T-cells and macrophages are a prominent component of the inflammation within active plaques. Reactive astrocytes are also prominent in plaques (*see* Bradley's NiCP, 7th edn, Ch. 51, pp. 676–695).

4. **A.** Molecular weight, charge, and lipid solubility are all important components of passive diffusion of a molecule across the BBB. Further, substances with specific transporters (e.g. amino acids) may cross. However, immunogenicity is not an important factor in BBB crossing (*see* Bradley's NiCP, 7th edn, Ch. 88, pp. 1261–1278).

5. **A.** This patient has an action tremor consistent with essential tremor and has tried and failed numerous medications. At this point, her quality of life is severely affected due to her dependence on others for feeding, clothing, and dressing. In the absence of medical contraindications, DBS could be considered. The most common target for essential tremor is the VIM nucleus of the thalamus. Both the GPi and the STN have been considered for the treatment of Parkinson disease. Generally, the GPi is considered for the treatment of dystonia (generalized and segmental). The CM thalamus is being evaluated in medically refractory tic disorders such as Tourette syndrome. The nucleus accumbens is being evaluated in medically refractory depression (*see* Bradley's NiCP, 7th edn, Ch. 37, pp. 401–406).

6. **C.** This pregnant patient has severe migraine headaches that are keeping her from working and taking care of her child. Generally migraine preventative medications are avoided during pregnancy, but in cases where patients are unable to perform their daily activities, the benefits of treatment may outweigh the risks. This patient's headaches are severe enough that postponing treatment would not be the best option. Propranolol is regarded as reasonably safe during pregnancy and is class C. Valproic acid, although previously effective in this patient, is considered pregnancy class X for migraine headaches. Daily ibuprofen may be helpful, but can lead to medication overuse headaches and premature closure of the ductus arteriosus in the third trimester. Acetazolamide is used for idiopathic intracranial hypertension (IIH), which is more common in pregnancy. However, the patient's headaches are not characteristic of IIH, which would generally include nocturnal headaches, transient visual obscurations, and papilledema (*see* Bradley's NiCP, Ch. 112, pp. 1973–1991).

7. **C.** The muscle biopsy shows variation in fiber size, central nuclei, and increased endomysial fibrous tissue and fat, which are consistent with Duchenne muscular dystrophy. Steroid myopathy is characterized by diffuse necrosis, with fiber atrophy worse in fast fibers on ATPase staining. Inclusion body myositis is notable for a mixture of myofiber degeneration and inflammation, with accumulation of myelinoid bodies and amyloid deposition, vacuoles with basophilic granules, and lymphocytic infiltration into myofibers. A biopsy from polymyositis would show lymphocyte and macrophage infiltration of the endomysium (between and around individual myofibers) (*see* Bradley's NiCP, 7th edn, Ch. 110, pp. 1915–1954). Figure from Ferri FF 2009 *Ferri's Color Atlas and Text of Clinical Medicine*, Elsevier, with permission.

8. **A.** Hyponatremia may be related to the syndrome of inappropriate antidiuretic hormone secretion, cerebral salt wasting, medication effect, or excessive intake of hypotonic fluids (as in alcoholism or psychogenic polydipsia). Overly rapid correction of severe hyponatremia may lead to central pontine myelinolysis (or osmotic demyelination). As such, hypertonic saline should only be used with great caution in the setting of severe and symptomatic hyponatremia with correction not to exceed 10–12 mEq/L per day. Hypernatremia is most commonly seen with diabetes insipidus or medication effect and is associated with intravascular volume depletion and dehydration. The threat of osmotic demyelination is significantly lower with correction of hypernatremia. The risk of overly rapid correction of hypokalemia is mainly cardiac, rather than neurological. Hypocalcemia may lead to alteration of consciousness, but correction of calcium levels is not associated with demyelination. Finally, hypoglycemia should be corrected rapidly, as

prolongation of hypoglycemia may cause permanent neuronal injury. However, when safely and quickly possible, patients should be given thiamine before dextrose-containing fluids in order to reduce the risk of Wernicke encephalopathy (*see* Bradley's NiCP, 7th edn, Ch. 58, pp. 814–834).

9. A. This patient has multifocal motor neuropathy (MMN) with conduction block. This is commonly misdiagnosed as amyotrophic lateral sclerosis (ALS) because it is a pure motor disorder with fasciculations. The keys to discerning MMN from ALS include a lack of upper motor neuron findings in MMN and key electrodiagnostic findings. The electrodiagnostic hallmark of MMN is normal sensory responses with at least two motor nerves with conduction blocks outside of typical areas of entrapment. Approximately 50% of these patients have anti-GM1 antibodies. MMN responds to intravenous immunoglobulin and not plasmapheresis or steroids. Cytoalbuminological dissociation is present in chronic inflammatory demyelinating polyneuropathy (CIDP), and is not typically present in MMN. Although MMN is an autoimmune neuropathy, it is considered a distinct entity from CIDP. Polio is in the Picornaviridae family and causes a pure motor neuropathy, but there would be no conduction blocks on nerve conduction studies (*see* Bradley's NiCP, 7th edn, Ch. 98, pp. 1484–1518).

10. C. The combination of optic neuritis and transverse myelitis is commonly seen in neuromyelitis optica (NMO, previously known as *Devic disease*). NMO is associated with antibodies against aquaportin-4. Anti-GQ1b antibodies are associated with Miller-Fisher syndrome, a variant of Guillain-Barré syndrome. Although sensorimotor problems may present with Miller-Fisher syndrome, there is no mention of the classical triad in this stem, which is ophthalmoplegia, ataxia, and areflexia. Pathergy is a phenomenon associated with Behçet's disease in which minor cutaneous trauma is associated with robust inflammatory response, often with ulceration. The pathergy test is, therefore, merely pricking the skin with a needle to evaluate for this reaction as evidence of Behçet disease. Although HTLV-1 infection may cause a viral myelitis, it is not commonly associated with recurrent symptoms, nor with ocular symptoms. Anti-GM1 antibodies are associated with multifocal motor neuropathy. This disease is an autoimmune motor neuropathy that may mimic amyotrophic lateral sclerosis, but should not cause sensory loss or sphincter dysfunction (*see* Bradley's NiCP, 7th edn, Ch. 80, pp. 1159–1186).

11. D. The patient's symptoms fit anatomically with a radial neuropathy at the spiral groove. In lesions at the spiral groove, distal radial muscles are affected (as outlined in the stem) and sensation loss is confined to the region supplied by the superficial radial sensory nerve (as outlined in the stem). Notably, triceps strength is spared. A lower trunk plexopathy would affect median and ulnar muscles, such as the first dorsal interosseous muscle and abductor pollicis brevis, and cause numbness in the medial forearm. Clinically, a lower trunk plexopathy can look similar to a C8 radiculopathy, but they are differentiated on nerve conduction testing by normal sensory studies in a C8 radiculopathy but abnormal ulnar and medial antebrachial cutaneous sensory responses in a lower trunk plexopathy. Posterior interosseous neuropathy does not affect the brachioradialis or cause changes in sensation, because it is a purely motor nerve. A posterior cord plexopathy affects both the axillary and radial nerves, and results in deltoid weakness and numbness over the shoulder in addition to radial motor and sensory deficits (*see* Bradley's NiCP, 7th edn, Ch. 107, pp. 1791–1866).

12. A. Fragile X syndrome (FXS) is an X-linked dominant disease caused by CGG triplet repeats within the *FMR1* gene. There is no parental imprinting in this disease, although this phenomenon may be seen with Prader-Willi and Angelman syndromes. Autism spectrum disorder is commonly seen with FXS, but is not always present. An increased risk of leukemia is seen with various genetic disorders, especially Down syndrome, although not necessarily with FXS (*see* Bradley's NiCP, 7th edn, Chs. 50, pp. 648–675 and 90, pp. 1301–1323).

13. D. Sodium channels are clustered in the nodes of Ranvier, whereas potassium channels are under the myelin sheath. This clustering of sodium channels allows depolarization to occur at the nodes, leading to saltatory (not statutory) conduction, which flows from one nodal region to the next. Normal myelinated fiber conduction speeds are in the range of 40–60 m/s (*see* Bradley's NiCP, 7th edn, Chs. 34–35, pp. 349–391).

14. D. The patient scores 2 points for opening eyes to painful stimulation, 2 points for incomprehensible sounds, and 4 points for withdrawal to painful stimulation. The full scale is shown here (*see* Bradley's NiCP, 7th edn, Ch. 55, pp. 742–758).

TABLE FOR ANSWER 4.14 Glasgow coma scale for assessment of coma and impaired consciousness

Eye opening	Best motor response	Best verbal response
4 = Spontaneous	6 = Obeying	5 = Oriented
3 = To speech	5 = Localizing	4 = Confused
2 = To pain	4 = Withdrawing	3 = Inappropriate
1 = None	3 = Flexing	2 = Incomprehensible
	2 = Extending	1 = None
	1 = None	

Data from Teasdale G, Jennett B 1974 Assessment of coma and impaired consciousness. Lancet 2: 81–84.

15. B. The high-pass filter, also known as the low-frequency filter, reduces the amplitude of waveforms below the selected frequency, but only reduces the selected frequency's amplitude in the range of 50%. Low-frequency waveforms on EEG are usually artifacts, with a major artifact coming from sweat. This results in waves that are usually 0.5 Hz or less. A standard low-frequency filter is usually set at 0.5 Hz or 1 Hz. Increasing this filter will further reduce the low-frequency sweat artifact. EMG artifact is typically very fast, in the range of 30 Hz or greater. To reduce this artifact, the low-pass filter (high-frequency filter) can be reduced to 30 or 35 Hz from a standard of 70 Hz. Electrode impedance is a measure of resistance between the skin and the electrode. This is usually increased by poor electrode–skin contact, either from improper attachment or lack of conducting gel (*see* Bradley's NiCP, 7th edn, Ch. 34, pp. 348–365).

this personal relationship will affect professional judgment, referral to another physician could be considered.

30. E. Hydrocodone is the most appropriate medication in this case for a severe headache. Other options include acetaminophen, tramadol, and mild opiates. Ibuprofen and ketorolac should not be used in the third trimester due to the risk of early closure of the ductus arteriosus. Valproic acid has the most risk in early pregnancy due to neural tube defects, but there are concerns with long-term cognitive effects if used later in pregnancy. Sumatriptan can be used during pregnancy, but is considered a second- or third-line agent after acetaminophen or mild narcotics because vasoconstriction may put the mother at a higher risk of stroke or heart attack, and vasoconstriction of the placenta may result in relative ischemia to the fetus (*see* Bradley's NiCP, 7th edn, Ch. 112, pp. 1973–1991).

31. D. IRBs are committees empowered to ensure the safe performance of human research, for which minimal risk must be matched by sufficient benefit to patients, human rights are respected, and informed consent is obtained. IRBs are governed by the Office of Human Research Protections within the Department of Health and Human Services. Although IRBs do review the scientific method posed for a given research study, in order to ensure that a scientifically sound result may be achieved, the specific analyses thereof may be outside the scope of an IRB.

32. C. Adjustment disorders involve the development of behavioral symptoms within 3 months of a stressor. The behavioral symptoms (either anxiety or depression) typically cause significant functional impairment and seem to be out of proportion to the expected response. Death of close friends or family members can result in significant distress and even occasional hallucinations in normal bereavement. However, in this case the stressful event was not closely related to her. One would expect sadness from a tragedy such as a plane crash but not an inability to continue with her regular life. An acute stress disorder must begin within 4 weeks of a stressful event and involves flashbacks, recurrent thoughts, symptoms of increased anxiety and arousal, and significant clinical impairment. Posttraumatic stress disorder involves similar clinical symptoms to an acute stress disorder, except the symptoms must be present for >1 month. MDD can involve a low mood, anhedonia, feelings of worthlessness, suicidal ideation, guilt, helplessness, decreased libido, and changes to appetite and sleep. Notably, though, MDD is not usually in response to a particular stressful event.

33. A. McArdle disease is type V glycogenosis, an autosomal-recessive disorder caused by a defect in myophosphorylase. This results in a buildup of glycogen below the sarcolemma, which stains brightly with PAS staining. Becker muscular dystrophy is associated with atrophic fibers, hypertrophic fibers, and fibrosis. Polymyositis is associated with an endomysial inflammatory infiltrate with CD8+ lymphocytes. Myotonic dystrophy is associated with variation in fiber sizes and central nuclei but has no characteristic pathological features. The diagnosis of myotonic dystrophy is usually made by testing the *DMPK* gene on chromosome 19 for CTG repeats. Charcot-Marie-Tooth 1a is a hereditary demyelinating polyneuropathy that can cause fiber type grouping and group atrophy on muscle biopsy and onion bulbs on nerve biopsy (*see* Bradley's NiCP, 7th edn, Ch. 110, pp. 1915–1955). Figure from Klatt EC 2014 *Robbins and Cotran Atlas of Pathology*, 3rd edn, Saunders, with permission.

34. E. In general, neurogenic bladder dysfunction can be grouped by lesion location. Suprapontine lesions (as seen with stroke) are often associated with urinary frequency and urgency due to detrusor overactivity, with normal flow and minimal postvoid residual. Lesions below the level of the pons but above the sacrum (as seen with spinal cord injury) are associated with urinary frequency and urgency due to detrusor overactivity, but may also have interrupted stream and incontinence due to detrusor-sphincter dyssynergia (poorly coordinated activity of detrusor and sphincter muscles). These lesions may or may not result in elevated postvoid residual. Infrasacral lesions, or those at the conus medullaris or cauda equina, are associated with detrusor underactivity, resulting in hesitancy, poor stream, and notably large postvoid residual volumes (*see* Bradley's NiCP, 7th edn, Ch. 47, pp. 605–621).

35. D. There are three neurons in the major pathway of sensation for joint position sensation and vibratory sensation. The first-order neuron is the actual sensory receptor in the skin, which houses its cell body in the dorsal root ganglion. These cells have a central projection that bypasses synapses in the spinal cord and forms the dorsal columns. These neurons synapse in the medulla at the nucleus gracilis (for the legs) and nucleus cuneatus (for the arms). The second-order neurons form the medial lemniscus, which decussates and travels to the ventral posteromedial nucleus of the thalamus. Third-order neurons go from the thalamus to the primary sensory cortex. The anterior commissure of the spinal cord crosses the midline of the spinal cord anterior to the gray matter of the cord. This carries pain and temperature sensation to the contralateral side to form the anterior spinothalamic tract. The substantia gelatinosa of the spinal cord is located in the head of the dorsal horn, which receives a variety of mechanical and sensory information to relay to the cerebellum or thalamus. Rexed lamina VI receives information from the muscle spindles, which are the interneurons that synapse on motor neurons to make spinal reflexes (*see* Bradley's NiCP, 7th edn, Ch. 26, pp. 273–278).

36. D. The clinical scenario describes Dejerine-Roussy syndrome, also known as *thalamic pain syndrome*, a condition developing weeks to months after a thalamic stroke. Patients tend to have severe and chronic pain out of proportion to the environmental stimulus (allodynia), often described as burning, tingling, and hypersensitivity to little or no stimuli. This syndrome is thought to stem from a stroke-induced miscommunication between the afferent pathway and the somatosensory cortex. Unfortunately, thalamic pain is very challenging to treat, and often involves trials of multiple agents, including opiates, tricyclic antidepressants, anticonvulsants such as gabapentin or pregabalin, or topical analgesics such as lidocaine patches. Research is ongoing with regard to the use of deep brain stimulation to modulate pain in thalamic pain syndromes. The reason this scenario does not represent a new stroke is that new infarcts develop acutely and tend to cause "negative symptoms" such as

numbness. Similarly, the history and localization are not consistent with a peripheral cause of pain in this case. Although poststroke patients can develop headaches or migraines after their infarct, a thalamic pain syndrome is the most likely etiology in this case. Melkersson-Rosenthal syndrome is characterized by recurring facial paralysis, swelling of the face and lips, and a furrowed tongue, usually seen in the pediatric population (*see* Bradley's NiCP, 7th edn, Ch. 30, pp. 314–323).

37. C. Clean nerve transection, as with a knife or scalpel, is generally repaired immediately due to the relatively clean and well-perfused injury. More ragged nerve tears, as with a propeller, generally need to be surgically debrided first. Nerve endings may be tacked to fascia so that they can be easily identified in 2–3 weeks for primary nerve graft repair. Compressive neurapraxia does not require surgical repair, except in the case of compartment syndrome, in which case fasciotomy should be performed (but not primary nerve repair). Stretch injury similarly would not be benefitted by surgical nerve repair. If meaningful nerve regeneration is not seen by 5 months after humerus fracture, repair is indicated, and generally has best results before 6 months (*see* Bradley's NiCP, 7th edn, Ch. 64, pp. 903–919).

38. A. For the long-term prevention of episodic cluster headaches, verapamil is generally considered first-line therapy. Although inhaled oxygen is efficacious for abortive therapy for cluster headaches, this is not useful for preventive therapy. Although paroxysmal hemicrania, another of the trigeminal autonomic cephalgias, is exquisitely sensitive to indomethacin, cluster headaches are generally not responsive to indomethacin. Amitriptyline is often beneficial in the prevention of other headache types, such as migraine, but is generally not helpful for cluster headaches. Levetiracetam has little evidence in headache prevention (*see* Bradley's NiCP, 7th edn, Ch. 103, pp. 1686–1719).

39. E. The length of the triplet repeat in the *Huntingtin* gene is associated with age of symptom onset. Further, the triplet repeat length increases over subsequent generations, leading to earlier disease onset. This phenomenon is known as *genetic anticipation*. Parental age of onset may provide a rough guide for a patient, but genetic anticipation means that the patient will generally have earlier onset than the parent. Neither the gender of the patient nor of the affected parent (parental imprinting) affects symptom onset in Huntington disease. The cause of Huntington disease is a specific CAG triplet repeat, not a point mutation (*see* Bradley's NiCP, 7th edn, Ch. 96).

40. D. The next best step in this case is to obtain a noncontrast head CT to rule out cerebral hemorrhage and to ensure there is not already major ischemic change or structural lesions. Laboratory tests such as a point-of-care glucose and international normalized ratio (INR) should be immediately obtained. If the patient is within 4.5 hours of the last known normal and is without exclusion criteria, then IV tPA should be considered at a dose of 0.9 mg/kg, with a 10% bolus initially, and the rest given over 1 hour, but not without first obtaining a noncontrast head CT to rule out hemorrhage. Examples of exclusions include, but are not limited to, intracranial hemorrhage, rapidly improving symptoms, platelet count <100,000, INR >1.6, major surgery or head trauma in the last 2 weeks, stroke within the last 3 months, systolic blood pressure > 185 mm Hg, and known arteriovenous malformation or aneurysm. The risk of bleeding is around 1%–6%, and the risk of death is similar, with or without treatment. In general, those who receive IV tPA earlier have a better prognosis than those who receive it later. Although aspirin is needed, this should not be administered before a CT of the brain. In addition, if IV tPA is given, aspirin should not be administered for at least 24 hours. Nicardipine is an option to decrease blood pressure, but it would only be needed if the blood pressure were above 185 mm Hg systolic or 110 mm Hg diastolic, if IV tPA is to be given, or if above 220 mm Hg systolic otherwise. There is no evidence for impending herniation in this particular case, but the patient would be at risk of intracerebral swelling in the next week if there were a large territory stroke (malignant cerebral edema; *see* Bradley's NiCP, 7th edn, Ch. 65, pp. 920–967).

41. A. DiGeorge syndrome results from a deletion on chromosome 22q11, and is commonly inherited in an autosomal-dominant pattern. It is associated with various anomalies, including facial deformities like cleft palate and cardiac anomalies like tetralogy of Fallot. Additionally, anomalies of the third and fourth branchial pouches during embryogenesis lead to congenital absence of the thymus and parathyroid (*see* Bradley's NiCP, 7th edn, Ch. 50, pp. 648–675).

42. C. Telling patients to learn to deal with a given issue is not advocating for them, but rather tolerating a problem. All of the other items listed in the answer choices are routes to advocating for patients.

43. B. The case is one of mononeuritis multiplex, and the image shows an epineural blood vessel with fibrinoid necrosis of its wall and perivascular and transmural inflammation, consistent with a vasculitic process (*see* Bradley's NiCP, 7th edn, Ch. 107, pp. 1791–1866). Figure from Daroff RB, Jankovic J, Mazziotta JC, Pomeroy SL 2016 *Bradley's Neurology in Clinical Practice*, 7th edn, Elsevier, with permission.

44. E. The history and MRI are compatible with radiation necrosis. On imaging, this can present as diffuse, heterogeneous enhancement with fluid attenuated inversion recovery (FLAIR) signal change. Notably, radiation necrosis tends to be less nodular than tumor, although clear differentiation is often difficult by MRI alone. Photon scatter from high-dose radiation for head and neck cancers often leads to adjacent cerebral necrosis. Generally such effects are long-term complications, occurring a few years or, rarely, decades after radiation therapy. If symptomatic, radiation necrosis can first be treated with steroids. Antiangiogenic therapy (with bevacizumab) has been useful in some cases; otherwise, surgical resection may be considered. Although observation alone might be appropriate if radiation necrosis is found incidentally, it would not be appropriate in this case given that the patient is symptomatic. There is little to suggest a fungal infection in this case, so antifungal therapy would not be necessary. Radiation therapy would likely exacerbate the problem. There is no suggestion of paraneoplastic disease in the case description, nor do paraneoplastic diseases often cause such focal, enhancing lesions (*see* Bradley's NiCP, 7th edn, Ch. 75,

pp. 1065–1083). Figure from Winn H 2011 *Youmans Neurological Surgery*, Saunders, with permission.

45. A. Blink reflexes are uncommonly used tests that check the function of cranial nerves (CN) V and VII and the brainstem relay systems. In this testing, each supraorbital nerve is stimulated independently with recording electrodes over the orbicularis oculi. The two responses seen are the R1 and R2 responses, which are electromyography responses from the orbicularis oculi. R1 is seen ipsilateral to stimulation, whereas the R2 response is seen both ipsilaterally and contralaterally in a normal response. In the given example, with right-sided stimulation there is a normal ipsilateral R1 response, a normal ipsilateral R2 response, and a delayed low-amplitude contralateral R2 response. This shows the right-sided CN V and VII are both working, whereas the output of CN VII on the left seems to be affected. With left-sided stimulation there is an almost-absent R1 response, a delayed and low-amplitude ipsilateral R2 response, and a normal robust R2 response contralaterally. This demonstrates that the left CN V and brainstem are working because of the robust contralateral R2 response, but the left CN VII is not working well because of the poor ipsilateral R1 and R2 responses. Absent responses with unilateral stimulation but normal responses on the other side would indicate a trigeminal neuropathy on the side with absent responses. Trigeminal neuralgia and internal capsule strokes would not cause blink reflex abnormalities. Pontine strokes can cause various patterns of abnormalities—usually the loss of R2 responses or significant delay in R2 responses bilaterally with stimulation of the affected side (*see* Bradley's NiCP, 7th edn, Ch. 35, pp. 366–390). Figure from Aminoff M 2012 *Aminoff's Electrodiagnosis in Clinical Neurology*, 6th edn, Saunders, with permission.

46. A. Fatal familial insomnia is an autosomal-dominant genetic prion disease associated with mutations in the *PRNP* gene. Patients generally present with progressive, severe insomnia and dysautonomia, including tachycardia, hyperhidrosis, and hyperpyrexia. Motor and cognitive symptoms tend to come later in the disease course, with an average survival of about 1.5 years (*see* Bradley's NiCP, 7th edn, Ch. 94, pp. 1365–1379).

47. C. Central retinal artery occlusion classically presents with a sudden, profound, painless vision loss in one eye. The two most common causes are vasculitis or atherosclerosis, as is most likely in this case. Fundoscopy is often associated with a cherry-red spot surrounded by retinal whitening. Management may involve ocular massage or tissue plasminogen activator. Immediate stroke evaluation is important due to risk of unstable plaque in the carotid artery. Central retinal vein occlusion is often acute and painless, but generally a moderate decrease in visual acuity (as opposed to profound vision loss with CRAO). Fundoscopy shows tortuosity and dilation of retinal veins, with flame hemorrhages. Paraneoplastic retinopathy is associated with antiretinal antibodies, but generally has a more gradual onset of vision symptoms. Optic neuritis is generally associated with subacute central vision loss. The most common causes of optic neuritis include multiple sclerosis or neuromyelitis optica. Anterior ischemic optic neuropathy (AION) may be either arteritic or nonarteritic. Nonarteritic AION is more common, and may present similarly to CRAO, including sudden, painless vision loss, although this may be severe blurring rather than darkness. Further, often only part of the visual field is affected in the eye, generally in an altitudinal pattern. Fundoscopy with nonarteritic AION generally reveals optic disc edema and hyperemia, with occasional flame hemorrhages. Arteritic AION is associated with giant cell arteritis. The vision loss can be transient or acute and persistent, often with contralateral vision loss within 14 days, if left untreated. Fundoscopy in arteritic AION is likely to show an edematous, pale disc with retinal whitening and/or cotton wool spots (*see* Bradley's NiCP, 7th edn, Ch. 17, pp. 163–178). Figure from Duker JS, Waheed NK, Goldman D 2014 *Handbook of Retinal OCT: Optical Coherent Tomography*, Saunders, with permission.

48. D. The correct answer, only 3 days after the accident, is brief psychotic disorder. Her psychosis started after witnessing a horrible accident and consists of visual hallucinations with disorganized behavior. In order to meet criteria for brief psychotic disorder, she needs to have one or more delusions, hallucinations, disorganized speech, and/or grossly disorganized or catatonic behavior. The duration is >1 day but <1 month, and the symptoms are not accounted for by mood or substance exposure. Schizophreniform disorder is characterized by psychosis for >1 month but <6 months, and schizophrenia for 6 months or more. Schizoaffective disorder has prominent mood symptoms and at least 2 weeks of psychotic symptoms in the absence of mood symptoms. The presence of psychosis precludes bereavement. Typically, there is a return to the premorbid psychiatric state after a brief psychotic disorder.

49. C. Lewy bodies are relatively large, round, eosinophilic cytoplasmic inclusions formed from the aggregation of alpha synuclein and ubiquitin. These are seen most often in dementia with Lewy bodies, but can also be seen in Parkinson disease. Neurofibrillary tangles are most often seen in Alzheimer disease and are elongated filamentous intracellular inclusions made of tau protein. Negri bodies are small intracellular inclusions seen in rabies. Spongiform changes are seen in prion diseases and involve the presence of many large extracellular vacuoles, giving the tissue a spongelike appearance. Cowdry A inclusions are eosinophilic inclusions seen in the nucleus of a neuron in herpes simplex virus or varicella zoster virus (*see* Bradley's NiCP, 7th edn, Ch. 95, pp. 1380–1421). Figure from Kövari E, Horvath J, Bouras C 2009 Neuropathology of Lewy body disorders. *Brain Research Bulletin* 80(4–5): 203–210, with permission.

50. C. The branches from the internal carotid (in order from proximal to distal; see the figure) are the ophthalmic artery, posterior communicating artery, anterior choroidal artery, and then bifurcation into the anterior and middle cerebral arteries (*see* Bradley's NiCP, 7th edn, Ch. 65, pp. 920–967).

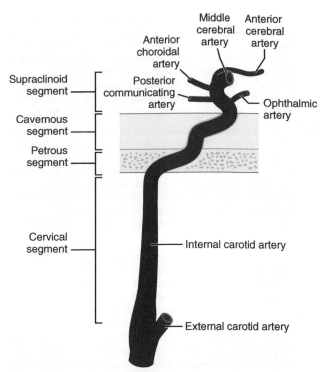

Figure for Answer 4.50 (*from Caplan LR 2009* Caplan's Stroke: A Clinical Approach, *4th edn, Elsevier, with permission.*)

51. A. Febrile seizures occur in 2%–4% of children younger than 5 years of age and are generally associated with a systemic infection. They are divided into either simple or complex categories. Simple febrile seizures are characterized by no more than one seizure in a 24-hour period, which lasts less than 15 minutes and has no focal postictal features. The diagnosis of simple febrile seizures is contingent upon a normally developed child with no neurological abnormalities and no family history of seizures. Notably, simple febrile seizures are usually generalized, with no focal features or preceding automatisms. Complex febrile seizures are diagnosed in anyone who does not meet the aforementioned criteria, including patients with developmental abnormalities, family history of seizure, focal seizures, prolonged postictal period, or more than one seizure per 24-hour period. In patients with complex febrile seizures, the likelihood of an underlying diagnosis of epilepsy or central nervous system infection is relatively higher than with simple febrile seizures, and more elaborate workups may be pursued, including lumbar puncture and/or electroencephalogram. Seizure prophylaxis is generally not needed for simple febrile seizures, but may be considered in complex febrile seizures (*see* Bradley's NiCP, 7th edn, Ch. 101, pp. 1563–1614).

52. C. The patient is in the midst of an acute manic episode with history of depressive disorder in the past that required hospitalization. To meet criteria for bipolar 1 disorder, one must have at least three or more of the following for at least 1 week in duration: decreased need for sleep, pressured speech, inflated self-esteem, flight of ideas, distractibility, increased goal-directed behavior, or excessive involvement with

pleasurable activities. The mood disturbance must be severe enough to cause impairment. Treatment involves mood stabilizers, antipsychotics, and selective serotonin reuptake inhibitors. Bipolar 2 disorder consists of hypomania, which usually has milder symptoms and lack of significant functional impairment in contrast to mania. The episode of acute mania would preclude a diagnosis of major depressive disorder. Conversely, a major depressive episode may be a part of bipolar disorder, but only if an episode of mania occurs. There is no psychosis in this case to suggest schizophrenia. Cyclothymic disorder is unlikely, as this patient has mania (not hypomania) and has met prior criteria for major depressive episode.

53. E. Vitamin B12 is a key cofactor to many biochemical reactions in the body, so its deficiency may cause many unwanted effects. Chief among these for the neurologist are demyelinating myeloneuropathy, causing loss of proprioception and ataxia, subacute combined degeneration of the spinal cord, and cognitive decline. Additional considerations include macrocytic anemia and hypercoagulability due to resultant hyperhomocysteinemia. Although depression can be seen with vitamin B12 deficiency, mania is not generally seen (*see* Bradley's NiCP, 7th edn, Ch. 85, pp. 1226–1236).

54. B. The MRI shown depicts schizencephaly, a developmental abnormality that consists of a cleft extending from the ependyma to the pia mater, lined with *gray* matter. There are two types of schizencephaly: open-lipped (shown) and closed-lipped. This is in contrast to porencephaly, which usually consists of cysts lined by *white* matter, caused by a toxic, ischemic, or developmental insult. Holoprosencephaly is caused by failure of the brain to divide into the left and right hemispheres. The alobar subtype is the most severe, followed by semilobar, then lobar. Holoprosencephaly can sometimes be associated with septooptic dysplasia. Polymicrogyria is a migrational abnormality that consists of multiple shallow gyri, usually associated with congenital cytomegalovirus or other developmental conditions such as Aicardi syndrome and DiGeorge syndrome. Periventricular nodular heterotopia is also a migrational abnormality that is associated with abnormally placed islands of gray matter near the ventricles, often resulting in seizures (*see* Bradley's NiCP, 7th edn, Ch. 89, pp. 1279–1300). Figure from Shimizu M, Maeda T, Izumi T 2012 The differences in epileptic characteristics in patients with porencephaly and schizencephaly. *Brain & Development* 34(7): 546–552, with permission.

55. D. The Purkinje cells are the major output cells of the cerebellum. They are located in the middle layer of the cerebellar cortex. Sensory information arrives through the mossy fibers and is first processed by granular cells and in the molecular layer by the stellate and basket cells layer, which in turn send signals to Purkinje cells. The Purkinje cells are GABAergic and send inhibitory signals to the deep cerebellum and brainstem. Purkinje cells are the main target in diseases like paraneoplastic cerebellar degeneration (*see* Bradley's NiCP, 7th edn, Ch. 97, pp. 1461–1483).

56. E. Haloperidol is one of the typical antipsychotics whose mechanism of action involves blocking the D_2

receptor. It is one of the high-potency D_2 antagonists, as opposed to chlorpromazine and thioridazine, which are two low-potency agents. The high-potency agents are good for injection and for reducing positive psychotic symptoms acutely. However, there is also a high potential for acute extrapyramidal side effects such as acute dystonic reactions (responsive to benztropine or diphenhydramine), as well as chronic extrapyramidal symptoms such as tardive orofacial dyskinesia or dystonia. The low-potency agents have a lower risk of extrapyramidal side effects, but higher anticholinergic properties.

57. E. Deep cerebellar nuclei transmit information back to the cerebrum, generally through excitatory output transmitted through mossy and climbing fibers. The main efferent pathway from the cerebellum is the superior cerebellar peduncle. The dentate is the most lateral nucleus, and controls voluntary movement planning and initiation. The emboliform is immediately medial to the dentate, and projects to the red nucleus and lateral thalamic nucleus, modulating voluntary movements. The globose is immediately medial to the emboliform, and is involved in posture control and voluntary movement. Together, the emboliform and globose are known as the *interposed nuclei*. The fastigial is the most medial deep cerebellar nucleus and receives input from the vestibular system, ultimately contributing to the corticoreticulospinal and vestibulospinal systems, leading to modulation of posture and proximal limb movements. The orientation of the deep cerebellar structures is demonstrated in the figure.

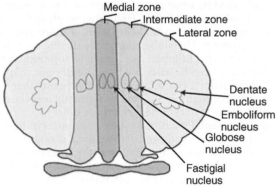

Figure for Answer 4.57 *(from Umphred DA, Lazaro RT, Roller M, Burton G 2013* Neurological Rehabilitation, *6th edn, Elsevier, pp. 631–652, with permission.)*

58. A. There are five primary urea cycle disorders, with OTC deficiency being the most common. Others include carbamoyl phosphate synthetase deficiency, argininosuccinic acid synthetase deficiency, argininosuccinic acid lyase deficiency, and arginase deficiency. All of these are autosomal recessive except for OTC deficiency, which is X-linked. Although OTC deficiency is X-linked, women can also have symptoms, including intermittent headache, vomiting, or eye movement abnormalities, especially in the postpartum state. Most urea cycle disorders present in the newborn period with the triad of hyperammonemia, encephalopathy, and respiratory alkalosis. Other symptoms may include vomiting, hypothermia, coma, or seizures (and may be confused with sepsis). The

clinical approach to urea cycle disorders includes the avoidance of dietary protein, as well as treatment with arginine, sodium benzoate, or sodium phenylacetate. Hemodialysis may also be helpful to remove excessive ammonia. Cerebral edema can be treated with mannitol. Even those infants treated early are still highly likely to develop mental retardation (*see* Bradley's NiCP, 7th edn, Ch. 91, pp. 1324–1341).

59. D. Pregabalin's exact mechanism is not known, but it binds calcium channels in the central nervous system, leading to antiepileptic and antinociceptive effects. Clonazepam and phenobarbital bind GABA receptors, increasing GABA activity. Vigabatrin irreversibly inhibits GABA metabolism to increase GABA activity. Tiagabine inhibits the reuptake of GABA into presynaptic terminals (*see* Bradley's NiCP, 7th edn, Ch. 101, pp. 1563–1614).

60. A. This patient has a lesion on the left side of her cervical spinal cord resulting in Brown-Seqúard syndrome, which involves ipsilateral weakness, ipsilateral loss of vibration and position sensation, and contralateral loss of sensation to temperature and pin prick below the level of the lesion. Central cord syndrome involves weakness of both upper extremities more so than the lower extremities, urinary retention, and sensory dysfunction of varying degrees, which can result in a capelike loss of sensation with cervical lesions. Lesions of the posterior columns cause loss of position and vibratory sensation bilaterally without loss of strength. When it occurs in the setting of B12 deficiency, this is called *subacute combined degeneration*. A lesion of the left side of the pons would cause ipsilateral facial weakness and contralateral extremity weakness. A lesion on the right side of the cervical cord would cause right-sided weakness, right-sided loss of vibration/proprioception, and left-sided loss of pin prick and temperature sensation (*see* Bradley's NiCP, 7th edn, Ch. 26, pp. 273–278).

61. B. Denial is considered the first stage in the Kübler-Ross stages of grief. In this stage, people will choose to ignore the loss or live in an alternate reality. Anger is the second stage in which they become easily frustrated or question why this loss has befallen them. Bargaining is the third stage in which people try to make deals to take away the loss that they have suffered. The fourth stage is depression, and the fifth stage acceptance.

62. B. Wernicke-Korsakoff syndrome is caused by a thiamine deficiency (vitamin B1) leading to the triad of memory loss, ataxia, and ophthalmoplegia. It is commonly seen in alcoholics or patients with decreased dietary intake or absorption of thiamine (especially after gastric bypass surgery). Wernicke-Korsakoff syndrome can be acutely precipitated by administering glucose without thiamine in an emergent setting. If left untreated, the syndrome will progress to encephalopathy and even death. Response to treatment is variable, but ocular symptoms tend to resolve quickly, whereas memory and ataxia take much longer to improve. Many patients are left with Korsakoff syndrome, which involves anterograde and retrograde amnesia, confabulation, and disorientation. Magnetic resonance imaging abnormalities include FLAIR or T2 hyperintense lesions in the periaqueductal gray matter, tectal plates, medial thalami, and bilateral mammillary bodies. The APOE4 allele is associated

with an increased risk of developing Alzheimer disease and has no known association to Wernicke-Korsakoff syndrome (*see* Bradley's NiCP, 7th edn, Ch. 85, pp. 1226–1236).

63. A. The patient likely has a West Nile virus infection causing diffuse central nervous system symptoms, including encephalitis, and either rhombencephalitis or myelitis. Texas is a common location for this virus, and the summer months present the greatest incidence due its mosquito vector. Treatment is supportive, and mortality is low, although deficits may persist. Poliovirus infections are exceedingly rare in the United States, and this individual has been vaccinated, making this unlikely. Guillain-Barré syndrome may be difficult to discern from West Nile virus, but does not usually have confusion, stiff neck, or ongoing fever. Similarly, ADEM may follow illness, but rarely has ongoing fever and would be apparent on MRI. Botulinum toxin ingestion may cause flaccid weakness, but is usually accompanied with bulbar weakness, autonomic disturbance (including loss of pupillary responsiveness), and constipation (*see* Bradley's NiCP, 7th edn, Ch. 78, pp. 1121–1146).

64. D. The relationship between physicians and nurses should be focused on appropriate care of the patient. Nurses are justified in questioning orders by physicians, especially if these orders are out of usual care. Nurses also have the obligation to not provide care they believe is inappropriate. The best response is to educate the nurse on why certain medications are necessary, not changing orders to appease her concerns. There is no need to contact the risk management team or report the nurse to her charge nurse. Demanding the nurse give medications that she is uncomfortable giving is an abuse of power within the physician–nurse relationship (AMA Code of Medical Ethics).

65. D. Dravet syndrome (early-onset epileptic encephalopathy) is associated with early generalized tonic-clonic seizures, followed by additional seizure types later in early childhood. Additionally, cognitive function declines as seizures become intractable. Dravet syndrome is associated with *SCN1A* mutations. Rett syndrome is a neurodevelopmental disorder usually found in females with normal development early on, but later milestone loss and loss of functional movements of the hands. Rett syndrome is associated with *MECP2* mutations. West syndrome represents the triad of infantile spasms, interictal electroencephalograph abnormality known as *hypsarrhythmia*, and mental retardation. West syndrome has been associated with *ARX* mutations on the X chromosome in some cases. Landau-Kleffner syndrome, also known as *epileptic aphasia*, is an autosomal-dominant focal epilepsy with continuous spike and wave discharges in the dominant temporal lobe during sleep that causes speech delay or regression. Landau-Kleffner syndrome is associated with *GRIN2A* mutations. GEFS+ is a condition in which febrile seizures continue beyond 6 years of age or develop into epilepsy without regard to fever. It is associated with mutations in the sodium channel–encoding gene *SCN1B* (*see* Bradley's NiCP, 7th edn, Ch. 101, pp. 1563–1614).

66. B. The patient has several features that point to a diagnosis of Guillain-Barré syndrome (GBS), including history of preceding diarrheal illness, absent reflexes, and absent F waves on nerve conduction studies. Generally, nerve conduction abnormalities are not seen for the first several days with GBS, and up to 2 weeks may pass before abnormal spontaneous activity is seen. Reduced recruitment should be seen immediately in weak muscles from GBS, but unfortunately this patient could not activate any units. Polymyositis would have no effect on F waves. Further, motor units should be activated and would be of short duration and low amplitude, and significant positive waves and fibrillations would be present. Myasthenia gravis would not have changes in reflexes or F waves. If the exacerbation is severe enough, motor units may not be seen, but there should be no spontaneous activity or recruitment changes. Critical illness neuropathy can cause diffuse weakness and loss of reflexes; however, this develops during a prolonged intensive care unit stay. Acid maltase deficiency is a treatable metabolic myopathy in which there is a deficiency of alpha-glucosidase. This disorder can present with precipitous respiratory failure. Nerve conduction studies would be expected to be normal, although EMG would show diffuse spontaneous activity, including prominent myotonia and small-amplitude, short-duration motor units (*see* Bradley's NiCP, 7th edn, Ch. 55, pp. 742–758 and Ch. 107, pp. 1791–1866).

67. D. The patient has an acute onset of movement disorder, which corresponds temporally with a new stressor. Walking requires great effort, and she has a Hoover sign (lack of leg extension into the bed while attempting to flex the contralateral leg against resistance) but no localizable neurological findings. Observation shows that even though the patient reports the inability to lift her legs, she does so when moving about in bed. Given these findings, along with a history of physical and sexual abuse, conversion disorder is most likely. Keep in mind that a preceding stressor no longer is required to meet criteria for conversion disorder. Treatment is aimed at treating comorbid depression with selective serotonin reuptake inhibitors, cognitive behavioral therapy, and intense physical therapy. A flaccid paralysis from an anterior horn cell injury (i.e. West Nile virus) would not be intermittent and not have normal tone and reflexes. Conus medullaris syndrome would be expected to have low back pain with decreased perianal sensation, bowel/bladder changes, and possibly bilateral lower extremity (true) weakness. After 1 month of symptoms, one would expect tone abnormalities (upper motor neuron signs). There is no indication of dysmetria; ataxic dysarthria; truncal instability; or wide-based, ataxic gait to suggest a diagnosis of cerebellar ataxia. Finally, somatization is not likely given the patient's examination and symptoms are mostly neurological in nature rather than multisystemic as in somatization disorder.

68. B. This patient has a contrast-enhancing lesion on her MRI, which is located in the periphery near the gray-white junction. This lesion is small, round, and associated with significant edema. This is most consistent with a metastatic lesion. Choriocarcinoma is a rare cancer that frequently metastasizes to both the lungs and the brain. It commonly occurs after a spontaneous abortion, premature labor, or a molar pregnancy. The tumor can occur in the spine, lumbrosacral plexus, and the cauda equina. Glioblastomas are primary brain tumors, and would

not have spread to the lungs. Multiple sclerosis can cause round lesions that enhance with contrast, but they are not typically associated with significant edema, and usually have incomplete ring enhancement. Meningiomas are benign tumors outside of the parenchyma of the brain. These can cause cerebral edema if large enough and typically enhance homogenously with contrast. Ischemic strokes do not cause the pattern seen on the MRI. Subacute strokes (2–4 weeks old) may show enhancement, though not ring enhancement, and most edema would be resolved at that point (*see* Bradley's NiCP, Ch. 112, pp. 1973–1991). Figure from Kang TW, Kim ST, Byun HS, et al. 2009 Morphological and functional MRI, MRS, perfusion and diffusion changes after radiosurgery of brain metastasis. *European Journal of Radiology* 72(3): 370–380, with permission.

69. C. Deep inhibitory postsynaptic potentials cause a positive charge to develop in the body of the neuron, making the more superficial portion of the neuron appear more negative, and therefore the EEG electrode records a negative potential. The same is seen with superficial excitatory postsynaptic potential, which causes negativity in the superficial portion of the neuron and is recorded as a negative scalp discharge. Vertically oriented dipoles are recorded well on scalp electrodes, whereas radial-oriented dipoles are not seen well (*see* Bradley's NiCP, 7th edn, Ch. 34, pp. 348–366).

70. D. Susac syndrome is a small-vessel vasculitis that commonly presents with sensorineural hearing loss, branch retinal artery occlusions, and encephalopathy. MRI classically shows "cannonballs" of T2 hyperintensity within the corpus callosum related to demyelination. Multiple sclerosis causes T2 hyperintense areas of demyelination throughout the brain, commonly including the corpus callosum. Although optic neuritis is associated with multiple sclerosis, this does not generally cause partial field cuts and has no associated hearing loss. Marchiafava-Bignami disease is a progressive demyelinating disease that generally affects the corpus callosum of alcoholics. Although the cause is not known, it is believed to relate to a nutritional deficiency. There is no specific association of hearing loss or vision loss. Creutzfeldt-Jakob disease is a prion-related spongiform encephalopathy that may cause rapidly progressive dementia. MRI findings include T2 hyperintensity in the basal ganglia, thalamus (pulvinar sign), and insula, as well as restricted diffusion along the cortex. Manganism is an accumulation of manganese in the basal ganglia, which may present with parkinsonism. MRI demonstrates accumulation of manganese, which may be hyperintense on both T1 and T2 (*see* Bradley's NiCP, 7th edn, Ch. 65, pp. 920–967). Figure from Allmendinger A, Mallery RM, Magro CM, et al 2014 Cauda equina involvement in Susac's syndrome. *Journal of the Neurological Sciences* 337(1–2): 91–96, with permission.

71. A. Dementia with Lewy bodies is marked by fluctuating levels of wakefulness and alertness, visual hallucinations, mild parkinsonian features, and memory loss. Although brain biopsy is the only definitively diagnostic test for dementia with Lewy bodies, FDG PET scans can provide important clues, including characteristic hypometabolism in the occipital lobes. Hypometabolism in the temporal and parietal lobes can be seen in dementia with Lewy bodies and Alzheimer disease, but Alzheimer disease does not typically affect the occipital lobes. Hypometabolism of the anterior temporal lobes and frontal lobes is seen in frontotemporal dementia. Hypometabolism of the striatum is commonly seen in Huntington disease (*see* Bradley's NiCP, 7th edn, Ch. 41, pp. 486–503).

72. E. Temozolomide is *not* a common cause of chemotherapy-induced peripheral neuropathy. The other answer choices mentioned are common culprits for a peripheral neuropathy, but different chemotherapeutic agents can lead to different neuropathic syndromes. For example, paclitaxel and bortezomib often lead to a painful sensory neuropathy. Vincristine may be associated with a relatively painless sensorimotor and autonomic neuropathy. Cisplatin may lead to a relatively painless large-fiber and/or sensory ganglionopathy. The neuropathy can occur at any point in time while on the chemotherapy, but occurs usually in a dose-dependent fashion and worsens when the patient has other factors or conditions that can predispose to nerve injury (such as diabetes mellitus). The neuropathy generally improves when the offending agent dose is lowered or discontinued. Most of the time, the neuropathy improves after the chemotherapy has stopped and can be treated with the same agents that treat other painful peripheral neuropathies (gabapentin, pregabalin, nortriptyline, venlafaxine). No trials have shown clinically meaningful benefit for any agent to prevent chemotherapy-induced peripheral neuropathy (*see* Bradley's NiCP, 7th edn, Ch. 107, pp. 1791–1866).

73. B. Fingolimod is one of the newer disease-modifying treatments for multiple sclerosis. It is a sphingosine-1-phosphate analog that binds to the sphingosine-1-phosphatase enzyme, resulting in sequestration of lymphocytes into lymph nodes. Natalizumab is a monoclonal antibody that binds to the alpha-4-integrin adhesion molecule, preventing lymphocytes from crossing the blood–brain barrier used in the treatment of multiple sclerosis. Teriflunomide is a dihydroorotate dehydrogenase inhibitor used in the treatment of multiple sclerosis that works by inhibiting synthesis of pyrimidines. Pyridostigmine is a reversible acetylcholinesterase inhibitor and has no role in the treatment of multiple sclerosis, but is used in myasthenia gravis. Rituximab is a CD20 monoclonal antibody originally used in the treatment of lymphoma, but is now also used in neuromyelitis optica, multiple sclerosis, myasthenia gravis, and other B-cell–mediated autoimmune neurological conditions (*see* Bradley's NiCP, 7th edn, Ch. 80, pp. 1159–1186).

74. C. This patient presents with a history of kidney failure, strokes, angiokeratomas, and neuropathy at a young age. This presentation should be concerning for Fabry disease. This disorder is caused by a deficiency in a lysosomal enzyme, α-galactosidase A. *PMP22* duplication causes Charcot-Marie-Tooth type 1a, whereas the deletion causes hereditary neuropathy with predisposition to pressure palsies. Metachromatic leukodystrophy is associated with an arylsulfatase-A deficiency. Phytanic acid accumulation occurs in Refsum disease, which causes night blindness, visual field abnormalities, hypertrophic palpable nerves, distal leg weakness, hearing loss, and

cardiomyopathy (*see* Bradley's NiCP, 7th edn, Ch. 107, pp. 1791–1867).

75. C. According to the 2015 American Academy of Neurology consensus guidelines regarding concussion and traumatic brain injury, there are several clear risk factors for sport-related concussion. The type of sport is highly associated with concussion risk, and is greatest in football, rugby, hockey, and soccer. Gender is also associated with risk, but differs by sport, with greater risk in females playing soccer and basketball. History of prior concussion is strongly associated with risk for additional concussions, possibly within 10 days of the first. There is moderate evidence that certain well-fitted helmets effectively reduce the risk of concussion, whereas soft head protectors provide no benefit in sports such as soccer or basketball. However, there is insufficient data to date to establish position played as a risk factor in specific sports. Similarly, there are insufficient data that age or competition level contributes to overall concussion risk (*see* Bradley's NiCP, 7th edn, Ch. 61, pp. 860–866).

76. A. Proprioception is transmitted through afferent A alpha fibers, and somatic motor innervation is sent through the efferent A alpha fibers. Touch and pressure are transmitted through afferent A beta fibers, and efferent A beta fibers contribute to somatic motor innervation. Pain, cold, and touch are transmitted through afferent A delta fibers. The A gamma fibers are specialized efferent fibers, sending input to intrafusal muscle fibers and muscle spindles. Group B fibers are preganglionic autonomic nerves. Both group A and group B fibers are myelinated, but group B fibers are smaller and have a slower conduction velocity. Group C fibers are small and unmyelinated, and therefore have slow conduction velocity. They are involved in pain, temperature, and reflex responses in the dorsal spinal roots, as well as postganglionic sympathetic output.

77. C. The patient in this question most likely has anorexia nervosa. This is a disorder that affects 1% of adolescent girls. Only 5%–10% of patients with anorexia nervosa are men. Most have weight loss associated with a fear of being overweight that often leads to starvation and excessive exercise. Patients refuse to maintain body weight at or above the normal weight for age, and also have an altered perception of their body weight. In those who have begun their menstrual cycles, there is often amenorrhea, defined by the absence of three consecutive menstrual cycles. Patients with anorexia nervosa can also binge eat and purge, so long as they are still underweight. Alternatively, patients with bulimia nervosa must have recurrent episodes of binge eating (eating more than what others would eat in a discrete period) and purging (through vomiting, laxatives, diuretics, enemas or exercise), but have a normal body weight and generally poor control over eating habits. Binge eating and purging must occur at least two times per week for at least 3 months for bulimia nervosa. Treatment includes nutritional counseling, psychotherapy, and selective serotonin reuptake inhibitors.

78. A. The image depicts a crescent (or concave) hemorrhage located between the dura and the arachnoid, best known as a *subdural hematoma* (SDH). This is caused by tearing of bridging veins that drain into the dural venous sinuses. Most commonly, SDH is associated with trauma, especially in older or alcoholic patients with frequent falls. Radiographically, SDHs are not restricted by cranial sutures, but rather are restricted by dural reflections (such as the falx). Treatment depends on the patient's clinical status and the amount of mass effect from the bleed. This can include clinical observation, hematoma drainage through burr holes, or even evacuation by craniotomy. Epidural hematomas are convex hemorrhages that result from the tearing of the middle meningeal artery, usually due to a skull fracture in the temporal region. There is often loss of consciousness due to trauma followed by a lucid interval that precedes a period of coma. CAA usually results in a lobar hemorrhage, which is parenchymal. Hemorrhages can also occur as a part of venous sinus thrombosis, but are usually located in the deep regions of the brain or in the draining distribution of the sinus. Ruptured berry aneurysms usually lead to subarachnoid hemorrhages, not subdural hematomas (*see* Bradley's NiCP, 7th edn, Ch. 39, pp. 411–458). Figure from Johnstone EC, Owens DC, Lawrie SM, McIntosh AM, Sharpe MD 2010 *Companion to Psychiatric Studies*, 8th edn, Churchill Livingstone, with permission.

79. C. Emery-Dreifuss myopathy is most commonly inherited through an X-linked pattern, with autosomal-dominant transmission less frequent, and autosomal-recessive quite rare. The disease is caused by mutations in either the *EMD* or *LMNA* genes, which encode nuclear envelope proteins. The earliest symptom of Emery-Dreifuss myopathy is generally contractures of the elbows, ankles, and neck, followed by progressive weakness and cardiac arrhythmia. With a pacemaker preventing cardiac death, most patients live into adulthood, although some die prematurely from progressive cardiac or pulmonary disease (*see* Bradley's NiCP, 7th edn, Ch. 110, pp. 1915–1955).

80. E. The boy in this case has Tourette syndrome, manifested by both multiple motor tics and at least one phonic tic for at least 1 year in someone younger than 21 years of age. Notably, the question details the criteria for a tic, in that they are suppressible actions with a premonitory urge accompanied by a sense of relief after the action. Many times psychological conditions coexist with Tourette syndrome, including ADHD, poor impulse control, OCD, and self-injurious behavior. The treatment usually consists of tetrabenazine, topiramate, or antidopaminergic medications for the motor symptoms. Stimulants, clonidine, or guanfacine can be used to treat comorbid ADHD. Selective serotonin reuptake inhibitors are usually used to treat comorbid OCD (*see* Bradley's NiCP, 7th edn, Ch. 96, pp. 1422–1460).

81. A. The patient has central diabetes insipidus (DI) as a result of pituitary stalk compression from his Rathke cleft cyst. Urine osmolality is typically low (not high) in central DI, due to the pituitary's inability to release antidiuretic hormone (also known as *vasopressin*). Patients will often present with an increased sensation of thirst and polyuria with very dilute urine. Etiologies of central DI include cerebral hemorrhages, hypophysitis, compression by mass lesions such as craniopharyngiomas or Rathke cleft cysts, trauma, or postoperatively from sellar surgeries. Treatment includes desmopressin or thiazide diuretics (*see* Bradley's NiCP, 7th edn, Ch. 52, pp. 696–712).

82. D. Several items in this case point toward stroke as the etiology of his vertigo. First, one should recognize his stroke risk factors of age and heavy smoking history. Further, recurring episodes of vertigo over recent days is suggestive of transient ischemic attacks, and acute vertigo onset suggests a vascular cause. Finally, normal bilateral head thrust test is highly sensitive for stroke. In patients with a vestibular cause of vertigo, such as labyrinthitis or vestibular neuritis, individuals cannot maintain target fixation when the head is turned toward the affected side, although they perform normally when the head is turned toward the unaffected side. The key distinction between labyrinthitis and vestibular neuritis, both of which are generally viral in nature, is the presence or absence of hearing loss. Vestibular neuritis affects the vestibular nerve only, thereby causing vertigo and balance disturbance only, whereas labyrinthitis also affects the cochlear nerve and thereby causes hearing loss as well. BPPV is a condition caused by otolith malposition in the semicircular canals, and is associated with sudden, severe vertigo, prompted by movement of the head and lasting only a few minutes per episode. The findings of a Dix-Hallpike maneuver are often abnormal with posterior canal otolith displacement, which is the most common location. In such a case, otolith repositioning, such as with the Epley maneuver, may be therapeutic. Nicotine withdrawal may be associated with headaches, anxiety, depression, or difficulty with concentration. However, vertigo is not a common symptom (*see* Bradley's NiCP, 7th edn, Ch. 46, pp. 583–604).

83. A. Tauopathies include Alzheimer disease, progressive supranuclear palsy, frontotemporal dementia, and corticobasal degeneration. Alpha-synucleinopathies include Parkinson disease, dementia with Lewy bodies, and multiple system atrophy (*see* Bradley's NiCP, 7th edn, Ch. 96, pp. 1422–1460).

84. E. Restless legs syndrome (RLS) is diagnosed clinically when five criteria are met: (1) an often uncomfortable urge to move the legs (2) at times of inactivity (3) or in the evening (4) that is usually relieved by movement (5) and is not accounted for by another medical or behavioral condition. RLS is frequently associated with periodic limb movements of sleep. If she had pain and cramping in her legs with activity, rather than at rest, an arterial study could be helpful. RLS is not diagnosed by polysomnogram, but is rather a clinical diagnosis. Nerve conduction studies can help determine whether there is a neuropathy or radiculopathy present, but these conditions would not be common in a 23-year-old. Ropinirole or other dopamine agonists are the initial medical treatment for RLS, but this is not the next best course of action. Iron deficiency is the most common cause of secondary RLS. If the ferritin is <50, iron supplementation is recommended and could be curative (*see* Bradley's NiCP, 7th edn, Ch. 102, pp. 1615–1685).

85. B. Although the precise pathophysiology of migraine aura is not known, the phenomenon is cortical in origin. As such, common visual disturbances such as scintillating scotoma or fortification spectra are generally binocular but homonymous. However, similar to other homonymous symptoms, patients may erroneously report a monocular disturbance. Migraine auras may be preceded by up to 1 day of prodromal symptoms, including changes in mood, energy, hunger, or excessive yawning. The aura itself is usually <30

minutes and tends to dissipate as the headache begins. Although visual symptoms are the most common aura complaint, rarely patients may have any of the previously mentioned symptoms instead (*see* Bradley's NiCP, 7th edn, Ch. 103, pp. 1686–1719).

86. B. C fibers are unmyelinated fibers with a relatively small diameter and slow conduction velocity. These fibers are present in the dorsal root ganglia and transmit nociception in a nonspecific and poorly localized way. They are also present in postganglionic fibers in the autonomic nervous system. A-delta fibers are fast myelinated fibers that transmit sharp localized pain and temperature signals. A-alpha fibers include the alpha motor neurons involved in muscle contraction and sensory fibers to the muscle spindles. A-gamma fibers innervate the muscle spindle, which helps sense the level of muscle contraction (*see* Bradley's NiCP, 7th edn, Ch. 54, pp. 720–741).

87. D. The listed symptoms all localize to the cavernous sinus, including oculomotor, trigeminal, and facial nerves. A diagram of the cavernous sinus is shown here. Mucormycosis is associated with infiltrating cavernous sinus infections in immunocompromised patients, including diabetic patients. Poorly controlled diabetes is associated with embolic events in cranial nerves, although the likelihood of multiple involved nerves at once is unlikely. Hyperglycemia may cause focal neurological deficits, but is less likely to cause multiple ipsilateral cranial neuropathies. Tolosa-Hunt syndrome is an idiopathic, steroid-responsive granulomatous condition that affects the cavernous sinus, but would be less likely than an infectious process in this case. Viral infection may cause multiple cranial neuropathies, but not generally localized only to nerves traversing the cavernous sinus (*see* Bradley's NiCP, 7th edn, Chs. 79, pp. 1147–1158 and 104, pp. 1720–1735).

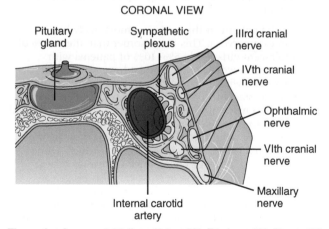

CORONAL VIEW

Figure for Answer 4.87 (*from Kaiser PK, Friedman NJ, Pineda II R 2014* Massachusetts Eye and Ear Infirmary Illustrated Manual of Ophthalmology, *Saunders, with permission.*)

88. A. Visual evoked potentials measure the conduction time of the visual system by stimulating the retina with either flashes of lights or, more commonly, a reversing checkerboard pattern on a screen. Responses are recorded over the occipital region, with the P100 as the main diagnostic waveform. This is a positive wave, which occurs approximately 100 ms after the stimulus. The eyes are stimulated independently and then responses are compared with each other. The visual

evoked potential demonstrates a delayed P100 wave in the right eye, whereas the left eye is normal. This is consistent with a prechiasmal lesion of the right optic nerve, such as optic neuritis. Other causes of a unilateral prolonged P100 include ischemic optic neuritis, nutritional or toxic optic neuropathies, hereditary neuropathies, optic nerve tumors, compressive tumors, refractive errors, glaucoma, and retinopathies. Bilateral delayed responses usually represent a lesion posterior to the chiasm but are not specific to the right or left occipital lobe. Hemifield stimulation, which is essentially never performed these days, can help localize postchiasmal lesions, but with the easy access to neuroimaging, this is of limited value today. Chiasmal lesions can show prolonged P100 or absent P100 bilaterally (*see* Bradley's NiCP, 7th edn, Ch. 34, pp. 348–366). Figure from Daroff RB, Jankovic J, Mazziotta JC, Pomeroy SL, editors, 2016 *Bradley's Neurology in Clinical Practice*, 7th edn, Elsevier, with permission.

89. C. At 2 years of age, most children will be able to name parts of the body, identify objects in pictures, say short sentences, and follow simple instructions. They are able to sort shapes, play make-believe, and build a tower of four or more blocks. Physically, children of this age are able to stand on their tiptoes, kick a ball, throw overhand, and begin running. Two-year-old children demonstrate parallel play in which they play next to other children, but not with other children. At 18 months a child will say single words, point to objects he or she wants, follow one-step commands, walk, eat with a spoon, and drink from a cup. At 1 year, a child will be nervous when away from parents or around strangers, play games like "peek-a-boo," use simple gestures to communicate, have very few words, rise to a sitting position without help, and may stand alone or even walk. At 3 years, children will copy friends and adults, show affection, take turns, follow two- to three-step commands, have mostly understandable speech, play make-believe, copy a circle, or build a tower of six blocks. Three-year-olds should be able to pedal a tricycle. At 4 years, a child should be able to play "mom" and "dad," would rather play with children than adults, has difficulty determining what's real or make-believe, can tell stories, understands time, remembers parts of a story, draws a person with two to four body parts, plays board games, and stands on one foot (*see* Bradley's NiCP, 7th edn, Ch. 8, pp. 66–72).

90. B. This patient presents with episodes that are consistent with frontal lobe seizures. These are usually brief episodes that arise out of sleep, and can involve bicycling of legs, kicking, thrashing, or other odd behaviors. At times, tonic posturing can be seen. Of the options mentioned, the syndrome of autosomal-dominant nocturnal frontal lobe epilepsy best fits with this patient's episodes. This disorder is genetically heterogeneous; however, the most common mutations affect the neuronal nicotinic acetylcholine receptor. This syndrome usually presents between 8 and 20 years of age, and is commonly misdiagnosed as a parasomnia, nightmares, or a psychogenic disorder. Seizures in juvenile myoclonic epilepsy can occur at night, but these tend to be generalized convulsions, not partial seizures with bicycling. Mesial temporal sclerosis can also cause nocturnal seizures, but these seizures involve automatisms such as lip smacking and picking movements, not bicycling movements (*see* Bradley's NiCP, 7th edn, Ch. 101, pp. 1563–1614).

91. D. Comprehension of death develops in a step-wise fashion for children. Before the age of 3 years, there is generally no understanding of death. Then, until around the age of 6 years, children often have magical thinking in which they believe that their own actions or thoughts caused another person's death and that death is a reversible process. Between the ages of 6 and 9 years, magical thinking is replaced by a greater understanding of the finality of death. Between the ages of 9 and 12 years, a child's understanding of death becomes similar to an adult's understanding thereof.

92. E. The most likely underlying diagnosis is tuberculous meningitis. The patient's risk factors include homelessness and immigration from India, where the incidence of tuberculosis (TB) is relatively higher. The right upper lobe consolidation on chest x-ray is also suspicious for TB. Tuberculous meningitis often causes a basilar meningitis, leading to cranial neuropathies as a presenting symptom. Common CSF findings include profound hypoglycorrhachia (low glucose), elevated protein, and pleocytosis with lymphocytic predominance. Although the Gram stain is negative in this case, the acid-fast stain would likely be positive. Proper treatment would include airborne isolation, given his cough and chest x-ray consolidation, and directed antituberculous therapy until confirmatory microbiology testing returns. Whole-body PET-CT would be reasonable if this patient had a new diagnosis of cancer, although a tissue diagnosis should be obtained (if possible) before beginning radiation or chemotherapy. Although fungal meningitis causes hypoglycorrhachia and lymphocytic pleocytosis, India ink staining is generally positive for these infections. Further, this patient has none of the usual risk factors for fungal meningitis, including human immunodeficiency virus, posttransplant immunosuppression, chronic steroids, or diabetes. Finally, oral antifungal therapy would be insufficient in a case of fungal meningitis; instead, one should use broad spectrum intravenous therapy until a source is identified. Although tertiary syphilis may cause basilar meningitis, it does not generally cause hypoglycorrhachia or such severe pleocytosis in the CSF. Although Bickerstaff encephalitis or Miller-Fisher syndrome (both of which may lead to respiratory muscle weakness) may be considered in this case, the lack of ataxia or motor disturbance argues against these diagnoses (*see* Bradley's NiCP, 7th edn, Ch. 79, pp. 1147–1158).

93. E. Porphyrias are a group of disorders resulting from various enzyme deficiencies in the breakdown of porphyrins to produce heme. A buildup of porphyrins results in multisystem dysfunction, including anemia, abdominal pain, cold-induced neuropathy (due to crystallization of porphyrins), seizure, and psychosis. Porphyria crises may be triggered by various medications that also lead to porphyrin precipitation from the blood, including certain anticonvulsants (carbamazepine, phenytoin), certain antibiotics, and other classes of medications. Although hypertension and vasospasm may occur with porphyria attacks, stroke is a rare symptom of this disease (*see* Bradley's NiCP, 7th edn, Ch. 10, pp. 92–114).

94. E. The history consists of a boy with history of infantile spasms, complex partial seizures, and language delay with autistic qualities. The image of his

skin shows hypopigmented macules (ash-leaf spots) and one area in the middle back consistent with a Shagreen patch; these are classic cutaneous manifestations of tuberous sclerosis (TS). TS is an autosomal-dominant disorder caused by mutations in either *TSC1* (encodes hamartin) or *TSC2* (encodes tuberin). Aside from the aforementioned cutaneous findings, clinical features include facial angiofibromas, subependymal nodules or giant cell astrocytomas, retinal hamartomas, cardiac rhabdomyoma, and subungual (fingernail or toenail) fibromas. Other neurological presentations include seizures (most often infantile spasms), mental retardation (MR), or autism-like behavior. Focal neurological deficits may occur due to brain tumors. Rapamycin is often used in the treatment of giant cell astrocytomas. Hypomelanosis of Ito is an autosomal-dominant disorder characterized by seizures, MR, and congenital abnormalities. Patients often have hypopigmented or white macules along the lines of Blaschko, usually covering more than two dermatomes, and fluorescing under a Wood lamp. Patients may also have malformations affecting the palate, limbs, hands, feet, nails, teeth, hair, or face/skull. Sturge-Weber syndrome is characterized by angiomas that involve the leptomeninges as well as the skin, usually in the V1 and V2 distributions of the trigeminal nerve. The classic cutaneous manifestation is a nevus flammeus (port-wine stain). Patients may have developmental delay, focal seizures, visual loss, glaucoma, and hemiparesis. Magnetic resonance imaging typically reveals hemiatrophy with leptomeningeal angiomatosis and calcifications ipsilateral to facial manifestation. Ataxia-telangiectasia is an autosomal-recessive disorder caused by a mutation in the *ATM* gene and is characterized by cerebellar ataxia, variable immunodeficiency with susceptibility to sinopulmonary infections, malignancies, and cutaneous manifestations, including ocular and cutaneous telangiectasias. Often alpha-fetoprotein is elevated. Von Hippel-Lindau disease is an autosomal-dominant disease characterized by visceral cysts and tumors, including retinal and central nervous system hemangioblastomas, pheochromocytomas, and multiple organ cysts, all of which have malignant potential (*see* Bradley's NiCP, 7th edn, Ch. 100, pp. 1538–1562). Figure from Aminoff MJ, Josephson SA 2014 *Aminoff's Neurology and General Medicine*, 5th edn, Academic Press, with permission.

95. C. Romantic or sexual relationships between medical supervisors and trainees are unacceptable, regardless of the situation. The appropriate response in this situation is to remove the physician from the supervisory role to avoid any conflicts of interest; otherwise, the relationship must end during the period of supervision. Ignoring the relationship or acknowledging it and asking for discretion still allows for conflicts of interest to be present. Although most facilities have policies regarding romantic relationships, there is no need for immediate dismissal of the student or the attending.

96. C. Vitamin B1 (thiamine) deficiency is associated with Wernicke-Korsakoff syndrome with bilateral mammillary body hemorrhages. Vitamin B12 (cobalamin) deficiency is associated with peripheral nerve and dorsal column demyelination. Vitamin B6 (pyridoxine) deficiency is associated with peripheral neuropathy. Vitamin D deficiency is associated with increased risk of central demyelination, as with

multiple sclerosis. Vitamin B_3 (niacin) deficiency is associated with pellagra (dermatitis, diarrhea, and dementia) but no specific pathological changes in the brain (*see* Bradley's NiCP, 7th edn, Ch. 39, pp. 411–458). Figure from Perkin DG, Miller DC, Lane RJM, Patel MC, Hochberg FH 2010 *Atlas of Clinical Neurology*, 3rd edn, Saunders, with permission.

97. D. Diabetes has a plethora of neuromuscular complications, including distal sensory polyneuropathy, small fiber neuropathy, diabetic amyotrophy, diabetic cachexia, and insulin neuritis, to name a few. Insulin neuritis presents with rapid-onset painful paresthesias and hyperalgesia in the distal fingers and toes in the setting of rapid control of previously high glucose. EMG and nerve conduction tests are normal unless there is an underlying neuropathy already present. Distal sensory polyneuropathy involves paresthesias and numbness beginning in the toes and moving higher over the course of years until eventually involving the hands. EMG and nerve conduction studies show a length-dependent sensorimotor axonal polyneuropathy. Diabetic amyotrophy presents with rapid painful weakness of one limb, usually a leg, and significant weight loss, typically occurring in patients with poorly controlled diabetes. EMG and nerve conduction studies show findings consistent with a lumbosacral plexopathy or brachial plexopathy, depending on the affected limb. Diabetic cachexia presents with significant unintentional weight loss and severe neuropathic pain in the setting of poorly controlled diabetes. It is often associated with autonomic involvement, depression, and truncal paresthesias, which help differentiate it from insulin neuritis. Metformin has many side effects, including severe lactic acidosis when combined with computed tomography contrast, but painful paresthesias are not seen (see Bradley's NiCP, 7th edn, Ch. 107, pp. 1791–1866).

98. A. An internuclear ophthalmoplegia (INO) is characterized by impaired adduction of the affected eye, with abduction nystagmus of the opposite eye. The lesion responsible for an INO is generally within the ipsilateral medial longitudinal fasciculus (same side as the adduction deficit). A PPRF lesion generally causes slow or weak saccades toward the side of the lesion. The Edinger-Westphal nucleus is a parasympathetic nucleus of the oculomotor nerve; a lesion here disrupts the parasympathetic (constrictive) outflow to the pupillary constrictors in the light reflex. Lesions of the oculomotor nucleus would cause ipsilateral ptosis and weakness of adduction, with a "down and out" position of the affected eye on primary gaze. Lesions of the abducens nucleus cause weakness of abduction in the ipsilateral eye (*see* Bradley's NiCP, 7th edn, Ch. 44, pp. 528–572). Figure from Kanski JK, Bowling B 2011 *Clinical Ophthalmology: A Systematic Approach*, 7th edn, Saunders, with permission.

99. E. The superior division of the middle cerebral artery supplies the lateral frontal lobe, which involves Broca's area. The inferior division of the middle cerebral artery supplies the lateral temporal lobe and Wernicke's area. No aphasia is noted with strokes to the anterior cerebral artery. The artery of Heubner is a branch off of the anterior cerebral artery that supplies the caudate and anterior portion of the internal capsule. The lenticulostriate arteries are small arteries off of the middle cerebral artery that pass into the caudate,

posterior internal capsule, and lentiform nucleus. Strokes to the artery of Heubner and lenticulostriate arteries do not cause aphasia (*see* Bradley's NiCP, 7th edn, Ch. 13, pp. 128–144).

100. A. Cyclophosphamide is a nitrogen mustard alkylating agent used in the treatment of various malignancies, as well as various autoimmune disorders (including paraneoplastic disorders). For about 24 hours around the time of cyclophosphamide infusion, there is a risk of hemorrhagic cystitis. To prevent this, most institutions use prophylactic mesna, which binds to and detoxifies the bladder-toxic cyclophosphamide metabolite. Immunosuppression is common after cyclophosphamide, and often the goal of therapy for autoimmune disorders. Long-term risks of cyclophosphamide include infertility and secondary malignancies such as leukemia, lymphoma, skin cancer, and bladder cancer. Osteopenia is not associated with cyclophosphamide use, although it is often seen with steroids (*see* Bradley's NiCP, 7th edn, Ch. 109, pp. 1896–1914).

101. C. Balo's concentric sclerosis generally appears with concentric rings of hyperintensity and isointensity or hypointensity on T2/fluid attenuated inversion recovery, with associated ringlike enhancement. The presence of these rings makes this more likely than any of the other options. Balo's is a rare variant of multiple sclerosis, and is often quite aggressive. Metastatic lung cancer may have multiple lesions with ring enhancement, although it would generally be associated with significantly more mass effect than is shown. ADEM is most common in children after infection or vaccination. Imaging often shows bilateral white matter lesions with ring or incomplete ring enhancement and occasionally with hemorrhage. Tumefactive multiple sclerosis may be difficult to differentiate from the other listed lesions, although it is generally associated with significant mass effect. Abscesses are generally ring enhancing with central hypointensity and marked mass effect (*see* Bradley's NiCP, 7th edn, Ch. 80, pp. 1159–1186). Figures from Kreft KL, Mellema J, Hintzen RQ 2009 Spinal cord involvement of Balo's concentric sclerosis. *Journal of the Neurological Sciences* 279(1–2): 114–117, with permission.

102. B. This patient has botulism, which can come from ingestion of spores that are in various foods such as honey. This presents with diffuse weakness, cranial nerve abnormalities, autonomic dysfunction, ileus, and dilated pupils. There are several different botulinum toxins, each with its own target. These target SNARE proteins (SNAP25, synaptobrevin, syntaxin, or vesicle-associated membrane protein) are involved in vesicular binding to the presynaptic membrane. When these proteins are damaged by a botulinum toxin, this stops the release of acetylcholine from the synapse, leading to weakness. The other answers point toward spinal muscular atrophy (*SMN1* gene), Guillain-Barré (conduction blocks and elevated CSF protein), mitochondrial myopathy (biopsy with ragged red fibers), and myotonic dystrophy (autosomal-dominant disorder with anticipation). These disorders could cause some of the symptoms, but would not cause pupillary abnormalities like botulism does (*see* Bradley's NiCP, 7th edn, Ch. 109, pp. 1895–1914).

103. B. Pyridostigmine is a reversible acetylcholinesterase inhibitor used in the treatment of myasthenia gravis. Other reversible acetylcholinesterase inhibitors include donepezil, galantamine, rivastigmine, neostigmine, and carbamate insecticides. Irreversible inhibitors include organophosphate insecticides like malathion and parathion, and nerve agents like sarin gas. Nicotinic receptor antagonists include curare. Muscarinic antagonists include atropine. Voltage-gated calcium channels do not have any specific agonists because they are opened by a change in membrane potential, not ligand binding (*see* Bradley's NiCP, 7th edn, Ch. 109, pp. 1896–1914).

104. D. Normal cerebral blood flow at rest is 50–55 mL/100 g/min. In experimental models, blood flow between 8 mL/100 g/min and 18 mL/100 g/min is the threshold for electrical failure. This is the penumbra range, so neurons quit functioning, but are not irreversibly damaged. Blood flow below a rate of 8 mL/100 g/min can result in cell death if blood flow is not returned in a timely fashion (*see* Bradley's NiCP, 7th edn, Ch. 65, pp. 920–968).

105. B. Prosopagnosia is the inability to recognize faces, which commonly comes from bilateral temporoparietal lesions, although right-sided lesions in the fusiform gyrus (shown in the figure below) can cause the syndrome. This disorder makes patients unable to recognize family members or the faces of famous people unless they are able to memorize certain details about each face, like the haircut. Recognition usually comes from voice. Optic aphasia is the inability to name an object with retained ability to demonstrate or describe the use of the object. Anomic aphasia is the inability to name objects or people. Cortical blindness involves bilateral occipital lobe lesions, leading to an inability to see. Some patients are unaware of their deficits and will confabulate when asked to describe different visual stimuli (known as *Anton syndrome*). Aphemia is a variant of Broca aphasia in which the patient is initially mute, but recovers the ability to speak with phoneme substitutions and pauses (*see* Bradley's NiCP, 7th edn, Ch. 12, pp. 122–127).

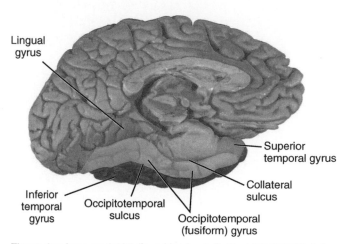

Figure for Answer 4.105 *(from Vanderah T, Gould D 2016 Nolte's The Human Brain, 7th edn, Elsevier, with permission.)*

Test Five

QUESTIONS

1. A 53-year-old man with a history of hypertension is admitted to the hospital for surgical repair of a descending aortic dissection. Upon awakening from surgery, he cannot move his legs when prompted by physical therapy. Neurological examination demonstrates flaccid paralysis of his lower extremities with absent reflexes. He has sensory loss to pin prick and temperature below his midabdomen; however, vibration and proprioception are intact. Which of the following is the most likely diagnosis?

   A. Acute inflammatory demyelinating polyradiculoneuropathy (AIDP)
   B. Diabetic radiculoplexopathy
   C. Conversion disorder
   D. Anterior spinal infarct
   E. Transverse myelitis

2. A 42-year-old woman with relapsing remitting multiple sclerosis was previously treated with mycophenolate and now with natalizumab over the last 3 years. She presents with 1 month of progressive headaches, confusion, and left hemiparesis, and felt under the weather just before symptom onset. T2/fluid attenuated inversion recovery (FLAIR) and postgadolinium T1 magnetic resonance images (MRIs) are shown. Which is the likely cause of the demonstrated problem?

   A. Ischemic stroke
   B. Human immunodeficiency virus (HIV) encephalitis
   C. Acute multiple sclerosis flare
   D. Acute disseminated encephalomyelitis
   E. John Cunningham (JC) virus reactivation

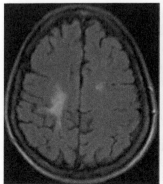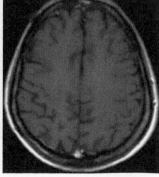

Figure for Question 5.2.

3. Which is the best treatment for the condition described in Question 5.1?

   A. Intravenous (IV) corticosteroids
   B. Plasma exchange
   C. Antiviral therapy
   D. Highly active antiretroviral therapy (HAART)
   E. Anticoagulation

4. Which of the following neurotransmitters is considered neurotoxic at excessive concentrations?

   A. Acetylcholine
   B. Glutamate
   C. Dopamine
   D. Serotonin
   E. Norepinephrine

5. A 54-year-old man suffers a cardiac arrest in the emergency room after having a myocardial infarction. He is resuscitated and placed in the intensive care unit for further monitoring. Gradually, he is extubated and his mental status improves to the point of discharge. He is referred to neurology because of sudden jerks in his legs upon gait initiation. There is no evidence of seizures. Which of the following medications is most indicated for his movement disorder?

   A. Carbidopa/levodopa
   B. Carbamazepine
   C. Clonazepam
   D. Clozapine
   E. Carvedilol

6. A 27-year-old female who is currently 8 weeks pregnant presents with a severe headache. The headache is located over the right side of her head with a severe, throbbing pain associated with nausea, photophobia, and phonophobia. Her neurological examination is normal. She has an urgent magnetic resonance imaging of the brain that is also normal. Which of the following would be a reasonable first-line agent to treat her headache?

   A. Sumatriptan
   B. Oral morphine
   C. Ergotamine
   D. Intravenous valproic acid
   E. Acetaminophen

7. The pathology sample shown here was taken from a 30-year-old woman with an incidental mass found on headache evaluation. Which of the following pathological hallmarks is demonstrated in the photomicrograph?

A. Pseudopalisading necrosis and microvascular proliferation

B. Meningothelial nests and whirls

C. Rosenthal fibers

D. Pseudorosettes

E. Homer Wright rosettes

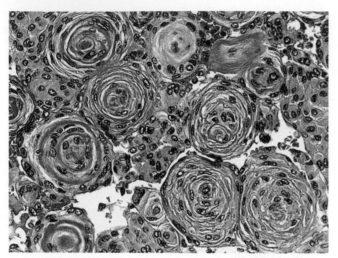

Figure for Question 5.7.

8. An 18-year-old man presents to the emergency room with several weeks of progressive tingling in his feet and legs, followed by gradual onset of weakness in the legs, poor balance, and falls. On examination, he has moderately reduced sensation to temperature and pinprick in a length-dependent fashion in his legs and arms, with a profound loss of joint position sense and vibration sensation in the legs and arms. He has ataxia on both finger to nose and heel to shin, and bilateral Babinski signs are present. Routine blood studies are normal except for an increased red blood cell size. He divulges that in his job as a barista, he has been inhaling nitrous oxide daily from whipped cream canisters. Which of the following most likely describes his underlying problem?

A. Low copper level

B. High calcium level

C. Low thiamine level

D. Low vitamin B12 level

E. Low vitamin E level

9. Which of the following electrodiagnostic findings would be expected in a C8 radiculopathy?

A. Ulnar compound muscle action potential distal latency prolongation

B. Ulnar sensory nerve action potential distal latency prolongation

C. Small-amplitude, short-duration motor units in the first dorsal interosseous (FDI)

D. Reduced recruitment in the biceps

E. Normal radial sensory response

10. A 44-year-old male presents to your outpatient clinic with a 6-month history of dysphagia and dysarthria. On examination he has mild upper and lower facial weakness, tongue atrophy with fasciculations, and bilateral proximal arm weakness. His reflexes are normal throughout, and sensory examination is unremarkable. He has noted mild gynecomastia, impotence, and testicular atrophy. Which of the following is true of this condition?

A. The most common genetic cause of this disease is a mutation in the *C9ORF72* gene.

B. This is a trinucleotide repeat disorder inherited in an X-linked recessive manner.

C. This is an autoimmune condition caused by antibodies to the muscle-specific receptor tyrosine kinase (MUSK) protein.

D. This is a trinucleotide repeat disorder inherited in an autosomal-dominant manner.

E. This disorder is treated with chelation therapy with penicillamine.

11. All of the following interventions have been proven to prolong survival in amyotrophic lateral sclerosis (ALS) *except*?

A. Riluzole

B. Treatment in a multidisciplinary clinic

C. Bilevel positive airway pressure when forced vital capacity is below 50%

D. Percutaneous endoscopic gastrostomy (PEG) tube

E. Dextromethorphan and quinidine

12. Which of the following is *not* true of children with Edwards syndrome?

A. Caused by trisomy 18

B. Majority die around 10 years old

C. Frequent arthrogryposis

D. Frequent micrognathia

E. Risk increases with greater maternal age

13. Which of the following ions has a higher intracellular concentration compared with the extracellular fluid?

A. Sodium

B. Chloride

C. Potassium

D. Calcium

E. Glucose

14. All of the following are characteristics of a persistent vegetative state *except*?

A. No sustained voluntary responses to stimuli

B. No evidence of language comprehension

C. Evidence of sleep/wake cycles

D. Preserved cranial nerve reflexes

E. Preserved bowel and bladder continence

15. Which of the following is demonstrated in the highlighted portion of this electroencephalogram (EEG)?

A. Subclinical rhythmic EEG discharges of adulthood (SREDA)

B. Right temporal theta

C. Mu rhythm

D. Lambda waves

E. Right central partial seizure

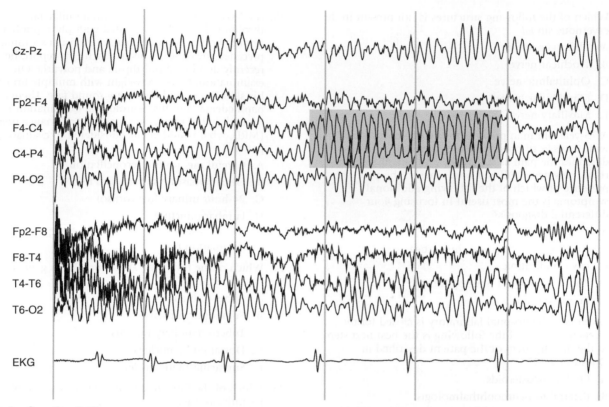

Figure for Question 5.15.

16. A mother brings her 17-year-old daughter into clinic because of concerns for depression. The patient quickly moves from one mood to the next. At times she praises her mother for being the best mother in the world, and other times she is cursing her mother for being too controlling. She has been pulled over for speeding several times and frequently changes boyfriends. Her mother became worried when she caught the patient cutting her forearm with scissors. Which of the following is the most likely diagnosis?

    A. Narcissistic personality disorder

    B. Bipolar 1 disorder

    C. Major depressive disorder

    D. Borderline personality disorder

    E. Histrionic personality disorder

17. A 2-year-old boy presents to the neurology clinic with gait difficulty. His mother reports that he always had difficulty walking and was "not like the other kids." Further questioning reveals a history of epilepsy, cognitive decline, and difficulty with swallowing. Examination is remarkable for a developmentally delayed child with macrocephaly, diffuse weakness, hyperreflexia, and spasticity. He also has profound dysarthria and mild ataxia. There is no family history of similar conditions. His magnetic resonance image (MRI) is shown. What is the most likely diagnosis based on the clinical history and the MRI?

    A. Alexander disease

    B. Pelizaeus-Merzbacher disease

    C. Young-onset Huntington disease

    D. Adrenoleukodystrophy

    E. Metachromatic leukodystrophy

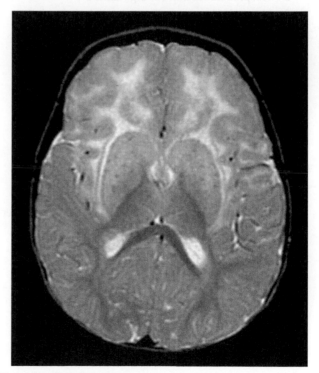

Figure for Question 5.17.

18. Which of the following structures is not present in the cavernous sinus?

    A. Abducens nerve

    B. Trochlear nerve

    C. Ophthalmic nerve

    D. Mandibular nerve

    E. Maxillary nerve

19. A 73-year-old man presents to the neurology clinic with 3 weeks of progressively severe headaches. He describes the pain as superficial and lateralized to the right. He's never suffered headaches in the past. The presence of which of the following additional symptoms is the most useful in focusing your differential diagnosis?

    A. Ocular pain

    B. Lateralized tearing and rhinorrhea

    C. Jaw claudication

    D. Photophobia and phonophobia

    E. Pulsatile tinnitus

20. Given that the hospital laboratory is closed for the weekend, which of the following is the best next step in the management of the patient described in Question 2.19?

    A. Oral corticosteroids

    B. Referral to neuroophthalmologist

    C. Schedule temporal artery biopsy

    D. Hospital admission for ergotamine

    E. Urgent brain magnetic resonance imaging (MRI)

21. Failure of the posterior portions of vertebral elements to fuse without protrusion of meninges or neural elements is called what?

    A. Meningomyelocele

    B. Meningocele

    C. Spina bifida occulta

    D. Syringohydromyelia

    E. Spina bifida cystica

22. Which of the following technical measures is insufficient for determination of brain death by electroencephalogram (EEG)?

    A. Interelectrode distances should be 10 cm or greater

    B. Sensitivity must be set to 5 μV

    C. Recording time of at least 30 minutes

    D. High-frequency filter set at 30 Hz or higher

    E. Interelectrode impedance <10,000 ohms

23. A 63-year-old man presents with a unilateral, throbbing headache associated with photophobia, phonophobia, and mild nausea. A visual scotoma preceded the onset of his headache. By report, he has recently developed polydipsia and polyuria. On examination, he is overweight with multiple bruises on his skin, striae, and has a very round face. There is no papilledema, and his neurological examination is normal. Other than brain magnetic resonance imaging (MRI), what would *not* be considered in evaluating this patient?

    A. Careful medication reconciliation

    B. Dexamethasone suppression test

    C. 24-hour urinary-free cortisol

    D. Lumbar puncture

    E. Corticotropin-releasing hormone (CRH) stimulation test

24. Which of the following anatomical areas generates norepinephrine?

    A. Locus ceruleus

    B. Supraoptic nucleus

    C. Tuberomamillary nucleus

    D. Dorsal raphe nucleus

    E. Suprachiasmatic nucleus

25. Which of the following would *not* be an example of a cognitive behavioral technique?

    A. Employing distraction techniques during the warning signs of a nonepileptic attack

    B. Gradually increasing the exercise of a functionally weak limb, avoiding focus on deficits

    C. Slapping one's wrist with a rubber band to avoid compulsive thoughts

    D. Taking lorazepam at the initiation of a nonepileptic attack

    E. Gradually increasing exposure to an item of irrational fear in order to overcome the fear

26. A 14-year-old male presents with a single generalized convulsion. A sleep segment from his electroencephalogram (EEG) is shown. Which of the following medications would be the best initial treatment?

    A. Ethosuximide

    B. Clonazepam

    C. Carbamazepine

    D. Lacosamide

    E. Valproic acid

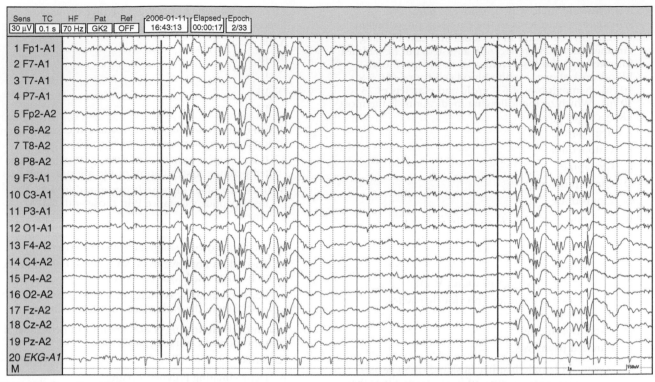

Sens	TC	HF	Pat	Ref	2006-01-11	Elapsed	Epoch
30 µV	0.1 s	70 Hz	GK2	OFF	16:43:13	00:00:17	2/33

1 Fp1-A1
2 F7-A1
3 T7-A1
4 P7-A1
5 Fp2-A2
6 F8-A2
7 T8-A2
8 P8-A2
9 F3-A1
10 C3-A1
11 P3-A1
12 O1-A1
13 F4-A2
14 C4-A2
15 P4-A2
16 O2-A2
17 Fz-A2
18 Cz-A2
19 Pz-A2
20 EKG-A1
M

Figure for Question 5.26.

27. Which of the following was likely present in the fetus shown here?

    A. Ventricular agenesis
    B. Agenesis of the corpus callosum
    C. Holoprosencephaly
    D. Polymicrogyria
    E. Lissencephaly

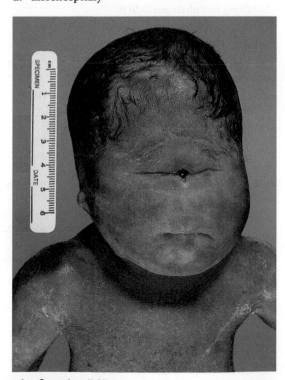

Figure for Question 5.27.

28. Which of the following nerves is responsible for taste on the anterior portion of the tongue?

    A. Lingual nerve
    B. Hypoglossal nerve
    C. Glossopharyngeal nerve
    D. Mandibular branch of trigeminal nerve
    E. Facial nerve

29. A 25-year-old mildly intellectually disabled patient with a history of intractable seizures presents to the clinic for an evaluation. During discussion of treatment options with the patient's parents, a randomized controlled trial of an investigational drug is discussed. The patient is not interested in the study, but his parents, who are his medical decision makers, would like him to participate. Which of the following is the best response?

    A. Enroll the patient in the trial with consent of the parents.
    B. Respect his wishes to remain out of the trial.
    C. Promise the patient he will improve on the study drug.
    D. Withhold other treatments unless the patient participates in the study.
    E. Place the patient on the study drug with his parents' knowledge but without his knowledge.

30. A 36-year-old male with a history of refractory schizophrenia presents to the emergency department with bright red blood in his stool and easy bruising. His medications were recently adjusted, but he had not followed up with his psychiatrist in the last month. Blood work shows a white blood cell count of $0.5 \times 10^3/\mu L$, hemoglobin of 6.7 g/dL, and platelets of $25 \times 10^3/\mu L$. Which of the following medications is the most likely culprit?

    A. Risperidone

    B. Haloperidol

    C. Clozapine

    D. Quetiapine

    E. Ziprasidone

31. Which of the following is a reimbursement model in which providers are paid based on meeting prespecified quality metrics?

    A. Fee for service

    B. Accountable care organization (ACO)

    C. Value-based purchasing (previously pay for performance)

    D. Capitation model

    E. Bundled payments

32. A 75-year-old female lost her husband of 50 years 1 week ago after a long course of lung cancer. Since that time she has felt immensely sad and has isolated herself at home. She feels that life is meaningless and has even wanted to die so she could be with her husband. At night she hears his voice in the house. Which of the following is the most likely diagnosis?

    A. Normal bereavement

    B. Brief psychotic disorder

    C. Major depressive disorder

    D. Adjustment disorder

    E. Schizophrenia

33. An experimental blood test for diagnosing Parkinson disease has a specificity of 90% and a sensitivity of 50%. Which of the following statements regarding this test is true?

    A. A positive result has a low probability of Parkinson disease.

    B. A negative result has a high probability of Parkinson disease.

    C. This test has a low false-positive rate.

    D. This test has a low false-negative rate.

    E. Increasing specificity decreases the false-negative rate.

34. Which of the following is *not* a recommended nonpharmacological approach to neurogenic bladder dysfunction?

    A. Pelvic floor exercises

    B. Fluid restriction

    C. Crede maneuver

    D. Suprapubic vibration

    E. Timed toileting

35. All of the following fiber types involve myelinated fibers *except*?

    A. Ia

    B. Ib

    C. II

    D. III

    E. IV

36. Which of the following is *not* true about complex regional pain syndrome (CRPS) type 1?

    A. It is common to have skin discoloration as well as temperature dysregulation of the affected limb.

    B. There are often increased concentrations of neuropeptide substance P in those with CRPS type 1.

    C. The pain that occurs with CRPS type 1 is often in the pathway of a single peripheral nerve.

    D. There does not have to be an inciting event in order to be diagnosed with CRPS type 1.

    E. Bone scintigraphy is useful in the diagnosis of CRPS, especially in the early stages of the condition.

37. Which of the following is not a common neurological complication of cardiac bypass?

    A. Stroke

    B. Demyelinating polyneuropathy

    C. Brachial plexopathy

    D. Encephalopathy

    E. Seizure

38. Which of the following is true of paroxysmal hemicrania, but not cluster headache or short-lasting unilateral attacks with conjunctival injection and autonomic symptoms (SUNCT)?

    A. Strong male predominance

    B. Attacks last 2–30 minutes each

    C. Strong circadian periodicity

    D. Improves with oxygen

    E. Improves with sumatriptan

39. Based on the Optic Neuritis Treatment Trial (ONTT), which of the following is true?

    A. Treating optic neuritis with intravenous (IV) methylprednisolone leads to more rapid vision improvement than with oral prednisone.

    B. Treating a multiple sclerosis flare with plasma exchange is associated with shorter length of stay than with IV methylprednisolone.

    C. Bilateral optic neuritis should prompt initiation of disease-modifying therapy.

    D. The risk of developing multiple sclerosis after optic neuritis depends on the patient's visual acuity at presentation.

    E. Thinning of the retinal nerve fiber layer is seen with history of optic neuritis.

40. A 53-year-old man presents with right-sided weakness. Which of the following is the most likely etiology of his computed tomography scan findings?

    A. Venous sinus thrombosis

    B. Atrial fibrillation

    C. Chronic hypertension

    D. Anticoagulation

    E. Amyloid angiopathy

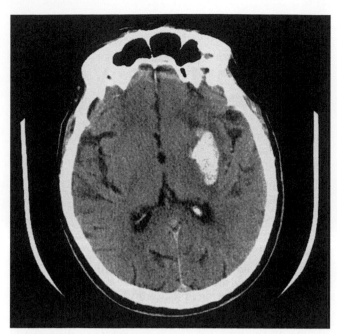

Figure for Question 5.40.

A. Health management organization (HMO)

B. Preferred provider organization (PPO)

C. Point-of-service plan (POS)

D. Indemnity plan

E. Accountable care organization (ACO)

43. The image on the right shows electron microscopy of a neuromuscular junction from a patient, and the image on the left shows a normal neuromuscular junction. Which of the following is the likely underlying diagnosis?

    A. Curare toxin exposure

    B. Duchenne muscular dystrophy

    C. Myasthenia gravis

    D. Diabetic neuropathy

    E. Succinylcholine exposure

44. A thin 26-year-old woman on no medications presents with 6 months of progressive headaches and decreased sense of smell. On examination she has a large blind spot in the center of her left eye vision, left optic disc atrophy, and right papilledema. Which of the following most likely represents the cause of her symptoms?

    A. Foster Kennedy syndrome

    B. Complicated migraine

    C. Venous sinus thrombosis

    D. Conversion disorder

    E. Idiopathic intracranial hypertension

45. The nerve conduction studies in the following table are obtained on a 53-year-old female with arm numbness. Which of the following is the correct interpretation?

    A. Chronic inflammatory demyelinating polyneuropathy

    B. Multifocal motor neuropathy

    C. Median neuropathy at the wrist

    D. Martin-Gruber anastomosis

    E. Ulnar neuropathy at the elbow

41. Which disease is associated with multinucleated globoid cells on brain biopsy?

    A. Niemann-Pick disease

    B. Canavan disease

    C. Krabbe disease

    D. Fabry disease

    E. Metachromatic leukodystrophy

42. Which of the following is a group of physicians and hospitals that share responsibility for providing care to a group of patients, with a link between reimbursement and patient safety and cost containment?

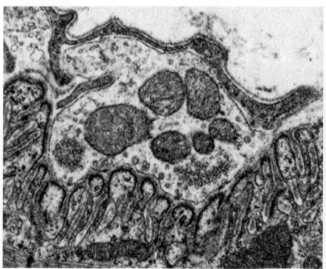

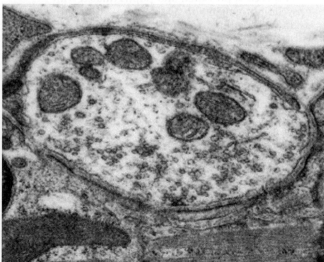

Figure for Question 5.43.

TABLE FOR QUESTION 5.45

Motor nerve	Location	Latency (ms)	Amplitude (mV)	Velocity (m/s)
Median	Wrist	3.5	6.0	
	Forearm	7.0	9.0	55
Ulnar	Wrist	2.5	10.0	
	Below elbow	7.9	6.0	53
	Above elbow	9.5	6.0	52
Sensory nerve	Location	Latency (ms)	Amplitude (mV)	Velocity (m/s)
Median (D2)	Wrist	3.1	37	55
Ulnar (D5)	Wrist	2.4	22	52

46. Which of the following is *false* regarding the thymus?

    A. Removal results in 80%–90% remission rate of myasthenia gravis

    B. Plays an important role in T-cell education in developing humans

    C. Removal is not recommended for prepubertal patients

    D. Removal results in significantly increased risk of infections

    E. Thymoma is associated with a variety of paraneoplastic syndromes

47. A 45-year-old woman on prolonged multidrug treatment for tuberculosis presents with an enlarging black spot in her central vision bilaterally. Additionally, she has noted difficulty discerning colors. Which of the following is the most likely cause of her symptoms?

    A. Vitamin B6 deficiency

    B. Ethambutol toxicity

    C. Hereditary optic neuropathy

    D. Ocular tuberculosis

    E. Methanol toxicity

48. A 41-year-old man is brought to the emergency room after being found by the police, walking the streets and yelling at other citizens. On examination, he is hypertensive to 195/99 and tachycardic to 120 bpm. His speech is pressured and pupils dilated with psychomotor agitation and constant scratching at his skin because there are "ants crawling all over him." He also has mild choreiform movements. What is the most likely diagnosis?

    A. Schizophrenia

    B. Huntington disease

    C. Amphetamine intoxication

    D. Heroin intoxication

    E. Cannabis intoxication

49. A 52-year-old female presents to the office for evaluation of memory problems. She has developed progressive memory loss in the last 6 months. Her family says she is quite confused and has visual hallucinations. She has a history of human immunodeficiency virus (HIV), and she has not been compliant with appointments. Magnetic resonance images (MRI) of her brain and lumbar puncture are normal. All of the following are true of this condition *except*?

    A. It is associated with an increased viral load.

    B. It is associated with a low CD4 count.

    C. Delirium with psychosis is a common presentation.

    D. Highly active antiretroviral therapy (HAART) should improve memory loss.

    E. Magnetic resonance (MR) spectroscopy shows a decreased N-acetylaspartate peak.

50. Which of the following structures encompasses the striatum?

    A. Caudate, putamen

    B. Putamen, globus pallidus

    C. Thalamus, mammillary bodies

    D. Red nuclei, inferior olivary nuclei

    E. Ventral posterolateral thalamic nucleus, medial lemniscus

51. A 1-year-old girl was brought to the emergency room by her parents for a spell of altered consciousness. The patient was playing in the yard when she was told to come inside. She then began crying hysterically, which was followed by bluish discoloration of her face leading to loss of consciousness. While on the ground, she had a brief jerking of her arms and legs followed by return to consciousness. She continued to cry and quickly came back to her baseline. Which of the following is most likely the diagnosis?

    A. Cataplexy

    B. Seizure

    C. Prolonged QT syndrome

    D. Sandifer syndrome

    E. Breath-holding spell

52. A 22-year-old woman is brought to the clinic by her husband for excessive worrying. She has always been an anxious person, but her symptoms have become more severe lately, causing her to lose her job. For example, she will worry that her husband will be unsafe while commuting to work each day. As a result, she frequently calls him and his work to ensure he made it safely, despite reassurance from both the husband and his co-workers. She also worries that someone will steal her identity and withdraw money from her savings account, leading her to check her bank account at least three to four times per day. The stress of her worrying results in strained muscles and frequent episodes of anxiety. What is most likely the diagnosis?

    A. Hypochondriasis

    B. Panic disorder

    C. Generalized anxiety disorder (GAD)

    D. Major depressive disorder

    E. Obsessive-compulsive disorder (OCD)

53. Which of the following is not a monoamine catabolized by monoamine oxidase-A (MAO-A)?

    A. Serotonin

    B. Melatonin

    C. Norepinephrine

    D. Glutamate

    E. Dopamine

54. Which of the following is *not* true regarding the condition depicted in the image?

    A. It can be associated with *LIS1* mutation.

    B. It can be associated with *DCX* mutation.

    C. Females with the *DCX* mutation have a magnetic resonance image (MRI) similar to the one shown, but males show subcortical-band heterotopia.

    D. Seizures are a common manifestation of this condition.

    E. It is associated with congenital muscular dystrophies.

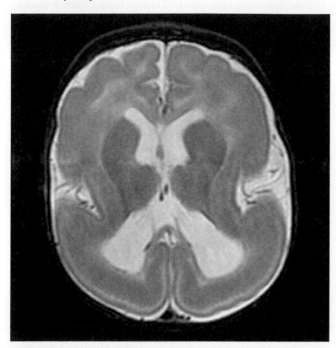

Figure for Question 5.54.

55. Which of the following cerebellar nuclei is most directly involved with planning and initiation of voluntary movements?

    A. Dentate nucleus

    B. Fastigial nucleus

    C. Globose nucleus

    D. Emboliform nucleus

    E. Red nucleus

56. Which of the following is true of the atypical antipsychotics?

    A. The atypical antipsychotics are stronger antagonists of the D_2 receptor than the typical antipsychotics.

    B. Clozapine is safe in those with intractable epilepsy.

    C. Clozapine and quetiapine are associated with fewer extrapyramidal side effects than other antipsychotics.

    D. Olanzapine is the least likely to be associated with weight gain.

    E. Ziprasidone is only helpful with the positive symptoms of schizophrenia.

57. The fascicles of the facial nerve travel around which structure before exiting the brainstem?

    A. Medial longitudinal fasciculus

    B. Trigeminal spinal tract

    C. Corticospinal tract

    D. Vestibular nucleus

    E. Abducens nucleus

58. A 5-month-old infant is brought to the neurologist because of failure to thrive and seizures. Additionally, he is delayed in reaching motor milestones. On examination, the child has hypotonia and is unable to hold up his head. Also, his skin is light, and his hair seems fragile and colorless. Which of the following is *not* true regarding Menke syndrome?

    A. Some symptoms may be mistaken for nonaccidental trauma.

    B. Diagnosis usually involves low serum copper and elevated ceruloplasmin.

    C. The inheritance is X-linked recessive.

    D. Osteoporosis is common.

    E. Connective tissue abnormalities are common.

59. An 82-year-old female with a history of stroke, memory problems, and seizures presents with multiple breakthrough seizures despite compliance with her levetiracetam therapy. Imaging of her brain demonstrates evidence of her prior infarct, but no acute findings. A complete blood count, complete metabolic profile, and urine analysis are all normal. Notably, she was recently placed on a new medication; which of the following would be the most likely cause of her seizures?

    A. Clopidogrel

    B. Donepezil

    C. Warfarin

    D. Verapamil

    E. Rifampin

60. All of the following are true regarding cauda equina *except*?

    A. Progresses in an insidious manner, unless caused by acute trauma

    B. Reflexes are preserved

    C. Causes weakness and sensory loss

    D. Sphincter dysfunction is common late in the course

    E. Involves compression of nerve roots below termination of the spinal cord

61. A 16-year-old male presents to the office for evaluation of weakness. He is active in football, but has noted that he cannot run as fast as before, and he cannot jump as high. On neurological examination, he is noted to have normal strength throughout but no deep tendon reflexes. With repeated contraction of the quadriceps, the patient's patellar reflex returns. Nerve conduction studies show a normal sural response, but a very low-amplitude peroneal motor response. After brief exercise the peroneal motor response amplitude increases by 300%. Which of the following is the most likely diagnosis?

    A. McArdle disease

    B. Myasthenia gravis

    C. Lambert-Eaton myasthenic syndrome

    D. Charcot-Marie-Tooth type 2a

    E. Becker muscular dystrophy

62. All of the following are risk factors for the development of thiamine deficiency *except*?

    A. Hyperemesis gravidarum

    B. Chronic alcoholism

    C. Treatment of tuberculosis

    D. Hemodialysis

    E. Bariatric surgery

63. A 60-year-old man receives a corneal transplant from a donor who died from a mysterious, rapidly progressive dementia. About 6 months after his vision is restored, he begins to suffer cognitive decline. A magnetic resonance image (MRI) of the brain is obtained and shown here. Based on the underlying diagnosis, which of the following is most likely to be seen on brain biopsy?

    A. Reactive gliosis

    B. Diffuse demyelination

    C. Negri bodies

    D. Cowdry type A bodies

    E. Spongiform changes with vacuolization

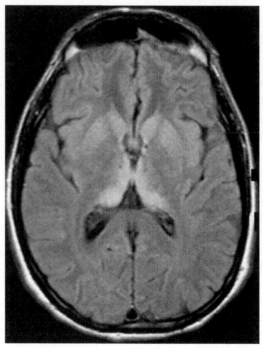

Figure for Question 5.63.

64. Which of the following is *not* necessary when performing procedures on medical students for educational purposes?

    A. Complete explanation of procedure and exposure

    B. Students should have free choice in participation

    C. Grading must be tied to participation

    D. Reasons for nonparticipation need not be disclosed

    E. Abnormalities found remain confidential

65. For which of the following hereditary neuropathies is an enzyme replacement therapy available?

    A. Refsum disease

    B. Porphyria

    C. Fabry disease

    D. Hereditary neuropathy with liability to pressure palsies (HNPP)

    E. Charcot-Marie-Tooth disease (CMT)

66. All of the following are features of critical illness polyneuropathy and myopathy *except*?

    A. Intensive care unit (ICU) stay longer than 2 weeks

    B. Distal-to-proximal gradient of symptoms

    C. Hyperglycemia is a risk factor

    D. Increased risk in patients treated with intravenous (IV) steroids

    E. Facial weakness

67. A 26-year-old woman is involved in a motor vehicle accident after another person runs a stop sign and T-bones her car. Thankfully, the other person is not injured, but the patient states that she is unable to walk effectively and has intractable neck pain preventing her from holding a normal job. As a result, she is seeking compensation for all of her medical bills, lost wages, and pain and suffering. However, she is seen riding roller coasters at a theme park. Which is the correct diagnosis?

    A. Conversion disorder

    B. Somatization disorder

    C. Factitious disorder

    D. Hypochondriasis

    E. Malingering

68. A 37-year-old female presents to the emergency department with a severe headache. She has a history of migraine headaches and delivered her fourth child 2 weeks ago. Her current headache is different from her previous headaches. It started midmorning and reached peak intensity very quickly. It hurts predominantly behind her eyes. She has had associated nausea, vomiting, and photophobia. Her husband says she has been disoriented with this headache. She is afebrile. Her neurological examination reveals mildly reduced sensation on the left side of her face and arm, as well as disorientation to place and time, but is otherwise normal. Which of the following test results would be most likely in this patient?

    A. Computed tomography (CT) angiogram showing beading of multiple intracranial blood vessels

    B. Lumbar puncture (LP) demonstrated a cerebrospinal fluid (CSF) opening pressure of 2 cm H_2O

    C. LP demonstrating a white cell count of 500 and protein of 100

    D. Magnetic resonance image (MRI) of the brain demonstrating an enlarged pituitary with a low T1 signal and ring enhancement

    E. MRI with fluid attenuated inversion recovery (FLAIR) abnormalities in a fingerlike shape arising from the ventricles

69. Early treatment of status epilepticus is necessary because of alterations in the functional properties of which receptor?

A. N-methyl-D-aspartate (NMDA) receptor

B. Gamma aminobutyric acid A (GABA_A) receptor

C. Voltage-gated calcium channel receptor

D. Acetylcholine receptor

E. Alpha–2 receptor

70. Two months into chemotherapy treatment, a 66-year-old woman develops painful paresthesias in her hands and feet, as well as weakness when standing on her toes. Which of the following is the most likely agent to which these symptoms are attributable?

A. Bortezomib

B. Cisplatin

C. Bevacizumab

D. Temozolomide

E. Lomustine

71. A 52-year-old female presents with memory loss over the last several weeks. A magnetic resonance image is obtained, and a key diffusion weighted image is displayed here. Which of the following is the most likely diagnosis?

A. Frontotemporal dementia

B. Huntington disease

C. Creutzfeldt-Jakob disease

D. Alzheimer disease

E. Dementia with Lewy bodies

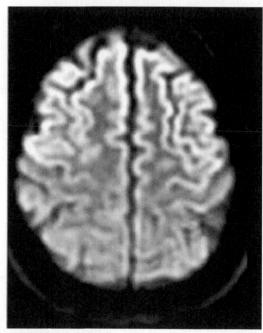

Figure for Question 5.71.

72. A 33-year-old man presents to the emergency room with shooting pain in his left cheek. He describes the onset as acute and severe, as if he's "chewing glass." Each pain lasts only seconds but occurs repeatedly. These attacks are often triggered by brushing his teeth. His neurological examination, including sensation in the left V2 distribution, is normal. Which of the following is true regarding the suspected condition?

A. These episodes are usually responsive to indomethacin.

B. Magnetic resonance imaging (MRI) is not indicated in all cases of this condition.

C. The masseter inhibitory reflex test is often abnormal.

D. Sodium channel blockers are usually ineffective for treating this condition.

E. Muscle relaxants are usually ineffective for treating this condition.

73. A 63-year-old female on treatment for small cell lung cancer presents with multiple falls. Her examination shows normal cranial nerve function except for sensation loss on her face. She has normal strength in her extremities. She has loss of sensation to pin prick, vibration, and proprioception in all extremities, and pseudoathetosis is present. Reflexes are absent in her extremities. Nerve conduction studies show absent sensory responses in all extremities, but normal motor responses. Which of the following medications is the most likely cause of her symptoms?

A. Cisplatin

B. Vincristine

C. Bortezomib

D. Rituximab

E. Methotrexate

74. A 36-year-old male presents to your office for evaluation of weakness. Over the last year he developed progressive weakness in his extremities. He has difficulties climbing up stairs and reaching his hands above his head. He can only walk 1 block before becoming short of breath. He has no numbness. Electromyography (EMG) demonstrates diffuse myotonia and myopathic motor units. Deltoid muscle biopsy demonstrates glycogen-filled vacuoles, which intensely stain for acid phosphatase. Which of the following is the most likely diagnosis?

A. Nonaka myopathy (hereditary inclusion body myositis)

B. McArdle disease (myophosphorylase deficiency)

C. Becker muscular dystrophy

D. Pompe disease (α-glucosidase deficiency)

E. Limb girdle muscular dystrophy type 1A (LGMD-1A; myotilin deficiency)

75. Which of the following is *not* an effective means of reducing intracranial pressure?

A. Elevate head of bed beyond 30 degrees

B. Tighten cervical collar to keep head straight

C. Sedation

D. Hyperventilation

E. Hyperosmolar therapy

76. Which of the following features of the sarcomere represents the whole of the thick filaments?
    A. A-band
    B. I-band
    C. Z-line
    D. M-line
    E. H-band

77. Which of the following is true regarding tricyclic antidepressants (TCAs)?
    A. They only have action at the serotoninergic receptors.
    B. They are used to treat severe depression and not used in other conditions.
    C. One cannot develop serotonin syndrome from TCAs.
    D. TCAs have a stimulating property, making them great for treating excessive daytime sleepiness.
    E. TCAs are metabolized via cytochrome P450 isozymes.

78. A 29-year-old man with Crohn disease has a 3-week history of diarrhea. His wife notices that he is now more somnolent and has a diffuse headache that worsens when lying down. His examination shows blurring of the optic nerve, as well as encephalopathy, but otherwise nothing focal. Computed tomography (CT) of the brain without contrast is unremarkable. What is the next best step to evaluate the etiology of this patient's symptoms?
    A. Lumbar puncture (LP)
    B. Administer trial of sumatriptan
    C. CT of the abdomen/pelvis
    D. CT venogram
    E. Magnetic resonance imaging (MRI) of the brain

79. Which is true of Fukuyama congenital muscular dystrophy?
    A. Causative gene not known
    B. Weakness is mild, so most can exercise normally
    C. Often associated with lissencephaly
    D. Inherited in an X-linked recessive manner
    E. Generally live into adulthood

80. A 63-year-old woman presents with frequent falls for the last year. Each fall is preceded by lightheadedness upon standing and walking. She has had several episodes of syncope with a negative cardiac workup, and even more episodes of presyncope. On examination, she has masked facies, stuttering speech, hypophonia, and a mixed resting and action tremor in both hands. Her strength is normal, but her legs are discolored with mild peripheral edema. Her magnetic resonance image is shown. Which of the following is the most likely diagnosis?
    A. Dehydration
    B. Postural orthostatic tachycardia syndrome (POTS)
    C. Lambert-Eaton myasthenia syndrome (LEMS)
    D. Multiple system atrophy
    E. Amyloidosis

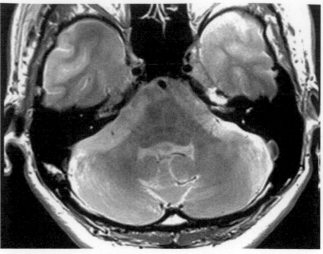

Figure for Question 5.80.

81. A 53-year-old woman presents to the emergency department with altered mental status. She has had no preceding infectious symptoms, although she has a history of medication noncompliance. On examination, she is hypothermic with mild hypotension and bradycardia. She has periorbital edema, cool skin, and diffuse lower extremity edema. Neurologically, she is somnolent and oriented only to person. She has diffuse weakness with poor effort and delayed relaxation of reflexes. Which of the following is the next best treatment for the patient's most likely condition?
    A. Intravenous immunoglobulin (IVIG)
    B. Plasma exchange
    C. Furosemide
    D. Naloxone
    E. Levothyroxine

82. On examination of a patient with unilateral hearing loss, you perform Weber and Rinne testing in the office. On Rinne testing, air conduction is greater than bone conduction bilaterally. On Weber testing, the tuning fork is loudest on the right. Which of the following describes the type of hearing loss from which this patient suffers?
    A. Right sensorineural hearing loss
    B. Left sensorineural hearing loss
    C. Right conductive hearing loss
    D. Left conductive hearing loss
    E. Selective hearing

83. An 82-year-old female with Parkinson disease presents to the office with her husband. Her husband complains of vivid dreaming, kicking movements, and even yelling during the night, but the patient has no memory of this. It has been bothersome enough that her husband sleeps in the next room. Which of the following is the most appropriate treatment?
    A. Reassurance
    B. Amitriptyline
    C. Zolpidem
    D. Clonazepam
    E. Trihexyphenidyl

84. All of the following are causes of circadian rhythm disorders *except*?

    A. Dementia

    B. Children with mental retardation

    C. Obstructive sleep apnea

    D. Blindness

    E. Travel across three time zones

85. After a diagnostic lumbar puncture, which of the following is *least* suggestive of a low-pressure headache?

    A. Responsiveness to caffeine

    B. Improvement with recumbency

    C. Enlarging physiological blind spot

    D. Duration of up to several weeks

    E. Dural enhancement on magnetic resonance imaging (MRI)

86. Which of the following opioid receptors is involved in analgesia, euphoria, respiratory depression, and opioid tolerance?

    A. Mu receptor

    B. Delta receptor

    C. Kappa receptor

    D. Alpha 2 receptor

    E. N-methyl-D-aspartate (NMDA) receptor

87. A 24-year-old man presents with several months of progressive tinnitus and hearing loss on the right and new right facial weakness. His mother is deaf and has poor balance for unknown reasons. Which is the most likely root cause of his symptoms?

    A. Genetic mutation in *NF2* gene

    B. Genetic mutation in *NF1* gene

    C. Recurrent viral infection

    D. Vascular abnormality

    E. Demyelinating disease

88. Which of the following anatomical structures corresponds to wave IV in brainstem auditory evoked potentials?

    A. Cochlear nerve

    B. Cochlear nucleus

    C. Lateral lemniscus

    D. Superior olive

    E. Inferior colliculus

89. At what age should a child be able to draw a person with two to four body parts, use scissors, play a board game, and stand on one foot?

    A. 18 months

    B. 2 years

    C. 3 years

    D. 4 years

    E. 5 years

90. A 25-year-old female presents with episodes of confusion. These episodes start with a rising feeling in her abdomen followed by anxiety and diaphoresis. Her family states she will mumble and hold her left arm stiff while her right arm picks at her shirt. These episodes will last for 45 seconds before resolving. She is tired and confused after these episodes have occurred. Which of the following is the most likely localization for her symptoms?

    A. Left orbitofrontal lobe

    B. Left lateral temporal lobe

    C. Right occipital lobe

    D. Right mesial temporal lobe

    E. Right dorsolateral frontal lobe

91. By what age should a child learn to play peek-a-boo?

    A. 2 months

    B. 4 months

    C. 6 months

    D. 9 months

    E. 12 months

92. A 50-year-old man with acquired immunodeficiency syndrome (AIDS) and chronic intravenous drug abuse presents with 2 days of progressive headache, confusion, and left hemiparesis. A magnetic resonance image (see figure) is obtained in the emergency room and T2, T1 with contrast, and diffusion weight imaging sequences are shown here. Beyond consideration of hyperosmolar or corticosteroid therapy, which of the following is the next best therapy?

    A. Emergent neurosurgical consult

    B. Initiate methotrexate therapy

    C. Initiate antiretroviral therapy

    D. Positron emission tomography (PET) scan to determine site of origin

    E. Lumbar puncture

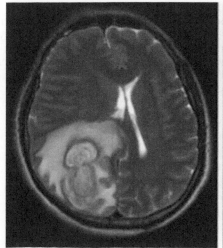 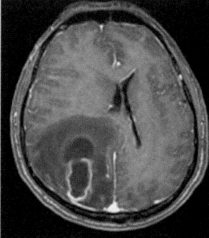 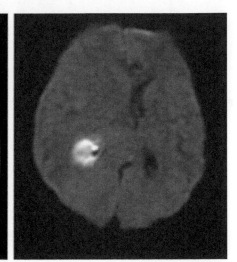

Figure for Question 5.92.

93 A 70-year-old woman has several months of progressive gait difficulty, trouble controlling her legs, and more recently, poor coordination in her arms. She additionally has tingling in her hands and feet. She denies any change in her bowel or bladder habits. On neurological examination, she has intact strength throughout, but severely impaired proprioception in the arms and legs. Her deep tendon reflexes are brisk, and she has bilateral extensor plantar reflexes. She reports normal dietary intake since getting her dentures fit more securely, with large quantities of an old supply of denture cream. Which of the following is the most likely cause of her symptoms?

A. Copper toxicity

B. Copper deficiency

C. Zinc deficiency

D. Vitamin B12 deficiency

E. Vitamin B12 toxicity

94. Which of the following is *not* true regarding the condition depicted in the figure?

A. It is usually associated with bilateral vestibular schwannomas.

B. This usually results from a mutation in the *NF1* gene on chromosome 17.

C. Clinical manifestations consist of café-au-lait macules, cutaneous neurofibromas and/or plexiform neurofibromas, iris hamartomas, and optic nerve gliomas.

D. Patients often have cognitive difficulties.

E. This condition is autosomal dominant in inheritance.

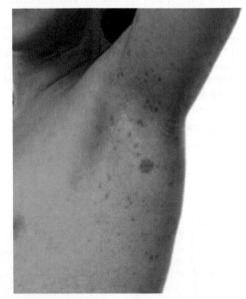

Figure for Question 5.94.

95. Which of the following does not constitute a conflict of interest?

A. Participating in a pharmaceutical medication study

B. Referring patients to a magnetic resonance imaging (MRI) center in which you are invested

C. Performing a procedure for higher reimbursement when medication would suffice

D. Prescribing pain medications to close family members

E. Initiating a sexual relationship with a patient

96. The photomicrograph depicts a subarachnoid specimen. Which of the following are indicated by the arrows?

A. *Streptococcus pneumoniae*

B. *Neisseria meningitidis*

C. *Rhizopus*

D. Herpes simplex virus

E. *Naegleria fowleri*

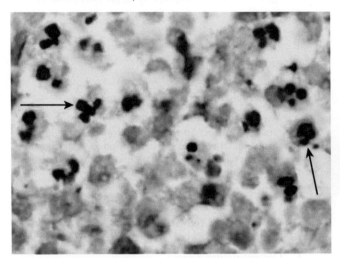

Figure for Question 5.96.

97. Which of the following is *not* true of phosphofructokinase deficiency (Tauri disease)?

A. Abnormal forearm ischemic lactate test

B. Exercise intolerance

C. Exercise-induced myoglobinuria

D. Autosomal recessive

E. Second wind phenomenon

98. In a healthy 30-year-old woman, painful obscuration of visual acuity and impaired color vision develop over the course of 1 day. She has a relative afferent pupillary defect in that eye. There is no family history of similar symptoms. Which of the following is true regarding her most likely diagnosis?

A. Ninety percent 5-year risk of developing multiple sclerosis

B. Greater risk of recurrence if treated with oral prednisone

C. Untreated vitamin A deficiency may lead to permanent blindness

D. This is a hereditary condition, passed on by mitochondrial genetics

E. The gene associated with this disease is *Rb*

99. A 35-year-old female presents for evaluation of an intention tremor that developed in the last 3 months and is severe enough that she cannot feed herself. Her mood has been labile, with episodes of extreme irritability and euphoria. She complains of excessive sweating and occasional confusion. She was recently fired from her job at the battery factory because her tremor interfered with work. A complete metabolic profile, thyroid-stimulating hormone, and urine drug screen are normal. A complete blood count shows mild anemia. Which of the following is the most likely cause?

  A. Functional or psychogenic tremor

  B. Mercury

  C. Lead

  D. Manganese

  E. Wilson disease

100. Which of the following is the target molecule of alemtuzumab?

  A. CD20

  B. CD52

  C. Vascular endothelial growth factor

  D. Cell adhesion molecule α4

  E. Sphingosine 1-phosphate receptor

Questions 101-105: Match the trinucleotide-affected protein to the appropriate disease.

101. Huntington disease

102. Myotonic dystrophy

103. Friedreich ataxia

104. Spinobulbar muscular atrophy (Kennedy disease)

105. Dentatorubropallidoluysian atrophy (DRPLA)

  A. Frataxin

  B. Myotonin

  C. Huntington

  D. Androgen receptor

  E. Atrophin-1

ANSWERS

1. D. This patient suffered an anterior spinal infarct, which is a relatively uncommon complication of aortic dissections, aortic surgery (whether stenting or an open surgery), prolonged clamping of the aorta above the renal arteries, or from embolism (either from atrial fibrillation or emboli dislodged from the aorta or branch arteries). Anterior spinal infarcts have prominent weakness associated with loss of sensation to temperature and pin prick, but the posterior column function remains preserved. Urinary and bowel dysfunction are common. Initially flaccid paralysis predominates, but over time, patients develop spasticity and hyperreflexia, as expected for a myelopathy. AIDP can occur postoperatively, but sensory loss usually doesn't spare certain modalities over others. Further, sensory levels are not a component of AIDP. Diabetic radiculoplexopathy occurs in cases of uncontrolled diabetes and involves pain and weakness with atrophy in one leg. Transverse myelitis may present similarly to this case, but the history of aortic dissection and repair is more suggestive of an anterior spinal infarct. Conversion disorder is unlikely given no mention of Hoover sign or other signs that may warn of a psychological disorder (*see* Bradley's NiCP, 7th edn, Ch. 69, pp. 1007–1014).

2. E. JC virus reactivation is associated with progressive multifocal leukoencephalopathy (PML). MRI often reveals multifocal, nonenhancing lesions affecting the white matter and U-fibers, generally sparing the cortex. The risk of PML is increased in individuals treated with natalizumab, especially if there was preceding immunosuppressive therapy or if natalizumab therapy continues for longer than 24 months. Ischemic stroke is rarely multifocal, unless embolic in nature, and would not spare the cortex. HIV encephalitis is unlikely without a listed diagnosis of HIV. Further, the associated FLAIR hyperintensity is generally periventricular and symmetric. An acute episode of demyelination is generally associated with contrast enhancement. Acute disseminated encephalomyelitis is generally associated with contrast enhancement. The mention of preceding illness is likely a red herring (*see* Bradley's NiCP, 7th edn, Ch. 80, pp. 1159–1186). Figures from Cinque P, Koralnik IJ, Gerevini S, Miro JM, Price RW 2009 Progressive multifocal leukoencephalopathy in HIV-1 infection. *Lancet Infectious Diseases* 9(10): 625–636, with permission.

3. B. Plasma exchange will remove the natalizumab from the circulating blood, thereby reversing the immunosuppression that led to John Cunningham (JC) virus reactivation. Immune reconstitution inflammatory syndrome (IRIS) is a risk with immunosuppression reversal and should be carefully monitored. IV corticosteroids would be appropriate for acute demyelination or acute disseminated encephalomyelitis (ADEM), but neither of those are the likely underlying disease process. No antiviral therapy has been proven effective for JC virus reactivation. HAART would be appropriate if this progressive multifocal leukoencephalopathy (PML) were associated with untreated HIV. However, given its association with natalizumab therapy (and no history of HIV infection), HAART is not likely to help. Anticoagulation would not be helpful

for PML (*see* Bradley's NiCP, 7th edn, Ch. 78, pp. 1121–1146).

4. B. Whereas glutamate is an excitatory neurotransmitter, excessive concentrations thereof (and therefore neuronal stimulation) may be toxic to neurons. Glutamate toxicity is one means by which damage is hypothesized in the penumbra after ischemic death of adjacent neurons and release of glutamate into the microenvironment (*see* Bradley's NiCP, 7th edn, Ch. 98, pp. 1481–1518).

5. C. This syndrome is known as *Lance-Adams syndrome* and is characterized by action myoclonus after hypoxic injury from cardiac arrest. Gait is usually affected if the myoclonus involves the legs. Medications that work on the gamma aminobutyric acid (GABA) receptor, such as clonazepam, are typically used for treatment of myoclonus, as well as levetiracetam, sodium valproate, zonisamide, and sodium oxybate. Although he may require a beta-blocker from a cardiac perspective, carvedilol is not likely to reduce his myoclonus. Carbamazepine is not indicated given there is no history of partial seizures. Carbidopa/levodopa is typically used to treat parkinsonism, not myoclonus. Clozapine is an atypical antipsychotic used to treat hallucinations and psychosis, especially in those with dementia of Parkinson disease (*see* Bradley's NiCP, 7th edn, Ch. 96, pp. 1422–1460).

6. E. Migraine treatments in pregnancy are limited. The first-line abortive treatment is always acetaminophen, which is pregnancy category C. Nonsteroidal anti-inflammatory drugs like ibuprofen, naproxen, and diclofenac can be used in the first and second trimesters, but should be avoided in the third trimester because they can cause premature closure of the ductus arteriosus. Sumatriptan is considered a third-line treatment and is pregnancy category C. Morphine and opioids can be used for severe headaches, but are reserved as a second- or third-line agent. Ergotamine and valproic acid are pregnancy category X and should be avoided at all costs (*see* Bradley's NiCP, Ch. 112, pp. 1973–1991).

7. B. Meningothelial nests and whirls are shown in the image and are pathologically diagnostic of meningioma. Whirls are the first step in the formation of concentric calcifications known as *psammoma bodies*. Pseudopalisading necrosis and microvascular proliferation are necessary findings for a diagnosis of glioblastoma. Rosenthal fibers are markers of long-standing gliosis and, among tumors, are characteristically found in pilocytic astrocytomas. Perivascular pseudorosettes are a spoke-wheel pattern of tumor cells around a blood vessel and are most commonly found in ependymomas, although they may also be seen in various other tumor types less commonly. Homer Wright rosettes are round structures with a central core of fiberlike structures and are most commonly found in medulloblastomas (*see* Bradley's NiCP, 7th edn, Ch. 72, pp. 1026–1044). Figure from Daroff RB, Jankovic J, Mazziotta JC, Pomeroy SL 2016 *Bradley's Neurology in Clinical Practice*, 7th edn, Elsevier, with permission.

8. D. Low levels of vitamin B12 (cobalamin) may lead to various medical and neurological complications. Most notably and severe among the neurological complications is subacute combined degeneration, a demyelinating syndrome of the dorsal columns of

the spinal cord and peripheral nerves. Additionally associated consequences of low B12 include confusion and macrocytic anemia. Laboratory testing reveals low vitamin B12 levels, along with high levels of methylmalonic acid and homocysteine. Whereas pathologically low vitamin B12 may be achieved through diet restriction (as in the case of veganism), autoimmune malabsorption (as in pernicious anemia), and structural malabsorption (as in gastrectomy or gastric bypass surgery), it is also important to note that nitrous oxide inhalation binds B12 and may produce rapid onset of symptoms related to deficiency. Low copper level is most commonly reported in association with excessive zinc intake, which prevents copper absorption. Most cases result from impaired absorption related either to gastric bypass or zinc toxicity (as with zinc-containing denture adhesives). Patients may present with a combination of myelopathy, neuropathy, and anemia, not dissimilar to cobalamin deficiency. Vision disturbance from optic neuropathy, however, may also be present. Another syndrome of copper deficiency is Menke disease, an X-linked recessive disorder in which copper absorption is profoundly impaired due to enzymatic deficiencies. In this disease, children develop weakness with hypotonia, intellectual disability, seizures, bony and vascular abnormalities, and the classic findings of kinky hair and blue sclera. Hypercalcemia is associated with many general medical symptoms, including renal calculi, bone pain, abdominal pain, and cardiac dysfunction. Neurologically, depression is present in a high number of patients with chronic hypercalcemia, with other psychiatric problems such as anxiety or confusion in smaller numbers. Low thiamine (vitamin B1) levels are most commonly associated with dietary deficiency, including malnutrition, alcoholism, or persistent vomiting. The most notable complications of thiamine deficiency are Wernicke encephalopathy or Wernicke-Korsakoff syndrome. These most commonly occur in alcoholics or after rapid correction of hypoglycemia without first administering thiamine. Wernicke encephalopathy is characterized by ophthalmoparesis or nystagmus, ataxia, and confusion. Without thiamine repletion (or sometimes in spite thereof), patients may deteriorate to Wernicke-Korsakoff syndrome in which they develop both retrograde and anterograde amnesia with confabulation. Outside of these syndromes, chronic thiamine deficiency is also associated with either wet or dry beriberi, both of which may include sensorimotor neuropathy. Low vitamin E levels may relate to poor absorption due to alpha-tocopherol transfer protein dysfunction or to abetalipoproteinemia. In either case, presentations are similar to Friedreich ataxia or spinocerebellar ataxia, including ataxia and myelopathy, with the addition of retinitis pigmentosa (*see* Bradley's NiCP, 7th edn, Ch. 85, pp. 1226–1236).

9. E. Typical electromyography (EMG) findings of radiculopathy include low-amplitude motor responses, normal sensory responses, and prolonged F waves. There should be no conduction blocks present or distal latency prolongation. EMG should show abnormalities in a root pattern. C8 muscles include the abductor pollicis brevis, extensor indicis proprius, extensor digitorum communis, and FDI. The biceps receive innervation from C5 and C6 (*see* Bradley's NiCP, 7th edn, Ch. 35, pp. 366–390).

10. B. The patient has Kennedy disease, also known as *spinobulbar muscular atrophy*. This is a lower motor neuron disease predominantly of the bulbar muscles that eventually causes proximal limb weakness. It can be difficult to distinguish initially from myasthenia, amyotrophic lateral sclerosis (ALS), or oculopharyngeal muscular dystrophy (OPMD). This is an X-linked disorder with a CAG repeat in the androgen receptor gene that leads to gynecomastia, infertility, impotence, and testicular atrophy, in addition to a lower motor neuronopathy. OPMD is an autosomal-dominant trinucleotide repeat condition on chromosome 14. ALS has several genetic causes, including *SOD1* and, more recently, *C9ORF72*. MUSK antibodies are associated with myasthenia gravis. Wilson disease is treated with chelation therapy such as penicillamine. It can cause dysarthria, but not typically fasciculations, testicular atrophy, or gynecomastia (*see* Bradley's NiCP, 7th edn, Ch. 98, pp. 1484–1519).

11. E. Dextromethorphan and quinidine are used in combination to treat pseudobulbar affect in ALS, which can improve quality of life, but have not been shown to improve survival. Riluzole, noninvasive positive ventilation, PEG tubes, and treatment in ALS multidisciplinary clinics have all been shown to have positive effects on survival in ALS patients, in addition to their benefits on quality of life (*see* Bradley's NiCP, 7th edn, Ch. 98, pp. 1484–1518).

12. B. Edwards syndrome is caused by chromosome 18 trisomy, and is associated with malformations in multiple organs, including ventricular septal defects, atrial septal defects, patent ductus arteriosus, omphalocele, and esophageal atresia. Craniofacial abnormalities include micrognathia, hypertelorism, cleft lip/palate, ptosis, low-set ears, and prominent occiput. Arthrogryposis is commonly seen due to muscular weakness. The risk of chromosomal imbalance disorders, such as trisomy 18, increases with increased maternal age. The majority of fetuses with Edwards syndrome die before birth (*see* Bradley's NiCP, 7th edn, Ch. 50, pp. 648–675).

13. C. Potassium is the only one of the choices that has a higher intracellular concentration. The difference between potassium, sodium, and chloride concentrations sets up the electrochemical gradient, which helps drive the flow of ions for action potentials. The Na-K pump forces sodium out of the cell and potassium into the cell against concentration gradients and requires the use of adenosine triphosphate to perform this (*see* Bradley's NiCP, 7th edn, Ch. 34–35, pp. 349–391).

14. E. Patients in a persistent vegetative state retain functions of the brainstem such as cardiac function, control of respiration, and blood pressure control. This state may have some spontaneous but nonpurposeful movements, evidence of sleep/wake cycles, and no response to outside stimulation. Cranial nerve reflexes remain intact. However, there is no control over bowel or bladder. The following chart displays important features of each level of consciousness (*see* Bradley's NiCP, 7th edn, Ch. 6, pp. 51–56).

TABLE FOR ANSWER 5.14 Comparison of disorders of consciousness

	Awareness	Wakefulness	Brain stem/ Respiratory	Motor	EEG	Evoked potentials	PET/FMRI	Comment
Brain death	Absent	Absent	Absent	Absent	ECS	Absent	Absent cortical metabolism	Legally dead in most jurisdictions
Coma	Absent	Absent	Depressed, variable	Reflex or posturing	Polymorphic delta, burst suppression	BAER variable; cortical ERPs often absent	Resting <50%	Prognosis variable
Vegetative state	Absent	Present, intact sleep/wake cycles	Intact	Reflex, nonpurposeful	Delta, theta, or ECS	BAER preserved; cortical ERPs variable	Resting <50%; primary areas stimulatable	Prognosis variable
Minimally conscious state	Intact but poorly responsive	Intact	Intact	Variable with purposeful movements	Nonspecific slowing	BAER preserved; cortical ERPs often preserved	Reduced; secondary areas also stimulatable	Prognosis variable

Data from Goldman L, Schafer A 2016 Goldman's Cecil Medicine, *Elsevier, with permission.*

15. C. A mu rhythm is a normal rhythm that is seen in the central region of the brain, usually unilaterally. These are archiform waveforms that occur at rest and resolve with contralateral limb movements or even thinking about contralateral limb movements. SREDA are bursts of rhythmic theta waves that have an abrupt onset and abrupt termination with no clinical changes. Although these appear seizure-like, they can be distinguished from a seizure by a lack of electrical buildup, the abrupt finish, and lack of slow waves. The rhythm shown here is seen in the central region of the brain and is at a rate of 8–9 Hz, so this would not be consistent with temporal theta. Lambda waves are seen posteriorly and are thought to be caused by visual fixation or reading. A focal seizure would have a buildup of synchronous activity, which eventually slows until stopping, whereas mu waves have no evolution in frequency, as well as an abrupt start and stop (*see* Bradley's NiCP, 7th edn, Ch. 34, pp. 348–365). Figure from Libenson MH 2010 *Practical Approach to Electroencephalography,* Saunders, with permission.

16. D. The patient demonstrates multiple behaviors classic for borderline personality disorder, including unstable relationships, rapid mood swings, impulsivity, splitting, and recurrent suicidal gestures (which are not common with other personality disorders). Narcissistic personality disorder involves a marked love of self, a grand sense of self-importance, fantasies of success, exploiting others to reach goals, and a lack of empathy for others. These patients react with intense emotion when criticized. Histrionic personality disorder involves excessive emotional lability and the need for attention (usually with provocative dress, seductive behaviors, or flamboyant behaviors). Major depressive disorder is marked by depressed mood or anhedonia and is associated with changes in sleep, appetite, interest in activities, psychomotor slowing, decreased libido, and suicidal thoughts. Bipolar 1 disorder is characterized by an episode of mania (inflated self-esteem, decreased sleep, pressured speech, flight of ideas, distractibility, and involvement in risky behaviors).

17. A. This patient has Alexander disease, a leukodystrophy caused by a mutation in the *GFAP* gene, and is associated with macrocephaly, psychomotor retardation, loss of developmental milestones, spasticity, and poor feeding. Seizures and hydrocephalus may also be present. Radiographic findings with Alexander disease include contrast-enhancing white matter signal change, which is predominantly in the frontal lobes and spares the U-fibers. There may also be periventricular rims of high T2 signal, as well as signal abnormalities in the basal ganglia and thalami. Most cases of Alexander disease arise spontaneously, although the less common adult-onset variety may be inherited in an autosomal-dominant pattern. The treatment for Alexander disease is supportive. The other answer choices have different MRI characteristics and presentations. Pelizaeus-Merzbacher and metachromatic leukodystrophy both have confluent white matter changes but are inherited in an X-linked and autosomal-recessive fashion, respectively. Huntington disease usually does not have confluent white matter pathology but instead has absent caudate. Adrenoleukodystrophy commonly has sparing of the frontal white matter and involves posterior white matter more commonly (*see* Bradley's NiCP, 7th edn, Ch. 91, pp. 1324–1341). Figure from Volpe JJ 2008 *Neurology of the Newborn,* 5th edn, Saunders, with permission.

18. D. The contents of the cavernous sinus are the oculomotor nerve, the trochlear nerve, the internal carotid artery, the ophthalmic nerve, the abducens

CORONAL VIEW

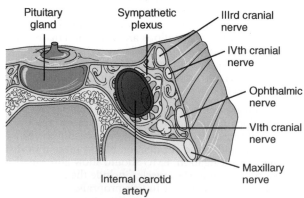

Pituitary gland — Sympathetic plexus — IIIrd cranial nerve — IVth cranial nerve — Ophthalmic nerve — VIth cranial nerve — Maxillary nerve — Internal carotid artery

Figure for Answer 5.18 *(from Kaiser PK, Friedman NJ, Pineda R 2014* Massachusetts Eye and Ear Infirmary Illustrated Manual of Ophthalmology, *Elsevier, with permission.)*

nerve, and the maxillary nerve. The mandibular branch of the trigeminal nerve is the only branch that does not traverse the cavernous sinus. The anatomical arrangement of the cavernous sinus is demonstrated in the figure (*see* Bradley's NiCP, 7th edn, Ch. 104, pp. 1720–1735).

19. C. The suspicion of giant cell arteritis (GCA) should be high in this elderly patient with new headaches and scalp tenderness. The presence of jaw claudication would most align with that theory and prompt further action. Other signs patients with GCA may describe include weight loss or painless vision loss, which often presents as unilateral and altitudinal, but may quickly involve both eyes in most untreated patients. Whereas the anterior ischemic optic neuropathy of GCA is painless, ocular pain would not be a relevant symptom here. Lateralized tearing and rhinorrhea are more common in trigeminal autonomic cephalgias, such as cluster headaches. Photophobia and phonophobia are common to migraine disorder, but not GCA. Pulsatile tinnitus is common to idiopathic intracranial hypertension, but not GCA (*see* Bradley's NiCP, 7th edn, Ch. 58, pp. 814–834).

20. A. Given sufficient suspicion of giant cell arteritis (GCA), the most important action is initiation of corticosteroid treatment in order to preserve vision. Although an elevated erythrocyte sedimentation rate or C-reactive protein would further motivate this treatment, the laboratory is closed in this case, and the prudent physician should act to prevent further potential harm. Neuroophthalmological evaluation may ultimately be helpful to ensure there is no ischemic injury or visual field deficit related to GCA, but this would not be the first necessary action. Temporal artery biopsy will likely provide the pathological proof of disease, but classic teaching says to begin steroids before the biopsy, given the risk of vision loss. Notably, the pathological findings of GCA are generally still apparent on biopsy for up to 2 weeks after steroid initiation. Ergotamine treatment is helpful for certain types of headaches, such as migraine, but would not be indicated in this instance. Brain MRI may be helpful for certain types of new headaches, but given the high suspicion of GCA in this case, MRI would not be immediately necessary (*see* Bradley's NiCP, 7th edn, Ch. 58, pp. 814–834).

21. C. There are several types of spinal dysraphism, with spina bifida occulta being the most common. In this defect, the posterior portions of the vertebrae do not develop completely, resulting in a bony defect over the posterior portion of the spine. However, there is no protrusion of the meninges or neural elements (either nerve roots or spinal cord, depending on the level) to result in significant neurological deficits. Most of the time this is asymptomatic, but occasional urinary or sphincter dysfunction or focal neurological deficits can come from this defect or associated spinal tethering. A dimple, hairy tuft, or even rudimentary tail could point toward spina bifida occulta. A meningocele involves a similar bony defect to occulta; however, there is protrusion of the meninges through the defect, whereas meningomyelocele involves protrusion of the neural elements and meninges into the defect, resulting in more dramatic neurological consequences such as paralysis. Spina bifida cystica is another name for meningomyelocele. Syringohydromyelia involves a cystic cerebrospinal fluid lesion in the central canal of

the spinal cord that can exert pressure on the spinal cord, causing central cord syndrome. These do not involve any defect in the overlying vertebrae (*see* Bradley's NiCP, 7th edn, Ch. 105, pp. 1736–1765).

22. B. When the EEG is used for assisting in brain death determination, certain standards must be met for determining electrocerebral silence. The EEG must have a full set of electrodes in standard positions. The montage used should have an interelectrode distance of at least 10 cm, and the recording time should be 30 minutes or greater. Sensitivity should be set at 2 μV. The high-frequency filter should be at 30 Hz or higher and the low-frequency filter at 1 Hz or lower. The system and recording integrity must be checked, and interelectrode impedance should be between 100 and 10,000 ohms.

23. D. The patient has clinical evidence of Cushing *syndrome*, which is associated with symptoms including moon facies, striae, thin skin, bruising, and weight gain. Most commonly, Cushing syndrome is associated with exogenous intake of glucocorticoids. Cushing *disease*, on the other hand, describes excess adrenocorticotropic hormone (ACTH) production from a pituitary tumor, most commonly a microadenoma (<10 mm). When evaluating someone with Cushing syndrome, an MRI of the brain should be obtained to evaluate for an adenoma. Further, a number of laboratory tests are important to consider, including a 24-hour urine cortisol collection or a 1-mg dexamethasone suppression test. If either of these is abnormal, confirmatory testing should be done with a late-afternoon ACTH level, as well as a CRH stimulation test. Occasionally, an abdominal computed tomography (CT) may be necessary to evaluate for an adrenal carcinoma if other symptoms suggest such pathology. In this particular case, the headaches are migrainous, and a lumbar puncture (LP) is not needed (*see* Bradley's NiCP, 7th edn, Ch. 52, pp. 696–712).

24. A. The locus ceruleus produces norepinephrine, which is one of the predominant neurotransmitters responsible for wakefulness. The supraoptic nucleus is responsible for antidiuretic hormone and oxytocin. The tuberomamillary nucleus is responsible for production of histamine, which is another important transmitter to maintain wakefulness. The dorsal raphe nucleus produces serotonin, which helps promote wakefulness. The suprachiasmatic nucleus in the hypothalamus generates melatonin (*see* Bradley's NiCP, 7th edn, Ch. 102, pp. 1615–1685).

25. D. Cognitive behavioral therapy (CBT) is a psychological technique used to build a set of skills to reshape negative thoughts, feelings, or emotions and allow an individual to see reality more clearly. Such reshaping generally allows patients to cope with symptoms in a more rational manner. CBT is often used in cases of functional neurological symptoms, obsessive compulsive disorder, and many others (*see* Bradley's NiCP, 7th edn, Ch. 113, pp. 1992–2008).

26. E. This patient presents with a single seizure, but has a very abnormal EEG. The EEG demonstrates generalized polyspike and wave abnormalities at a rate of 4–6 Hz consistent with a generalized epilepsy syndrome, likely juvenile myoclonic epilepsy (JME). Of the mentioned medications, valproic acid would be the most appropriate medicine to start for treatment of a generalized epilepsy. Other first-line considerations

could be levetiracetam, topiramate, or lamotrigine (although lamotrigine can worsen the myoclonus of JME). Whether or not the patient is a woman of childbearing age also determines which first-line treatment to initiate because valproic acid is highly teratogenic. Carbamazepine can worsen some generalized epilepsy syndromes. Ethosuximide is most effective for absence epilepsy, not a disorder involving generalized convulsions. Clonazepam and other benzodiazepines can be helpful in generalized seizure disorders; however, they are not considered first-line treatments. Lacosamide is approved for monotherapy in partial epilepsy syndromes, not primary generalized disorders (*see* Bradley's NiCP, 7th edn, Ch. 101, pp. 1563–1614). Figure from Werz MA 2010 Juvenile myoclonic epilepsy. *Epilepsy Syndromes* 28(S1): 21–23, with permission.

27. C. Holoprosencephaly is an incomplete separation of the two hemispheres of the cerebrum. It is often associated with other midline facial developmental abnormalities, including cyclopia, with or without proboscis (nose), and cleft lip or palate. Holoprosencephaly is associated with a variety of genetic abnormalities, including chromosomal imbalance events and multiple single-gene mutations (with *SHH* being the most common) (*see* Bradley's NiCP, 7th edn, Ch. 89, pp. 1279–1300). Figure from Finkbeiner WE, Ursell PC, Davis RL, Connolly AJ 2009 *Atlas of Autopsy Pathology*, 2nd edn, Elsevier, with permission.

28. E. Taste is provided to the anterior two thirds of the tongue by the facial nerve via the chorda tympani. General sensation is provided to the same region by the mandibular branch of the trigeminal nerve via the lingual nerve. The posterior tongue receives both taste and general sensation from the glossopharyngeal nerve. The hypoglossal nerve innervates the muscles of the tongue (*see* Bradley's NiCP, 7th edn, Ch. 104, pp. 1720–1734).

29. B. Clinical trials are important for advancing medical knowledge, and participation in trials requires informed consent from the patient and/or caregivers. No trials should be conducted on patients against their will, even if their caregiver consents to the study. Participation should be voluntary, so threatening to withhold other care from the patient or placing patients on medications without their consent is unethical. Promising improvement is misleading because the drug is unproven and the patient may end up on placebo.

30. C. Clozapine is an atypical antipsychotic that is usually reserved for refractory cases of schizophrenia and used in the treatment of severe hallucinations in Parkinson disease. It may be more effective than other antipsychotics, but is associated with a more severe risk profile, including agranulocytosis. As such, treatment with clozapine requires weekly complete blood count monitoring during the first 6 months, and continued frequent monitoring thereafter (*see* Bradley's NiCP, 7th edn, Ch. 10, pp. 92–114).

31. C. Value-based purchasing (previously known as pay for performance or P4P) is a model of payment in which physicians are not paid per procedure, but rather per successful achievement of prespecified metrics. An example of this would be maintaining a recent hemoglobin A1C on every diabetic patient in one's practice. Fee for service is the most common model of payment, in which each episode of care is reimbursed, regardless of quality metrics. ACOs are groups of physicians and hospitals that partner to provide care to a group of patients, with monetary incentives for safe and cost-containing care. Capitation is a payment model that was common in which (usually primary care) physicians were paid a flat rate for ongoing care of a patient, regardless of the number of visits or procedures performed. Bundled payments are meant to cover all costs for the uncomplicated treatment of a single disease and are most frequently used for acute and postdischarge care.

32. A. The patient is displaying characteristics of normal bereavement. This can involve intense sadness, preoccupation with the deceased or cause of death, emotional numbness, inability to reminisce positively about the deceased, excessive avoidance, a desire to die to be with the deceased, feeling of meaninglessness, reluctance to pursue interests, or loss of identity. Patients may even have hallucinations involving the deceased. A brief psychotic disorder is the sudden onset of delusions or hallucinations lasting less than a month and not associated with another mental illness or substance. Major depressive disorder involves low mood, anhedonia, feelings of worthlessness, suicidal ideation, guilt, helplessness, decreased libido, and changes to appetite and sleep, but the symptoms must last for at least 2 weeks and must be functionally disabling. Adjustment disorder involves a response of anxiety or depression out of proportion to a given stressor. Although the patient has auditory hallucinations, she does not have disorganized thinking or delusions (the hallmarks of schizophrenia), and is older than the expected age for new-onset schizophrenia.

33. C. Sensitivity and specificity are important concepts to understand and are easily confused. Specificity is the true negative rate, or the percentage of correctly identified negative patients. Specificity is calculated by dividing the number of true negative results by the total number of false-positive results plus true negative results. A high specificity means there is a low false-positive rate, so a positive result in a highly specific test helps rule in a disorder. Sensitivity is a measure of the true positive rate, or the percentage of correctly identified positive patients. It is calculated by dividing the number of true positives by the true positives plus the false negatives. A high sensitivity means most patients with a disorder are positive (low false-negative rate), so a negative test result helps rule out a disorder. The following chart shows how these calculations are made.

TABLE FOR ANSWER 5.33

	Disease is present	Disease is not present
Positive result	True positive (TP)	False positive (FP)
Negative result	False negative (FN)	True negative (TN)

Specificity = TN/(FP + TN)
Sensitivity = TP/(TP + FN)
Positive predictive value = TP/(FP + TP)
Negative predictive value = TN/(FN + TN)

34. C. The Crede maneuver (nonforceful suprapubic pressure) is not recommended for neurogenic bladder dysfunction, as it may result in elevated detrusor pressure and incomplete bladder emptying. The other methods listed in the question are all generally considered helpful

ways to cope (and retrain the bladder, in some cases) with neurogenic bladder dysfunction (*see* Bradley's NiCP, 7th edn, Ch. 47, pp. 605–621).

35. E. Type IV fibers (previously known as C fibers) are unmyelinated fibers that transmit pain and temperature signals at a speed of 0.5–2.0 m/sec. Type Ia fibers are large, well-myelinated fibers that transmit proprioception from muscle spindles to the spinal cord. Type Ib fibers transmit proprioception from Golgi tendon organs back to the spinal cord. Type II fibers are small, myelinated fibers that transmit pressure and touch sensation from the skin. Type III fibers are small, thinly myelinated fibers that transmit pain and temperature sensation (*see* Bradley's NiCP, 7th edn, Ch. 54, pp. 720–741).

36. C. CRPS is a disorder characterized by pain, swelling, skin changes, vasomotor instability, and patchy bone demineralization beginning after an injury, surgery, or vascular event. There are two types of CRPS: type 1 (previously called *reflex sympathetic dystrophy*) occurs without a definable nerve lesion, and type 2 occurs in a definable nerve lesion. Although the pathophysiology is incompletely understood, some studies suggest an increased level of neuropeptides such as substance P, interleukin-6, and tumor necrosis factor-alpha. There also appears to be a central maladaptive change in pain processing. Patients describe pain with burning, throbbing, aching, and sensitivity to cold and touch, as well as swelling of affected limbs with altered color and temperature (stage 1). Later, patients have more edema, thickening of skin, and muscle wasting (stage 2), and finally limitations in movement and contractures (stage 3). The diagnosis is made with a combination of history, autonomic testing (thermoregulatory sweat testing, resting skin temperature, and quantitative sudomotor axon reflex test), and imaging (magnetic resonance imaging and bone scintigraphy; *see* Bradley's NiCP, 7th edn, Ch. 54, pp. 720–741).

37. B. Demyelinating polyneuropathy is not commonly associated with cardiac bypass. Strokes in this setting are generally embolic, with risk varying by surgery type, as well as medical comorbidities. Brachial plexopathy is generally associated with traction or compression injury, causing upper extremity weakness and/or numbness. Acute encephalopathy may present in 3%–32% of patients after cardiac bypass, depending on the series. Chronic cognitive disturbance, sometimes known as *postpump syndrome*, may be identified in the first several weeks after bypass. Cognitive disturbance has been reported in 3%–79% of patients after bypass, depending on the series. Seizures are reported in 0.5%–3.5% of patients after coronary artery bypass surgery (*see* Bradley's NiCP, 7th edn, Ch. 58, pp. 814–834).

38. B. The attacks of paroxysmal hemicrania are generally 2–30 minutes in duration and occur up to 11 times per day, whereas cluster headache attacks are 30–180 minutes in duration and occur 1–8 times per day, and SUNCT attacks last 1–10 minutes and occur up to 100 times per day. The prevalence of paroxysmal hemicrania is roughly equal between genders, although cluster headaches are much more common in men than in women (3 : 1), and SUNCT slightly more common in men than in women (1.5 : 1). Cluster headaches often have both circadian and circannual periodicity, but not paroxysmal hemicrania or SUNCT. Cluster headaches improve with sumatriptan as an abortive therapy in up

to 90% of cases, but rarely do paroxysmal hemicrania or SUNCT improve with sumatriptan (*see* Bradley's NiCP, 7th edn, Ch. 103, pp. 1686–1719).

39. A. The ONTT demonstrated that high-dose IV methylprednisolone led to faster vision recovery than did oral prednisone. Additionally, this trial demonstrated a greatly increased risk of developing multiple sclerosis based on the presence and number of white matter lesions on initial magnetic resonance imaging (MRI). Although plasma exchange may be used in cases of refractory flares of demyelinating disease, it is not associated with shorter length of stay, and its efficacy over other treatments is not definitive. The ONTT did not specifically study bilateral optic neuritis, although we now know that this should prompt evaluation for aquaporin-4 antibodies (neuromyelitis optica). Although lesion burden on MRI does relate to the risk of developing multiple sclerosis, visual acuity does not relate to this risk. The retinal nerve fiber layer may thin (as seen on ocular coherence tomography) with history of optic neuritis, although this information was not a component of the ONTT.

40. C. The basal ganglia is a common location for primary intracerebral hemorrhage related to hypertension, which accounts for up to 10% of all strokes. Other common sites of hemorrhage include the pons, thalamus, cerebellum, and the deep subcortical structures. Pathologically, hypertension-related primary intracranial hemorrhages occur because of lipohyalinosis of the deep perforating arteries, which makes these small vessels highly sensitive to sudden changes in blood pressure. Venous sinus thrombosis can certainly lead to hemorrhage, but typically occurs in the territory of a draining vein. Atrial fibrillation could lead to hemorrhage, but most often is a secondary phenomenon after ischemia occurs. Anticoagulation can cause hemorrhage in any territory, but is a common cause for lobar hemorrhages and subdural hemorrhages. Amyloid angiopathy leads to amyloid deposition and microhemorrhages usually in the cortical regions of the brain (rather than the subcortical as in this case; *see* Bradley's NiCP, 7th edn, Ch. 66, pp. 968–990). Figure from Movalia M, O'Connell TX 2013 *Brochert's Crush Step 3*, 4th edn, Saunders, with permission.

41. C. Krabbe disease is a rare, autosomal-recessive sphingolipidosis, associated with *GALC* mutations, leading to a deficiency in the galactosylceramidase enzyme. Infants with Krabbe disease are generally normal at birth, but develop signs of progressive decline by 3 to 6 months of age, including irritability, spasticity, seizures, deafness, blindness, difficulty feeding, and developmental delay. The buildup of psychosine that results from this enzymatic deficiency causes demyelination and neuronal degeneration, and multinucleated globoid cells are commonly seen. Treatment is generally supportive for Krabbe disease, although there are early signs that bone marrow transplantation may be beneficial. Niemann-Pick disease is an autosomal-recessive deficiency in sphingomyelinase that is frequently seen in Ashkenazi Jews and leads to damaging accumulation of sphingomyelin, causing ataxia, dysarthria, dysphagia, dystonia, loss of milestones, and hepatosplenomegaly. Histologically, Niemann-Pick disease may show "sea-blue histiocytes" in the marrow due to lipid-laden

"foamy" macrophages. Canavan disease is an autosomal-recessive deficiency of the aminoacylase 2 enzyme that is commonly seen in Ashkenazi Jews, resulting in elevated levels of N-acetyl aspartate and resultant intellectual disability, motor milestone loss, paralysis, and blindness. Macrocephaly is commonly seen with Canavan disease, as well as vacuolization of white matter. Fabry disease is the only X-linked lipid storage disease, resulting from a mutation in the *GLA* gene that leads to alpha-galactosidase A deficiency. Symptoms are milder than the other diseases mentioned in the question, and include renal insufficiency, cardiomyopathy, cutaneous angiokeratomas, and painful neuropathy. Glycolipid storage can be seen in neurons pathologically. Metachromatic leukodystrophy is an autosomal-recessive mutation in the gene for the arylsulfatase A enzyme, leading to accumulation of cerebroside sulfate in the myelin of the brain and peripheral nerves. Symptoms include motor milestone regression in the second year of life, followed by spasticity, blindness, seizures, and ultimately coma and death around the age of 5 years. Pathologically, sulfatide deposits can be seen in the brain (*see* Bradley's NiCP, 7th edn, Ch. 91, pp. 1324–1341).

42. E. ACOs are a model of patient care in which physicians or hospitals join together to provide comprehensive care to a group of patients, with financial reimbursement tied to patient safety and cost containment. This model has been around for many years, but was recently made a greater priority through the Affordable Care Act. HMOs are a type of insurance plan in which patients are incentivized to receive as much of their care as possible from a single primary care provider, with a limited network of specialists available if a referral is made by the primary care provider. PPOs and POSs are similar types of insurance plans in which the network of covered specialists is larger and no referral is necessary for their consultation, but premiums tend to be higher than for HMOs. Indemnity plans are another type of insurance plan that provide more flexibility for which doctors the patient can visit, but pay only a percentage of the cost for a given visit or test. The cost of certain services is often higher with an indemnity plan, and there tends to be more paperwork required of patients.

43. C. Myasthenia gravis (MG) is caused by circulating antibodies against acetylcholine receptors, leading to complement-mediated destruction of acetylcholine receptors, as well as neuromuscular junctional folds in which the receptors are generally found. This results in a simplification of the postsynaptic region such that even with additional acetylcholine patients may not regain full strength. As such, treatment of the underlying autoimmune activity, as well as symptomatic treatment, is important in MG. The other listed diagnoses are not associated with specific electron microscopic changes in the neuromuscular junction (*see* Bradley's NiCP, 7th edn, Ch. 109, pp. 1896–1914). Figure from Mori S, Shigemoto K Mechanisms associated with the pathogenicity of antibodies against muscle-specific kinase in myasthenia gravis. *Autoimmunity Reviews* 2013; 12(9): 912–917, with permission.

44. A. Foster Kennedy syndrome is the constellation of headaches, ipsilateral central scotoma, ipsilateral optic atrophy, contralateral papilledema, and ipsilateral

anosmia. This is often related to an inferior frontal tumor, such as an olfactory groove meningioma. Although complicated migraine may involve headache and visual scotoma, it is unlikely to cause papilledema. The presence of papilledema and optic disc atrophy argue against conversion disorder, which should be reserved as a diagnosis of exclusion. Idiopathic intracranial hypertension generally causes bilateral papilledema, although vision loss may be either unilateral or bilateral. It is also associated with overweight individuals or those taking birth control or retinoic acid. Venous sinus thrombosis often presents similarly to idiopathic intracranial hypertension, with headaches, vision loss, and bilateral papilledema. Venous sinus thrombosis may be related to an underlying primary hypercoagulable disorder, pregnancy, birth control pills, severe dehydration, infection (in the case of Lemierre's syndrome, which is a gram-negative rod infection that travels from the oral cavity into the jugular vein and cephalad thereafter), or other causes (*see* Bradley's NiCP, 7th edn, Ch. 44, pp. 528–572).

45. D. This nerve conduction study demonstrates a Martin Gruber anastomosis (MGA), which is a normal variant. In this variant, ulnar nerve fibers travel with the median nerve proximally and cross over to the ulnar nerve in the forearm. This results in characteristic nerve conduction abnormalities that must be recognized, with a median compound muscle action potential (CMAP) that is of lower amplitude at the wrist than at the elbow, and the appearance of an ulnar conduction block in the forearm. This pattern emerges because median stimulation at the elbow stimulates both the median nerve and the extra ulnar fibers, resulting in a large response when recording over the thenar eminence. With median stimulation at the wrist, the ulnar fibers have crossed to rejoin the ulnar nerve, so the median CMAP recorded at the thenar eminence is significantly smaller. The ulnar response is large when stimulated at the wrist compared with the elbow because the fibers that traveled initially with the median nerve have rejoined the ulnar nerve at the wrist. This gives an apparent drop in amplitude with proximal stimulation, which can be confused with a conduction block (*see* Bradley's NiCP, 7th edn, Ch. 35, pp. 366–390).

46. D. Although congenital absence of the thymus is associated with profound immunodeficiency, postpubertal thymectomy patients do not have an increased risk of severe infections. Whereas the thymus plays an important role in T-cell education in developing humans, it is generally not recommended to remove it until after puberty. Thymoma is associated with various paraneoplastic syndromes, including paraneoplastic myasthenia gravis, Lambert-Eaton myasthenic syndrome, and sensory neuropathy. Regardless of whether thymoma is present or not, removal of the thymus is associated with an 80%–90% remission rate for myasthenia gravis (*see* Bradley's NiCP, 7th edn, Ch. 109, pp. 1896–1914).

47. B. Ethambutol is associated with a toxic optic neuropathy that may cause loss of visual acuity, field defects (including central scotoma), and dyschromatopsia (difficulty discerning colors). One should discontinue ethambutol immediately upon visual complaints, because further treatment may lead to progressive and possibly irreversible blindness.

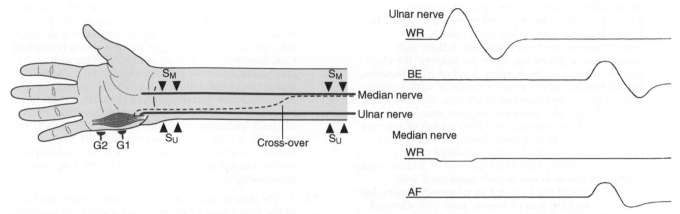

Figure for Answer 5.45 Crossover of median-to-ulnar fibers supplying the hypothenar muscles may occur in MGA. During routine ulnar motor studies, recording the abductor digiti minimi and stimulating the ulnar nerve (S$_U$) at the wrist (WR) and below-elbow (BE) sites, the ulnar CMAP amplitude with BE stimulation is lower than with WR stimulation. If an MGA is not recognized, a mistaken impression of a conduction block may occur. To demonstrate an MGA in this situation, the median nerve is stimulated (S$_M$) at the WR and antecubital fossa (AF) while recording the hypothenar muscles, looking for a CMAP stimulating at the AF that is not present stimulating at the WR. *(from Preston DC, Shapiro BE 2013* Electromyography and Neuromuscular Disorders, *Saunders, with permission.)*

Isoniazid, a perennial component of antituberculous therapy, competes with vitamin B6 as a cofactor of synaptic neurotransmission. Further, vitamin B6 levels may decrease while on this therapy. Although vitamin B6 deficiency may be associated with peripheral neuropathy, there is no such association with optic neuropathy or blindness. Hereditary optic neuropathy is an autosomal-dominant cause of slow, bilateral vision loss. In the absence of a reported family history, this choice is unlikely. Ocular tuberculosis generally results from untreated (or undertreated) systemic tuberculosis, and may cause chorioretinitis or choroiditis. Given that the patient is on therapy, this is less likely. Methanol may cause severe vision loss within 24 hours of ingestion due to toxic optic neuropathy from formaldehyde, the byproduct of alcohol dehydrogenase. However, no ingestion was mentioned in the question stem (*see* Bradley's NiCP, 7th edn, Ch. 17, pp. 163–178).

48. C. Amphetamine intoxication (i.e. meth, ice, speed) can lead to euphoria, impaired judgment, tachycardia, and pupillary dilation, as well as formication (sensation of crawling bugs). There is typically a high followed by a crash involving withdrawal symptoms, including depression, suicidal thoughts, and sleep disturbances. Other systemic effects include rhabdomyolysis, seizures, cerebral infarctions, cerebral hemorrhages, and movement disorders such as akathisia, chorea, and bruxism. Schizophrenia and Huntington disease may have hallucinations and chorea, respectively, but would not typically have the autonomic dysfunction seen in this case. Heroin intoxication would cause the clinical opposite of amphetamine intoxication, including hypotension, pinpoint pupils, and somnolence. Common heroin withdrawal symptoms include dysphoric mood, nausea, vomiting, lacrimation, rhinorrhea, pupillary dilatation, piloerection "goosebumps," and yawning. Cannabis intoxication typically causes a mellow high with conjunctival injection, increased appetite, dry mouth, memory impairment, decreased attention, and poor insight/judgment (*see* Bradley's NiCP, 7th edn, Ch. 87, pp. 1254–1260).

49. D. The patient presents with progressive memory loss and psychosis with HIV. Imaging and spinal fluid analysis rule out an opportunistic infection as the cause of her memory loss. This situation is most consistent with HIV dementia, which frequently presents with delirium, psychosis, and progressive memory loss. Patients with a high viral load, anemia, and low CD4 count are at greater risk of dementia. Highly active antiretroviral therapy may prevent the progression of the disease once it has begun, but it will not reverse prior damage. Although MRI should not show significant abnormalities other than atrophy, MR spectroscopy shows an increase in both myoinositol and choline with a relative decrease in N-acetylaspartate (*see* Bradley's NiCP, 7th edn, Ch. 77, pp. 1102–1120).

50. A. The striatum (also known as *striate nucleus*) is composed of the caudate and putamen, which are closely related embryologically. Physically, the caudate and putamen are separated by the internal capsule, although cellular bridges connect the two structures and give a striped appearance, leading to the structure's name. The striatum is the hub for nearly all input to the basal ganglia. The putamen and globus pallidus are together known as the *lentiform* or *lenticular nuclei*. The thalamus (specifically the anterior thalamic nucleus) and mammillary bodies are two components of the Papez circuit, a critical network for memory formation. The red nuclei and inferior olivary nuclei are two of three components of the triangle of Guillain-Mollaret (the third is the dentate), which is an important feedback circuit for modulating spinal cord motor activity. Additionally of interest, a lesion in the triangle of Guillain-Mollaret uniquely causes palatal myoclonus, one of the only movement disorders that does not disappear with sleep. The ventral posterolateral thalamic nucleus and medial lemniscus are two components of dorsal column sensory systems, which transmit vibration and joint position sense (*see* Bradley's NiCP, 7th edn, Ch. 96, pp. 1422–1460).

51. E. The patient most likely had a breath-holding spell. These are very common in infants and young children from 6 months of age to 6 years of age. Typically, the

child will become angry or upset in response to injury. There is usually a brief period of crying followed by breath holding with apnea and cyanosis. Loss of consciousness and hypotonia may follow with myoclonus or posturing. After the episode, the child quickly returns to the baseline level of consciousness. Breath-holding spells may be confused with seizures, but are generally provoked or elicited, whereas seizures are not. Video electroencephalogram monitoring is normal in these individuals. Other causes of syncope such as cardiac arrhythmias should be considered, especially if the episodes are prolonged or frequent or if there is a family history of syncope or sudden cardiac death. Cataplexy is not usually associated with discoloration of the face or loss of consciousness, but may have sudden loss of muscle tone with elevated emotions. There is no indication that these events occur after eating, which would be more common for Sandifer syndrome (*see* Bradley's NiCP, 7th edn, Ch. 2, pp. 8–16).

52. C. GAD is characterized by excessive anxiety and worry for at least 6 months in duration, along with difficulty controlling worry. At least three of the following symptoms must be present: restlessness, easy fatigability, decreased concentration, irritability, muscle tension, and sleep disturbance. GAD is more common in women than men and very common in the younger years. Treatment includes selective serotonin reuptake inhibitors, serotonin-norepinephrine reuptake inhibitors, beta-blockers, benzodiazepines, and psychotherapy, including insight-oriented therapy. Panic disorder is less likely, as the patient's worry is constant, whereas panic disorder is characterized by intermittent episodes. Although major depressive disorder may share similar features with GAD, many of the symptoms in GAD revolve around worry rather than severe mood symptoms, although the two may coexist. In OCD, the obsessions (intrusive thoughts) and compulsions (actions) are not simply excessive real-life worries, but may also involve behaviors such as turning a light on and off several times before exiting a room. In hypochondriasis, there is a preoccupation with developing a serious condition or disease for at least 6 months, often resulting from misinterpretation of minor symptoms.

53. D. MAO-A is an important enzyme in the oxidation of monoamines, and is found in neurons, glia, and various other organs. Monoamines oxidized by MAO-A include dopamine, serotonin, melatonin, epinephrine, norepinephrine, tyramine, and tryptamine. Monoamine oxidase inhibitors prevent these oxidation reactions, and thereby increase levels of serotonin, norepinephrine, and dopamine, and result in improved mood. Glutamate is broken down either by transamination or deamination for the production of alpha-ketoglutarate.

54. C. The MRI depicts lissencephaly, a migrational disorder during brain development that leads to few or no gyri. Clinical consequences of lissencephaly include seizures, developmental delay, failure to thrive, dysphagia, tone abnormalities, and weakness. There are multiple types of lissencephaly, ranging from toxic etiologies to genetic etiologies. Lissencephaly due to the *LIS1* gene mutation may be seen in isolation or as a part of Miller-Dieker syndrome, which is a larger deletion event consisting of lissencephaly, microcephaly, seizures, craniofacial abnormalities, and cardiac defects. Mutations in

doublecortin (*DCX*) also cause lissencephaly. If males have this mutation, they develop lissencephaly. If heterozygous females have this mutation, they develop subcortical-band heterotopia (double cortex syndrome). Cobblestone lissencephaly is a specific type with alternating regions of polymicrogyria and pachygyria with a thin cortex, which is associated with syndromic congenital muscular dystrophies (CMDs), including Fukuyama CMD, muscle-eye-brain disease, and Walker-Warburg syndrome (*see* Bradley's NiCP, 7th edn, Ch. 89, pp. 1279–1300). Figure from Mochida FH 2009 Genetics and biology of microcephaly and lissencephaly. *Seminars in Pediatric Neurology* 16(3): 120–126, with permission.

55. A. The dentate nucleus is the primary output nucleus of the cerebellum responsible for control of voluntary movement. The fastigial nucleus is involved with the vestibular nuclei controlling eye movements and estimating body movement in space. The globose and emboliform nuclei help coordinate agonist/antagonist pairs of muscles involuntarily. The red nucleus is not in the cerebellum, but is a relay center for many of the cerebellar paths, including the dentate nucleus, globose nucleus, and emboliform nucleus (*see* Bradley's NiCP, 7th edn, Ch. 97, pp. 1461–1483).

56. C. The atypical antipsychotics act similarly to the typical antipsychotics, though they usually have weaker affinity for antagonizing the D_2 receptor. The atypicals include aripiprazole, clozapine, quetiapine, olanzapine, risperidone, and ziprasidone. Aripiprazole is a partial agonist at D_2 and 5HT1A receptors, and an antagonist at 5HT2A receptors. It serves as a medium- to high-potency agent that is often used as an adjunct treatment in depression. Clozapine is a low-potency antipsychotic that has very little (if any) risk of extrapyramidal symptoms, and therefore is a good choice for treating psychosis associated with Parkinson disease. However, clozapine carries an increased risk of agranulocytosis, so blood counts must be collected weekly after starting this drug. Also, clozapine carries a risk of seizures and is therefore largely contraindicated in those with poorly-controlled epilepsy. Quetiapine is also a low-potency agent that, similar to clozapine, serves as a good agent for treating psychosis in those with Parkinson disease. Olanzapine is a medium- to high-potency agent that is known for causing weight gain, but causes fewer extrapyramidal symptoms than high-potency agents. Risperidone is a high-potency agent that can cause an increase in prolactin and sexual dysfunction. However, Risperdal works well for both positive and negative symptoms of schizophrenia. Ziprasidone is also good for both positive and negative symptoms, but can lead to QT prolongation.

57. E. The fascicles of the facial nerve exit the facial nucleus in the lower pons and travel anteriorly to wrap around the abducens nucleus before turning posterior laterally to exit the pons. This and surrounding structures are seen in the figure (*see* Bradley's NiCP, 7th edn, Ch. 104, pp. 1720–1735).

58. B. Diagnosis of Menke syndrome usually shows a *low* copper and *low* ceruloplasmin. Menke syndrome is an X-linked recessive neurodegenerative condition that results in the maldistribution of copper in the body due to a mutation in the *MNK* gene on the X chromosome. Ultimately, this leads to defective copper integration into copper-dependent enzymes. Clinically

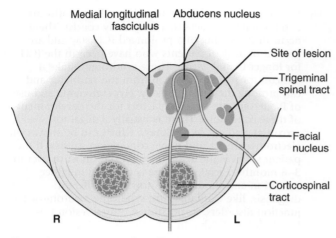

Medial longitudinal fasciculus

Abducens nucleus

Site of lesion

Trigeminal spinal tract

Facial nucleus

Corticospinal tract

R   L

Figure for Answer 5.57 *(from Tacik P, Alfieri A, Funke AD, Stock K, Kornhuber M 2013 Paradoxical activity of the masseter muscles due to upper motor neuron involvement. Clinical Neurology and Neurosurgery 115(4): 484–486, with permission.)*

patients have "kinky" hair that is often colorless and friable. Other manifestations include delayed milestones; hypotonia; seizures (focal clonic and infantile spasms); failure to thrive; skeletal abnormalities; ocular abnormalities such as iris hypoplasia and hypopigmentation; and vascular defects such as arterial rupture, aneurysms, and thrombosis. Spontaneous subdural hematomas can occur and may be mistaken for nonaccidental trauma. Treatment focuses on copper supplementation and genetic counseling. Unfortunately, despite the fact that body copper levels normalize with supplementation, the condition generally progresses and leads to infections, vascular complications, neurological degeneration, and ultimately death during childhood. Notably, Wilson disease relates to copper ATPase dysfunction and results in an accumulation of copper into tissues (*see* Bradley's NiCP, 7th edn, Ch. 91, pp. 1324–1341).

59. B. Donepezil is a predominantly centrally acting acetylcholinesterase inhibitor (AChEI) used in the treatment of Alzheimer-related dementia, and frequently used off-label in patients with other types of memory loss (although less proven and less effective). Common side effects include nausea, vomiting, anorexia, and weight loss. One of the rare, more severe, side effects is an increased risk of seizures. As such, donepezil should be used with caution in patients with a history of seizures. Further, it should not be combined with other AChEIs, including rivastigmine and galantamine, because this greatly increases the risk of seizures. Clopidogrel has no risk of seizures and would not lower the level of levetiracetam. Warfarin is commonly affected by hepatically metabolized antiepileptics, like phenytoin or carbamazepine, but it does not lower the level of levetiracetam. Verapamil is a potent hepatic enzyme inhibitor that can alter levels of some antiepileptics, but it would not affect levetiracetam because it is not hepatically metabolized. Rifampin is a potent hepatic enzyme inducer that can lower levels of antiepileptic drugs, but it would not affect levetiracetam (*see* Bradley's NiCP, 7th edn, Ch. 92, pp. 1342–1348).

60. B. Cauda equina and conus medullaris syndromes are similar lumbar spinal syndromes that are easy to

confuse. They can have the same etiologies such as lumbar disc disease or infections like abscesses, meningeal tumors, hematomas, or other mass lesions in the lumbar spinal region. Cauda equina is a syndrome of compression of nerve roots below the termination of the spinal cord with resulting weakness, numbness, and late-onset incontinence that progresses in a slow and insidious manner unless precipitated by acute trauma. Because this involves compression of nerve roots, reflexes are usually lost. Conus medullaris syndrome is a rapidly progressive syndrome of weakness, numbness, and very early sphincter dysfunction. Being a disease of the conus medullaris and not nerve roots, reflexes, particularly the patellar reflex, can be preserved. Conus medullaris syndrome is caused by infiltrative lesions of the conus medullaris itself, such as tumors like lymphoma, or external compression, such as by disc disease, or extramedullary tumors (e.g. dural-based; *see* Bradley's NiCP, 7th edn, Ch. 26, pp. 273–278).

61. C. Lambert-Eaton myasthenic syndrome (LEMS) typically presents as a paraneoplastic syndrome in middle-age adults in association with small cell lung cancer. This disorder can present in the young either as an autoimmune disorder or in association with testicular or ovarian cancers. LEMS is caused by voltage-gated P/Q calcium channel antibodies, which disrupt the presynaptic influx of calcium and lead to decreased acetylcholine release. With repeated contraction more acetylcholine is released, leading to a stronger contraction (facilitation). This may be seen on physical examination either by increasing strength with repeated contractions or by return of absent reflexes with repeated contraction. On nerve conduction studies, compound muscle action potentials (CMAPs) are generally very low amplitude and show facilitation (an increase in amplitude >200% baseline) with brief exercise or 50 Hz stimulation. Myasthenia, on the other hand, usually has normal reflexes, normal CMAPs, and worsening strength with repeated contractions. McArdle disease is a metabolic myopathy from excessive glycogen storage in the muscles, and clinically presents with cramps and weakness with short exercise followed by a "second wind" effect. Charcot-Marie-Tooth type 2a is a hereditary axonal neuropathy that generally has absent reflexes and abnormal low-amplitude nerve conduction studies in both motor and sensory nerves. Becker muscular dystrophy is a disorder with partially functional dystrophin, leading to progressive weakness. Testing would not show reflex abnormalities, and would not show facilitation (*see* Bradley's NiCP, 7th edn, Ch. 109, pp. 1896–1914).

62. C. Isoniazid, which is a common agent used in the treatment of tuberculosis, can precipitate a pyridoxine deficiency (B6) but not a thiamine (B1) deficiency. The rest of the listed conditions are all significant risk factors for thiamine deficiency. In addition to those listed in the question, other conditions associated with thiamine deficiency include prolonged intravenous feeding, systemic malignancy, anorexia, dieting, and acquired immunodeficiency syndrome (*see* Bradley's NiCP, 7th edn, Ch. 85, pp. 1226–1236).

63. E. The patient likely has Creutzfeldt-Jakob disease (CJD), a prion disease that leads to rapidly progressive dementia. The most common type of CJD is so-called *sporadic CJD* in 85% of cases, in which patients have no

risk factors for CJD. Hereditary CJD accounts for 5%–10% of cases, resulting from a genetic mutation. Finally, acquired CJD (as occurred after corneal transplant from an affected individual) describes transmission of CJD through exposure to brain or nervous system tissue, usually through certain medical procedures. The MRI pictured has classic fluid attenuated inversion recovery (FLAIR) hyperintensity in the thalamus (pulvinar sign). Other areas commonly seen with FLAIR hyperintensity include the cortex (especially insular) and the caudate. Pathologically, CJD is known for spongiform changes and extensive vacuolization, especially in the cortex and deep gray matter. Negri bodies are eosinophilic cytoplasmic inclusion bodies seen in rabies encephalitis. Cowdry type A bodies are eosinophilic nuclear inclusions seen in herpes infection (*see* Bradley's NiCP, 7th edn, Ch. 94, pp. 1365–1379). Figure from Bosque and Tyler Prions and prion disease of the central nervous system (transmissible neurodegenerative disease). In: Bennett J, Dolin R, Blaser M 2015 *Mandell, Douglas, and Bennett's Principles and Practice of Infectious Diseases*, 8th edn, Saunders, pp. 2142–2153, figure 181-3, with permission.

64. C. Procedures can be performed on medical students for educational purposes, but those students should be treated as if they are patients themselves. Participation in any procedure must be voluntary, not tied to evaluation, and students should not have to provide any reasons for nonparticipation. Before the procedure, there should be a thorough explanation of the testing, invasiveness, meaning of results, and how abnormal results will be handled. All results should remain confidential (AMA Code of Medical Ethics).

65. C. Fabry disease is an X-linked lipid storage disorder associated with alpha-galactosidase-A deficiency, leading to harmful buildup of lipids in various tissues, including peripheral and autonomic nerves. Treatment with recombinant alpha-galactosidase-A is available and helps symptoms of Fabry disease, though its effect on disease-related survival is not clear. Refsum disease is caused by deficiency of phytanoyl-CoA hydroxylase, leading to a buildup of phytanic acid in the plasma and symptoms of peripheral neuropathy, tinnitus, anosmia, night blindness, and ichthyosis. This disease is inherited in an autosomal-recessive disorder, and there are no enzyme replacements available to date. The porphyrias are composed of various disorders of heme breakdown leading to buildup of harmful by-products in various tissues (depending on the affected enzyme), which may include the peripheral nervous system, causing acute sensorimotor mononeuropathies. Depending on the causative gene, porphyria may be transmitted autosomal dominantly or recessively or X-linked. To date, no replacement therapies are available for any of the deficient enzymes that cause porphyria. HNPP is an autosomal-dominant neuropathy due to a deletion in the *PMP22* gene, which affects myelin function, causing increased sensitivity to pressure on nerves. There is no enzymatic contribution to HNPP. CMT is a group of diseases causing hereditary sensory and motor neuropathies autosomal dominantly, recessively, or X-linked, depending on the affected gene and neuropathy subtype. There are no enzyme treatments for CMT (*see* Bradley's NiCP, 7th edn, Ch. 107, pp. 1791–1866).

66. E. Critical illness polyneuropathy and myopathy are two separate disorders that frequently coexist. These occur in the setting of a prolonged ICU stay and are present in 50% of patients who have been in the ICU for longer than 2 weeks. These syndromes make it difficult for patients to wean from the ventilator and can prolong their hospital stay. Hyperglycemia and use of IV steroids are also risk factors for the development of these conditions. There is usually a distal-to-proximal gradient of weakness, which can be shown on electromyography and nerve conduction studies. If the patient survives the acute hospital stay, most recover in 3–6 months. Facial weakness is not seen in either condition and should point toward a different diagnosis, like Guillain-Barré syndrome, neuromuscular junction disorders, or possibly a central lesion (*see* Bradley's NiCP, 7th edn, Ch. 107, pp. 1791–1866 and Ch. 110, pp. 1915–1956).

67. E. The patient is feigning illness in hopes of having external secondary gain (money in this case), thus characterizing malingering. In factitious disorders symptoms are also intentionally feigned, but motivated by the satisfaction of being in the role of a patient. Munchausen's syndrome is a chronic form of factitious disorder. Munchausen's by proxy is the provocation of physical signs and symptoms in another individual for the satisfaction of the second person being a patient. Conversion disorder is the development of physical signs and symptoms at a subconscious or involuntary level. Somatization is the development of a number of somatic complaints involving pain in multiple systems (gastrointestinal, sexual, and neurological). These symptoms are also produced at the subconscious level. Hypochondriasis is a preoccupation with developing a serious condition or disease for at least 6 months, often resulting from misinterpretation of minor symptoms.

68. A. This patient presents with reversible cerebral vasoconstriction syndrome (RCVS). RCVS is also known as postpartum cerebral angiopathy, or Call-Fleming syndrome. This is a relatively uncommon condition that can occur in the first 4 weeks postpartum. It presents with a severe "thunderclap" headache that reaches peak intensity immediately. It can behave similar to a migraine with nausea, photophobia, and phonophobia. However, this is commonly associated with seizures, encephalopathy, ischemic strokes, and hemorrhagic strokes. This stem could also have easily been used to describe a cerebral venous sinus thrombosis, subarachnoid hemorrhage, and possibly eclampsia, but none of the answers were consistent with that possibility. Angiogram, whether CT, MR, or conventional, would show beading of blood vessels. MRI can show multifocal acute ischemic hemorrhagic strokes and subarachnoid hemorrhages. CSF low-pressure headaches are possible either from a spontaneous leak or continuous leak after epidural during delivery. An LP with high white cells and protein is suggestive of meningitis, which should also be a consideration, but this patient is afebrile without neck stiffness. Dawson's fingers are seen in multiple sclerosis, not RCVS. An enlarged pituitary gland with low T1 signal is consistent with Sheehan's syndrome, which would not cause encephalopathy or focal weakness (*see* Bradley's NiCP, Ch. 112, pp. 1973–1991).

69. B. Early treatment of seizures with benzodiazepines can stop seizure activity by activating inhibitory GABA$_A$ receptors. During prolonged seizures there is an alteration in the expression of GABA$_A$ receptors, reducing their functional ability, and therefore reducing the ability of benzodiazepines to stop prolonged seizures. NMDA, voltage-gated calcium channels, acetylcholine receptors, and alpha-2 receptors do not have a significant role in the refractory nature of status epilepticus (*see* Bradley's NiCP, 7th edn, Ch. 34, pp. 348–366).

70. A. Bortezomib, used to treat multiple myeloma and other hematological malignancies, is associated with painful sensorimotor neuropathy. Other agents that may cause similar symptoms include vinca alkaloids or taxanes. Although cisplatin causes painful sensory neuropathy, there is no associated motor component. Bevacizumab, temozolomide, and lomustine have no commonly associated neuropathies (*see* Bradley's NiCP, 7th edn, Ch. 107, pp. 1791–1866).

71. C. Few disorders can cause restricted diffusion to the gray matter (also known as *cortical ribboning*), and Creutzfeldt-Jakob disease is one of those causes. Other potential causes of cortical ribboning include anoxic injury, cortical stroke, postictal state, herpes simplex virus encephalitis, meningoencephalitis, and rarely, genetic conditions like mitochondrial myopathy, encephalopathy, and acidosis with strokelike episodes. Frontotemporal dementia, Huntington disease, Alzheimer disease, and dementia with Lewy bodies do not cause restricted diffusion (*see* Bradley's NiCP, 7th edn, Ch. 39, pp. 411–458). Figure from Wada R, Kucharczyk W 2008 Prion infections of the brain. *Neuroimaging Clinics of North America* 18(1): 183–191, with permission.

72. C. The patient has trigeminal neuralgia, a painful condition characterized by paroxysms of pain in the trigeminal nerve distribution, most often in the V2 distribution. The pain is short, stereotyped, and usually unilateral. Most cases are idiopathic, but some are secondary and attributed to a brain lesion (vascular compression, demyelinating lesion, or cerebellopontine lesion). MRI is recommended for all patients with pain in the trigeminal region associated with sensory loss, bilateral symptoms, or under the age of 40 years old. The diagnosis is mostly clinical, but trigeminal reflex testing is often abnormal with high sensitivity and specificity. Treatment usually involves sodium channel blockers such as carbamazepine or oxcarbazepine. If these do not work, other agents to consider include muscle relaxants such as baclofen. For refractory pain, botulinum toxin, rhizotomy, radiosurgery, or microvascular decompression are considered. Indomethacin is not generally helpful for trigeminal neuralgia (*see* Bradley's NiCP, 7th edn, Chs. 54, pp. 720–741 and 103, pp. 1686–1719).

73. A. Cisplatin is an alkylating agent used in the treatment of multiple types of cancers, including small cell lung cancer, sarcoma, and ovarian cancer. Cisplatin is toxic to the dorsal root ganglia and can lead to a sensory neuronopathy (ganglionopathy), as with the patient in this case. Vincristine and bortezomib are toxic to peripheral nerves, but typically cause painful peripheral neuropathies, not sensory neuronopathy. Rituximab is used in the treatment of lymphoma but is not toxic to peripheral nerves. It decreases B-cell populations and can increase the risk of infections, including progressive multifocal leukoencephalopathy. Methotrexate is used in a variety of cancers, including lymphoma, and it has central nervous system side effects, including encephalopathy, seizures, and aseptic meningitis, mostly if used intrathecally (*see* Bradley's NiCP, 7th edn, Ch. 107, pp. 1791–1866).

74. D. This patient presents with symptoms concerning for a myopathic process with proximal muscle weakness. His EMG confirms a myopathy, and his biopsy is diagnostic of Pompe disease, also known as *acid maltase deficiency* or *α-glucosidase deficiency*. This is an autosomal-recessive disorder with a deficiency of the enzyme α-glucosidase, which breaks down glycogen. This results in a large buildup of glycogen over time. There is a severe infantile form that can lead to death before the age of 2, a juvenile form, and an adult form that is often missed. In the adult version, patients generally have proximal muscle weakness, diaphragmatic weakness, elevated creatine kinase, and myopathic units on EMG. They can have significant myotonia on EMG. The biopsy demonstrates glycogen-filled vacuoles that intensely stain for acid phosphatase. This is an important diagnosis to consider because this is the only metabolic myopathy to date for which enzyme replacement therapy is available. Nonaka myopathy involves distal arm and leg weakness. The biopsy shows cytoplasmic inclusions and rimmed vacuoles. Becker muscular dystrophy has a biopsy similar to Duchenne, showing variation in the size of fibers, fibrosis, groups of basophilic fibers, and opaque or hypercontracted fibers. Special staining for dystrophin shows decreased levels. McArdle disease may show a buildup of glycogen and subsarcolemmal blebs with muscle necrosis. A stain for myophosphorylase activity would show reduced activity. This case is not McArdle because McArdle does not have myotonia on EMG and clinically presents with cramping and pain during brief episodes of exercise rather than a slowly progressive myopathy. LGMD-1A presents with proximal muscle weakness, and biopsy shows rimmed vacuoles along with dark green areas of amorphous material on Gomori trichrome stains, indicating loss of myotilin (*see* Bradley's NiCP, 7th edn, Ch. 110, pp. 1915–1955).

75. B. Keeping a patient's head straight is important to maintain adequate venous drainage bilaterally, although a tight cervical collar may impede jugular outflow and therefore increase intracranial pressure. All other techniques listed here are important tools for lowering intracranial pressure, either acutely (hyperventilation, head-of-bed elevation) or more continually (sedation, hyperosmolar therapy). Ultimately, if these measures are not sufficient, either ventricular drainage or craniectomy may be necessary to reduce intracranial pressure and prevent herniation (*see* Bradley's NiCP, 7th edn, Ch. 62, pp. 867–880).

76. A. The thick filaments, which are enriched with myosin, are represented by the A-band. The thin filaments, made of actin, are designated by the I-band. Although the length of the thick and thin filaments does not change with muscle contraction, the I-band and H-band shorten due to the binding of myosin to actin, after tropomyosin is removed from the actin-binding site. The Z-line is the border between

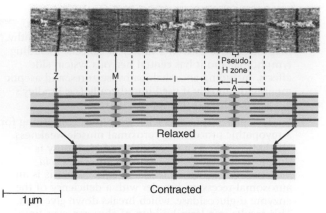

Figure for Answer 5.76 *(from Standring S (ed.) 2016* Gray's Anatomy, *41st edn, Elsevier, with permission.)*

sarcomeres and the base to which actin is bound. The M-line is a thin segment in the middle of the H-band that is the middle of the sarcomere, formed of cytoskeletal cross-connections. The H-band represents the portion of the thick filaments that is not superimposed by thin filaments (*see* Bradley's NiCP, 7th edn, Ch. 110, pp. 1915–1955).

77. E. TCAs antagonize the alpha$_1$-adrenergic receptors, muscarinic, and histaminergic receptors, each to a different degree. They also inhibit the reuptake of both serotonin and norepinephrine. Because of their broad mechanism of action, TCAs are used to treat a number of conditions, including depression, anxiety, bladder overactivity, insomnia, headache prophylaxis, and neuropathic pain. Also because of their broad mechanism of action, there are many side effects that include histaminergic effects (sedation, dry mouth and eyes, weight gain), antimuscarinic effects (constipation, tachycardia, blurred vision, and urinary retention), and alpha$_1$-adrenergic antagonism effects (postural hypotension). When combined with other serotonergic agents (selective serotonin reuptake inhibitors, tramadol, opioids, triptans, serotonin-norepinephrine reuptake inhibitors, trazodone, dextromethorphan), the risk of serotonin syndrome (altered mentation, myoclonus, autonomic instability, stiffness, mydriasis) should be considered. A few notable points regarding TCAs: (1) Nortriptyline has the least alpha$_1$-adrenergic antagonism and has the least orthostatic hypotension; (2) Imipramine is used to treat overactive bladder and enuresis; (3) Doxepin has high antihistamine activity and is the most sedating.

78. D. A CT venogram is the next best step to diagnosing the etiology of this patient's headache and optic nerve swelling. In the setting of a diarrheal illness, one should consider the possibility of cerebral venous sinus thrombosis. This is diagnosed most often on MR venogram or CT venogram. Aside from intravascular volume depletion, other predisposing factors include factor V Leiden (most common inherited cause of venous thrombosis), protein C and S deficiency, pregnancy, oral contraceptives, cancer, connective tissue disorders, and infections. Even postpartum patients are at high risk for venous sinus thrombosis. As a result of venous blockage, pressure can build up and result in infarcts in areas of mixed vascular territories and deep regions of the brain, leading to vision loss, hemorrhages, seizures, headache, and vomiting. In most cases,

anticoagulation should be started to prevent the further propagation of clot, even if hemorrhage is already present. Although an MRI of the brain would show restricted diffusion within venous territory and often suggest underlying venous sinus thrombosis, a venogram would clench the diagnosis. Although this particular patient has diarrhea, it is likely a Crohn's disease flare and would not warrant a CT of the abdomen/pelvis unless he had worsening abdominal symptoms to suggest perforation. Triptans should not be administered until the etiology of the headache has been determined, as labeling the symptoms migrainous would be erroneous in this case. An LP would be indicated if there was a suspicion of meningitis, encephalitis, or pseudotumor, but would not be the next best diagnostic study in this case (*see* Bradley's NiCP, 7th edn, Chs. 39, pp. 411–458 and 65, pp. 920–968).

79. C. Fukuyama congenital muscular dystrophy (also known as *muscle-eye-brain disease*) is an autosomal-recessive dystroglycanopathy related to mutations in the *FKTN* gene, encoding the protein fukutin. Symptoms are usually apparent in infancy, with hypotonia, weak cry, and poor feeding. Additionally, facial weakness is common, with ptosis and a perpetually open mouth. Children are often severely delayed in motor milestones and may never walk. Neuronal migration abnormalities are common, especially with lissencephaly. Eye malformations are common, with frequent retinal detachment. The prognosis for Fukuyama congenital muscular dystrophy is quite poor, with most dying before adulthood (*see* Bradley's NiCP, 7th edn, Ch. 110, pp. 1915–1955).

80. D. Multiple system atrophy is an alpha-synuclein neurodegenerative disease that usually presents in the sixth decade with profound autonomic dysfunction that can include orthostatic hypotension, urinary incontinence, urinary urgency, erectile dysfunction, decreased sweating, and constipation. Additionally, patients have parkinsonism, cerebellar findings, or both. The parkinsonism is often atypical, in that it presents bilaterally with a resting and action tremor (as opposed to a unilateral onset with a resting tremor in idiopathic Parkinson disease). Cerebellar findings can include hypermetric saccades, overshoot with finger follow, ataxic dysarthria, gait ataxia, nystagmus, vertigo, and dysmetria. Other associated features include inspiratory stridor, central sleep apnea, and hyperpigmentation of the distal legs. Typically, there is no family history. Imaging shows the "hot-cross bun sign" because of degeneration of the pontocerebellar fibers. There can also be increased signal lateral to the putamen on T2-weighted images, as well as pontine and/or cerebellar atrophy. A trial of levodopa could be considered, but typically the patient is unresponsive to dopamine. The mainstay of therapy is to address the autonomic dysfunction with fludrocortisone, midodrine, or droxidopa. Given the features of parkinsonism on examination and the delay in syncope, dehydration is much less likely, as this typically presents with orthostasis immediately upon standing. POTS has no features of parkinsonism, is usually associated with teenagers to young adults, and is associated with orthostatic tachycardia by more than 30 beats per minute in the absence of orthostatic hypotension. LEMS is a paraneoplastic phenomenon usually associated with small cell lung cancer associated with weakness and autonomic dysfunction.

Amyloidosis is typically associated with a small fiber peripheral neuropathy, autonomic dysfunction, and even multiorgan system involvement from amyloid deposition, but parkinsonism is not a typical feature (*see* Bradley's NiCP, 7th edn, Ch. 96, pp. 1422–1460). Figure from Kasaharaa S, Mikia Y, Kanagakia M, et al. 2012 "Hot cross bun" sign in multiple system atrophy with predominant cerebellar ataxia: a comparison between proton density-weighted imaging and T2-weighted imaging. *European Journal of Radiology* 81: 2848–2852, with permission.

81. E. The patient most likely has myxedema coma from severe hypothyroidism, with symptoms including hypothermia, bradycardia, hypotension, diffuse swelling, obtundation, and delayed relaxation of reflexes. This may relate to her medication noncompliance if there was a preexisting hypothyroid condition. Myxedema coma is considered a medical emergency, the best treatment for which is intravenous levothyroxine. Other symptoms of hypothyroidism include alopecia or coarse hair, constipation, heart block, hyponatremia, hypoglycemia, and activated partial thromboplastin time prolongation. IVIG and plasma exchange treat autoimmune conditions and Guillain-Barré syndrome, which would have absent reflexes and not likely affect the mental status. Naloxone is usually given for an opiate overdose, which would not usually have the physical findings on examination except for the mental status change. Furosemide is for symptomatic treatment only and would not reverse the underlying condition (*see* Bradley's NiCP, 7th edn, Ch. 52, pp. 696–712).

82. B. The Rinne test is performed by placing a vibrating tuning fork on the mastoid process until ringing is no longer heard (testing bone conduction). Immediately, the still-vibrating tuning fork is then placed next to the ear for the patient to hear the ringing (testing air conduction). Air conduction should last longer than bone conduction in a normally functioning ear. If there is conductive hearing loss, such as injury to the ossicles, bone conduction will be greater than air conduction. Sensorineural hearing loss, however, decreases both bone and air conduction equally, and so a Rinne test would still find air conduction greater than bone conduction on the affected side. The Weber test is performed by putting a vibrating tuning fork at the vertex of the skull or in the middle of the forehead. The sound should normally be equally loud in both ears, and a lateralization of the sound is abnormal. If the sound lateralizes to the hearing-impaired ear, this indicates conductive hearing loss. However, if the sound lateralizes away from the hearing-impaired ear, this suggests sensorineural hearing loss. In the event that the clinician does not know which ear is abnormal (such as in this case), combining the information from both the Rinne and Weber tests will localize the lesion (*see* Bradley's NiCP, 7th edn, Ch. 46, pp. 583–604).

83. D. Rapid eye movement (REM) sleep behavior disorder (RBD) involves the loss of REM hypotonia leading to patients acting out dreams, which can lead to injury to the patient or the patient's bed partner. This is seen in neurodegenerative conditions such as Parkinson disease, but also is seen with multiple system atrophy, progressive supranuclear palsy, corticobasal degeneration, and Alzheimer disease. RBD can be triggered by medications, including sedative hypnotics, tricyclic antidepressants, or anticholinergics.

Clonazepam is the first-line treatment and should be used when RBD becomes bothersome to the bed partner or dangerous to the patient. In this case, reassurance alone is not appropriate (*see* Bradley's NiCP, 7th edn, Ch. 102, pp. 1615–1685).

84. C. Circadian rhythm disorders are marked by a mismatch between the body's internal clock and the geophysical environment. The most common forms of this are jet lag or shift-work sleep disorder. Obstructive sleep apnea disturbs sleep by drops in oxygenation, leading to frequent arousals. This keeps patients from achieving deeper stages of sleep, but does not alter their circadian rhythm. Jet lag is bothersome when traveling either east or west and usually requires multiple time zones to be crossed. Shift-work sleep disorder involves working odd hours, particularly the third shift. Environmental signals tell the body that it should be asleep at night, yet these patients must adjust to sleep during the daytime. Frequently they will transition back to a normal schedule on off days or weekends, which can exacerbate insomnia and excessive sleepiness during awake time. Patients with dementia and mental retardation frequently have irregular circadian rhythms. Total sleep time in a 24 hour period may be normal, but it can be fragmented throughout the day. Patients with complete blindness can have free-running circadian rhythms because environmental cues such as sunlight do not synchronize their internal rhythms. These patients typically have a delay of sleep onset each day by 1 hour (*see* Bradley's NiCP, 7th edn, Ch. 102, pp. 1615–1685).

85. C. Enlargement of the physiological blind spot is concerning for increased intracranial pressure, rather than low intracranial pressure. This may also be associated with papilledema. Low-pressure headaches (or post–lumbar puncture headaches) are often improved with caffeine, when mild. They are generally worse when upright, and improve with recumbency. Although the duration of low-pressure headaches varies, they may last up to several weeks if the causative cerebrospinal fluid leak does not resolve either spontaneously or with intervention such as blood patching. Often MRI may demonstrate dural enhancement in the case of low intracranial pressure, as well as tonsillar sagging in the posterior fossa (*see* Bradley's NiCP, 7th edn, Ch. 103, pp. 1686–1719).

86. A. The main effect of opioids is on the mu receptor, which leads to analgesia, euphoria, respiratory depression, and opioid tolerance. The delta receptor has some antiinflammatory properties and can relieve bone pain. The kappa receptor is involved with visceral and neuropathic pain. The alpha-2 receptor is activated by epinephrine or norepinephrine and can lead to hypotension, sedation, and analgesia. The NMDA receptor is a glutamate receptor that opens an ion channel leading to neuronal activation (*see* Bradley's NiCP, 7th edn, Ch. 54, pp. 720–741).

87. A. *NF2* gene mutation is associated with development of vestibular nerve schwannomas. Given the proximity of the vestibular nerve to the facial nerve, patients often present with palsies of both nerves. Although *NF1* gene mutations are associated with nerve sheath tumors (generally neurofibromas), these are much less likely to affect cranial nerves. Recurrent varicella infection may cause symptoms such as Bell's palsy or

hearing loss, but is not generally progressive over several months. Vascular abnormalities may also occur in the cerebellopontine angle and affect the facial and vestibular nerves, but would be less likely due to the family history listed. Demyelinating disease would be more likely to present as a monophasic symptom rather than progressive (*see* Bradley's NiCP, 7th edn, Ch. 100, pp. 1538–1562).

88. C. Brainstem auditory evoked potentials can detect lesions in the auditory tract and brainstem when other testing is not available. Previously these were used to help in the diagnosis of multiple sclerosis, but with the advent of advanced imaging, they have less utility. They are frequently used in intraoperative monitoring, particularly in procedures involving the brainstem, such as microvascular decompression, cerebellar surgeries, or basilar artery aneurysm surgery. There are five prominent waves, although the main interpretation is based off of waves I, III, and V because II and IV are not always present (*see* Bradley's NiCP, 7th edn, Ch. 34, pp. 348–366).

TABLE FOR ANSWER 5.88

Wave	Anatomical location
I	Cochlea and cochlear nerve
II	Distal cochlear nerve, cochlear nucleus
III	Superior olive
IV	Lateral lemniscus
V	Inferior colliculus

89. D. At 4 years, a child should be able to stand on one foot, catch a bounced ball, play board games, copy capital letters, draw a person with two to four body parts, tell stories, play with other children, and have difficulty differentiating reality from make-believe. At 2 years of age, most children will be able to know names of body parts, identify objects in pictures, say short sentences, and follow simple instructions. They are able to sort shapes, play make-believe, and build a tower of four or more blocks. Physically, 2-year-olds are able to stand on tiptoe, kick a ball, throw overhand, and begin running. Two-year-old children demonstrate parallel play where they play next to other children, but not with other children. At 18 months, a child will say single words, point to objects he or she wants, follow one-step commands, walk, eat with a spoon, and drink from a cup. At 3 years, children will copy friends and adults, show affection, take turns, follow two- to three-step commands, have mostly understandable speech, play make-believe, copy a circle, and build a tower of six blocks. Three-year-olds should be able to pedal a tricycle. At 5 years, children like to sing, dance, act, show sympathy, are aware of gender, can tell what is make-believe and what is real, speak clearly, can tell a simple story, can draw a body with six or more parts, can print letters, can copy a triangle, and can skip (*see* Bradley's NiCP, 7th edn, Ch. 8, pp. 66–72).

90. D. Auras and physical findings during seizures can help localize seizures to certain lobes. This patient presents with classic symptoms of mesial temporal lobe sclerosis. This commonly presents with autonomic symptoms and a feeling of gastric rising. Psychiatric symptoms are also common. This seizure likely comes from the right side because of the dystonic left arm and ipsilateral automatisms. Occipital lobe seizures

typically have a visual aura. Lateral temporal lobe seizures can start with auditory hallucinations and visual misperceptions. Orbitofrontal seizures frequently present with gestural automatisms and olfactory hallucinations. Dorsolateral seizures present with versive eye and head movements with speech arrest (*see* Bradley's NiCP, 7th edn, Ch. 101, pp. 1563–1614).

91. D. By the age of 9 months, a child should learn to play peek-a-boo and should pick up items between the thumb and index finger. By the age of 2 months, a child should pay attention to faces, track objects, and recognize people from a distance. By 4 months, a child should reach for objects with one hand and express happy or sad emotions. By 6 months, a child should look at nearby objects, reach for items, and pass items between hands. By 12 months, a child should shake, bang, and throw items, and should begin using objects for their actual purpose (e.g. a cup for drinking) (*see* Bradley's NiCP, 7th edn, Ch. 8, pp. 66–72).

92. A. The image demonstrates a cerebral abscess in the right parietal lobe. The greatest imaging hint toward this diagnosis is the restricted diffusion and ring enhancement with central T1 hypointensity. Further, the sudden onset of symptoms argues toward an acute process rather than something more indolent such as a tumor. Although the presence of AIDS may increase the patient's risk of either infection or certain types of tumors, his intravenous drug abuse places him at risk of infections. Abscesses, such as the one shown in the image, should be emergently drained surgically, with concurrent systemic antibiotic therapy. Methotrexate therapy is used for central nervous system lymphoma. Although this is a possibility based on imaging alone, the patient should have surgery first to verify the diagnosis. Antiretroviral therapy should be considered after emergent treatment of the abscess and with drug abstinence. PET scan would be helpful if the cerebral lesion were a metastasis, although this is the less likely scenario as described earlier. Finally, lumbar puncture may be unsafe due to mass effect and risk of herniation, based on the imaging (*see* Bradley's NiCP, 7th edn, Chs. 77, pp. 1102–1120 and 79, pp. 1147–1158). Figure from Rath TJ, Hughes M, Arabi M, Shah GV 2012 Imaging of cerebritis, encephalitis, and brain abscess. *Neuroimaging Clinics of North America* 22(4): 585–607, with permission.

93. B. Copper deficiency classically leads to a myeloneuropathy that may mimic subacute combined degeneration. Copper deficiency may result from poor dietary absorption (e.g. after gastric bypass, or with celiac disease), or from excessive zinc ingestion. In the mid-2000s, the correlation between excessive zinc exposure (and, therefore, copper deficiency) and zinc-containing denture creams came to light, after which zinc was removed from these formulations. Copper toxicity would be similar to Wilson disease, with chronic liver dysfunction and progressive cognitive and movement disturbance. Zinc deficiency is rare in developed countries, and is associated with skin disorder, impaired immune function, and cognitive dysfunction. Vitamin B12 deficiency may present with a myeloneuropathy similar to the case presented, but because of the information about denture cream, this would not be the best answer. Vitamin B12 toxicity is not possible due to the fact that the vitamin is water soluble, so excess amounts are excreted in the urine (*see* Bradley's NiCP, 7th edn, Ch. 85, pp. 1226–1236).

94. A. The picture depicts axillary freckling, a cutaneous manifestation most often seen in neurofibromatosis type 1 (NF1). Other manifestations of this condition include multiple café-au-lait macules, cutaneous or subcutaneous neurofibromas, plexiform neurofibromas, optic nerve gliomas, iris hamartomas (Lisch nodules), migraines, cognitive dysfunction, and long-bone abnormalities. The disorder is caused by a mutation in the *NF1* gene on chromosome 17 and is inherited in an autosomal-dominant fashion. Neurofibromatosis type 2 (NF2) is an autosomal-dominant condition associated with a mutation in the *NF2* gene on chromosome 22. Unlike NF1, NF2 has a paucity of cutaneous manifestations. Instead, NF2 classically presents with bilateral vestibular schwannomas, as well as multiple other tumors, including lower cranial nerve or extracranial schwannomas, meningiomas, or ependymomas (*see* Bradley's NiCP, 7th edn, Ch. 100, pp. 1538–1562). Figure from Aminoff MJ, Josephson SA 2014 *Aminoff's Neurology and General Medicine*, 5th edn, Academic Press, with permission.

95. A. Conflicts of interest occur when the interest of the patient is in opposition to the interest of the physician. When physicians place their own financial or personal reward above patient care, conflicts occur. Participating in pharmaceutical medication studies is not inherently a conflict of interest because new medications can provide tremendous benefit to patients. However, these situations can become a conflict of interest by either coercing patients to participate (especially if it is more beneficial for the physician to enroll patients) or by investing in the company (which gives the physician more motivation for the trial to succeed). Referring patients to a third-party MRI center in which the physician is financially invested is considered a conflict of interest in most circumstances. The conflict of interest could be mitigated if there are no other facilities nearby, the recommended facilities have better equipment, or the radiologists are better. Performing procedures for financial gain when medical management would suffice is a conflict of interest because this places monetary gain ahead of patient care.

96. A. The image depicts gram-positive cocci in clusters that were identified within the subarachnoid space, classic for *Streptococcus meningitis*. Neisseria are gram-negative diplococci. Rhizopus is one of several fungi that constitute mucormycosis. It is generally filamentous with branching hyphae. Herpes simplex virus is visualized microscopically by presence of Cowdry type A intranuclear inclusions. *Naegleria fowleri* is an infectious amoeba that is found in the trophozoite stage when infecting brain tissue (*see* Bradley's NiCP, 7th edn, Ch. 79). Figure from McKeever PE 2012 Pathologic basis of central nervous system infections. *Neuroimaging Clinics of North America* 22(4): 773–790, with permission.

97. E. Phosphofructokinase deficiency is an autosomal-recessive glycogen storage disorder that is similar to McArdle disease with exercise intolerance, exercise-induced myoglobinuria, and an abnormal forearm ischemic lactate test, but notably does *not* have a second wind phenomenon, as is seen in McArdle disease (*see* Bradley's NiCP, 7th edn, Ch. 110, pp. 1147–1158).

98. B. The Optic Neuritis Treatment Trial demonstrated an increased risk of recurrent optic neuritis in patients with already diagnosed multiple sclerosis, as well as with oral prednisone treatment (compared with intravenous steroids). After a first episode of optic neuritis with otherwise no evidence of multiple sclerosis, the 5-year risk of developing multiple sclerosis is roughly 25%. Vitamin A deficiency is associated with dyschromatopsia (trouble discerning color) and night blindness. The patient in the question likely does not have vitamin A deficiency, given the asymmetry and rapid onset. Leber's hereditary optic neuropathy is an inherited disease that causes retinal degeneration and associated vision loss. It follows a mitochondrial inheritance pattern, and for unclear reasons the phenotype is much more penetrant in males. Retinoblastoma is an aggressive cancer of the retinae, about 50% of which are associated with an autosomal-dominant mutation in the *Rb* gene (*see* Bradley's NiCP, 7th edn, Ch. 17, pp. 163–178).

99. B. Mercury exposure can occur at battery factories, electronic factories, and mercury processing plants. Exposure can lead to hyperhidrosis, intention tremor, anemia, personality changes including irritability, euphoria, insomnia, and confusion or coma. With chronic exposure, patients develop progressive ataxia, constriction of visual fields, and central sensory disturbances. Acute lead toxicity typically starts with nausea, vomiting, and abdominal pain, and long-term exposure can lead to encephalopathy, seizures, behavioral changes, and motor neuropathy. Manganese toxicity most often occurs with chronic exposure in miners or welders, and results in headaches, dementia, behavioral changes, dystonia, and parkinsonism. Wilson disease is an autosomal-recessive disorder with a dysfunctional *ATP7B* gene leading to abnormal copper metabolism. This can present with psychosis, depression, impulsivity, tremor (particularly a wing-beating tremor), dystonia, and parkinsonism. Functional or psychogenic tremor may be a consideration, but organic disorders should be ruled out, especially considering her significant occupational exposure (*see* Bradley's NiCP, 7th edn, Ch. 86, pp. 1237–1253).

100. B. Alemtuzumab is an anti-CD52 monoclonal antibody with Food and Drug Administration approval for the treatment of relapsing forms of multiple sclerosis. CD52 is present on all lymphocytes; thus alemtuzumab is a B- and T-cell–depleting drug. CD20 is expressed on the surface of mature B-cells and is targeted by the monoclonal antibody rituximab. Vascular endothelial growth factor is the target of the monoclonal antibody bevacizumab, which is used in the treatment of glioblastoma. Cell adhesion molecule α4 is expressed on the endothelial lining of blood vessels and is used for white blood cells to extravasate into tissues like the brain. This is the target of the monoclonal antibody natalizumab, which is used in the treatment of multiple sclerosis. Sphingosine 1-phosphate is a major regulator of B- and T-cell trafficking, and is the target of fingolimod, which is used in the treatment of relapsing multiple sclerosis (*see* Bradley's NiCP, 7th edn, Ch. 80, pp. 1159–1186).

101. C. Huntington.

102. B. Myotonin.

103. A. Frataxin.

104. D. Androgen receptor.

105. E. Atrophin-1.

Test Six

QUESTIONS

1. A 32-year-old male presents to your office for complaints of muscle stiffness. After clenching his hands, they open slowly. On examination you note mild grip weakness, bilateral facial weakness, and frontal balding. On tapping the thenar eminence with a reflex hammer, he has a prolonged and involuntary contraction of the thenar muscles. Electromyography (EMG) demonstrates small motor units and spontaneous activity with a waxing and waning quality. Which of the following is true about the genetics of this disorder?

   A. This disorder is inherited in an autosomal-recessive pattern.

   B. *SOD1* gene mutations are responsible for this disease.

   C. This disorder is caused by a CTG triplet repeat.

   D. The responsible gene is located on chromosome 1.

   E. This disorder is inherited in an X-linked pattern.

2. Which of the following proteins is thought to be a primary candidate for the autoimmunity of multiple sclerosis and is the antigen targeted in experimental autoimmune encephalomyelitis (EAE)?

   A. Myelin basic protein

   B. Proteolipid protein

   C. Myelin-associated glycoprotein

   D. Myelin oligodendrocyte glycoprotein

   E. Cyclic nucleotide phosphodiesterase

3. Which of the following has *not* been putatively associated with an increased risk of multiple sclerosis (MS)?

   A. Smoking

   B. Vitamin D deficiency

   C. Certain infections

   D. Birth order

   E. Certain immune-associated genetics

4. Which of the following most closely approximates the volume of cerebrospinal fluid (CSF) in an adult?

   A. 500 mL

   B. 50 mL

   C. 100 mL

   D. 150 mL

   E. 250 mL

5. A girl was diagnosed with presumed cerebral palsy at 4 years old, when she began to toe-walk. Now, at 12 years old, she has worsening gait dysfunction and increased number of falls. She also complains of pain and cramping in her legs as the day goes on, which almost always improves after sleep. Her mother notices that she will occasionally have difficulty with writing due to curling of her fingers. Psychologically, she appears normal. What is the next best step in this case?

   A. Reassure the mother that this is a typical course for cerebral palsy

   B. Trial of carbidopa/levodopa

   C. Perform an electromyography

   D. Send to a genetic counselor

   E. Chelation therapy

6. A 32-year-old female who underwent a prolonged labor with epidural anesthesia presents to the office with weakness in her right leg 4 days postpartum. Her examination demonstrates weakness of the tibialis anterior and peroneus longus with normal strength of the medial gastrocnemius, tibialis posterior, quadriceps, hamstrings, and hip flexors. She has sensory loss over the lateral aspect of the lower leg and dorsum of the foot. Reflexes are normal, and Babinski response is negative. Electromyography (EMG) demonstrates reduced recruitment in the tibialis anterior and peroneus longus, but normal recruitment in the medial gastrocnemius, short head of the biceps femoris, and gluteus medius. No fibrillations or positive sharp waves were seen, including the lumbar paraspinal muscles. Which of the following is the most likely cause of her symptoms?

   A. Retroperitoneal hematoma

   B. Peroneal (fibular) compression at the fibular head

   C. Lumbar radiculopathy

   D. Spinal epidural hematoma

   E. Ischemic stroke

7. The image best represents which of the following tumors?

   A. Meningioma

   B. Pilocytic astrocytoma

   C. Central nervous system (CNS) lymphoma

   D. Schwannoma

   E. Oligodendroglioma

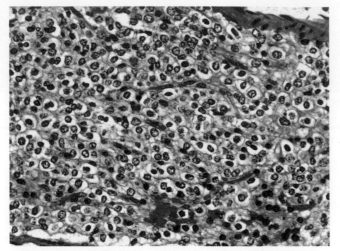

Figure for Question 6.7.

8. A 12-year-old boy of average stature presents to the hospital with an acute ischemic stroke. His only prior hospitalization was last year for unexplained, excruciating pain in his index finger, which resolved after several days of opiates and fluids. He is an only child, and neither of his parents has a history of early strokes or coagulopathy. Which of the following is the most likely test to identify his underlying stroke etiology?

A. Echocardiogram

B. *NOTCH3* genetic testing

C. Hemoglobin electrophoresis

D. Lipid screening

E. Mitochondrial genetic testing

9. A patient presents with a suspected C7 radiculopathy. Which muscles would be expected to show abnormalities on electromyography?

A. Biceps and brachioradialis

B. Triceps and flexor pollicis longus

C. First dorsal interosseous and abductor pollicis brevis

D. Extensor carpi radialis and anconeus

E. Extensor indices proprius and pronator quadratus

10. A 24-year-old female presents with new-onset headaches that occur mostly at night or in the early morning. These involve a dull frontal and occipital pain with associated tinnitus. Her physical examination demonstrates bilateral papilledema. Magnetic resonance imaging of her brain is normal. Which of the following is the most likely cause of her symptoms?

A. Topiramate

B. Acetazolamide

C. Recent weight loss

D. Snoring

E. Vitamin A supplements

11. A 22-year-old male presents to the office for evaluation of double vision, which has been present for the last several weeks. On examination, both eyes demonstrate limited vertical gaze, and the right eye also has severely limited abduction. The rest of his extraocular movements are intact. Pupils are equal and reactive, and no ptosis is present. The rest of his neurological examination is normal. A magnetic resonance image of his brain and a magnetic resonance angiogram of his head are both normal. He has also been followed by an ophthalmologist for pigmentary retinopathy, and he has noticed chronic hearing loss. Which of the following is the most likely diagnosis?

A. Oculopharyngeal muscular dystrophy

B. Myasthenia gravis

C. Kearns-Sayre syndrome

D. Mitochondrial encephalomyopathy, lactic acidosis, and strokelike episodes (MELAS)

E. Miller Fisher variant of Guillain-Barré syndrome

12. Which of the following is true of Rett syndrome?

A. Associated with abnormally large hands and feet

B. Most develop normal walking and talking, and then regress

C. Caused by mutations in *FMR1*

D. Majority are sporadic mutations

E. Associated with macrocephaly

13. Which of the following ion channels is the first to cause axonal depolarization leading to an action potential?

A. Voltage-gated K^+ channel

B. Slow calcium channel

C. Voltage-gated Na^+ channel

D. Ligand-gated chloride channel

E. Na-K ATPase pump

14. A 65-year-old female presents to the emergency room after a prolonged seizure, which was preceded by several days of fevers, headaches, and confusion. She had some hallucinations the day before her admission. On examination she was comatose, febrile to 101.5°F, with a stiff neck but with no focal findings. A lumbar puncture demonstrated 100 white blood cells with a lymphocytic predominance, a protein of 75, and a glucose of 45. Her electroencephalogram (EEG) is shown here. Which of the following is the most likely diagnosis?

A. Tuberculous meningitis

B. Strep pneumonia meningitis

C. Subacute sclerosing panencephalitis

D. Creutzfeldt-Jakob disease

E. Herpes encephalitis

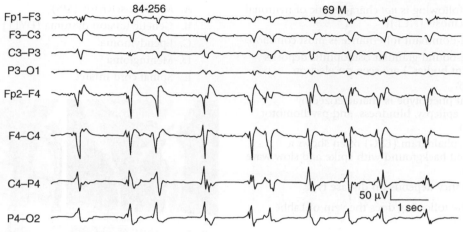

84-256   69 M

50 µV
1 sec

Figure for Question 6.14.

15. The following electroencephalogram (EEG) is typical in which condition?
    A. Subacute sclerosing panencephalitis
    B. Absence epilepsy
    C. Hepatic encephalopathy
    D. Herpes encephalitis
    E. Benign epilepsy with centrotemporal spikes

16. A 32-year-old male is evaluated in clinic because of concerns from his sister. Over the years, the patient has shown little to no interest in maintaining contact with his parents or his sister despite no serious disagreements. The patient is a computer programmer and rarely leaves his apartment, preferring isolation to groups. He is able to maintain eye contact and communicates well. On examination, his thought process is logical and he denies hallucinations. Which of the following is the most likely diagnosis?
    A. Avoidant personality disorder
    B. Schizoid personality disorder
    C. Schizophrenia
    D. Paranoid personality disorder
    E. Autism

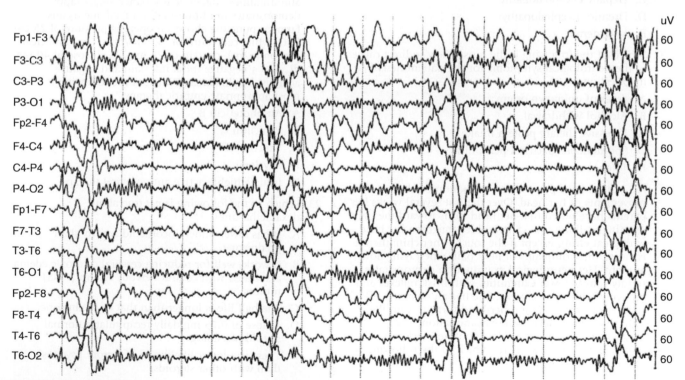

Figure for Question 6.15.

17. Which of the following is *not* characteristic of neuronal ceroid lipofuscinosis (NCL)?

    A. Autosomal-dominant inheritance is most common.

    B. Membrane-bound granular osmophilic deposits ("fingerprint bodies") are seen on electron microscopy.

    C. The clinical phenotype is characterized by myoclonic epilepsy, blindness, and psychomotor retardation.

    D. Electroencephalogram (EEG) often shows a disorganized background with spike and slow wave complexes.

    E. Life expectancy depends on disease type.

18. To which of the following does the vein of Labbé drain?

    A. Vein of Trolard

    B. Vein of Galen

    C. Superior sagittal sinus

    D. Inferior sagittal sinus

    E. Transverse sinus

19. A 55-year-old man with chronic alcoholism presents to the emergency room with increased confusion over the last 2 days, followed by difficulty waking. He has complained of increased abdominal girth over the last several months, and abdominal pain and fever over the last several days. On examination, he has a low-grade fever but otherwise normal vital signs. He awakens to loud stimulus, but is disoriented. He displays negative myoclonus, but no other motor symptoms. A plasma ammonia level is 55 μmol/L. Which of the following is the most likely source of his neurological decline?

    A. Hyperparathyroidism

    B. Intoxication

    C. Hepatic encephalopathy

    D. Uremic encephalopathy

    E. Myxedema

20. Which of the following is the most likely indirect cause of the neurological symptoms for the patient described in Question 6.19?

    A. Fever of unknown origin

    B. Alcohol withdrawal

    C. Excessive dietary protein intake

    D. Spontaneous bacterial peritonitis

    E. Tylenol overdose

21. A 5-year-old girl presents for evaluation of abnormal movements of her head. Over the last several weeks her parents have noted that her head turns toward the right seemingly all the time. She is able straighten her head with great effort, except if she touches her chin; then it is easier. She complains of neck pain when lying down at night. Her neurological examination demonstrates mildly spastic lower extremities with brisk reflexes and bilateral Babinski responses. She has an enlarged left sternocleidomastoid, and her head turns toward the right throughout most of the examination. The magnetic resonance image (MRI) of her neck was obtained and is shown here. Which of the following is the most likely diagnosis?

A. Multiple sclerosis (MS)

B. Genetic torsion dystonia (DYT1)

C. Ependymoma

D. Meningioma

E. Spinal cord infarct

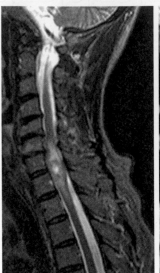
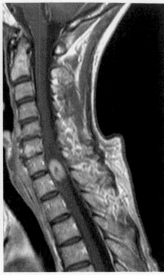

Figure for Question 6.21.

22. A 58-year-old male with a history of human immunodeficiency virus (HIV) presents to the emergency department because of a brief seizure that morning. He has had a several-week history of worsening headaches, memory loss, and neck stiffness. His neurological examination demonstrates a mild left-sided facial droop and right sixth nerve palsy. Magnetic resonance imaging demonstrates no acute abnormalities. Magnetic resonance angiography demonstrates multiple small cerebral aneurysms. Lumbar puncture shows an opening pressure of 25 cm H_2O, white cell count of 22 cells/mm³ (mononuclear predominant), protein of 75 mg/dL, glucose of 40 mg/dL, and a negative India ink stain and negative acid-fast bacilli smear. Which of the following is the most appropriate empiric therapy?

    A. Amphotericin B

    B. Penicillin G

    C. Vancomycin

    D. Acyclovir

    E. Initiate highly active antiretroviral therapy

23. Which of the following is *not* true about dexamethasone?

    A. It has lower mineralocorticoid activity than prednisone.

    B. It works well for reducing cerebral cytotoxic edema associated with central nervous system (CNS) tumors.

    C. The half-life is longer than that of prednisone.

    D. A dose of 0.75 mg daily recapitulates normal steroid physiology.

    E. There is a lower likelihood of steroid psychosis than with other steroids.

24. All of the following are risk factors for obstructive sleep apnea (OSA) *except*?

    A. Hypertension
    B. Menopause
    C. Male neck circumference >17 inches
    D. Alcohol use
    E. Male gender

25. An 80-year-old woman wakes in the night and screams when she sees a burglar in her room. Her son comes in to find that there was no burglar, but instead her robe was hanging from the door. Which of the following describes this phenomenon?

    A. Illusion
    B. Hallucination
    C. Dementia
    D. Delirium
    E. Delusion

26. All of the following factors predict success for temporal lobe epilepsy surgery *except*?

    A. Hippocampal sclerosis seen in magnetic resonance imaging (MRI)
    B. Unilateral ictal discharges
    C. Hypometabolism on positron emission tomography (PET) scan
    D. Etiology of head trauma
    E. Normal postoperative electroencephalogram (EEG)

27. The brain biopsy image shown here was taken from an elderly man with dementia. Which was his most likely underlying diagnosis?

    A. Pick disease
    B. Creutzfeldt-Jakob disease
    C. Parkinson disease
    D. Alzheimer disease
    E. Huntington disease

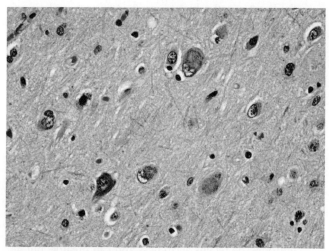

Figure for Question 6.27.

28. A 60-year-old woman presents with 3 days of fever followed by acute, constant vertigo, nausea, and hearing loss on the right. Which is the most likely etiology?

    A. Vestibular neuritis
    B. Vestibular schwannoma
    C. Labyrinthitis
    D. Ischemic stroke
    E. Aneurysmal rupture

29. Which of the following is an example of the principle of beneficence?

    A. Stopping a medication due to side effects
    B. Discussing causes of migraines
    C. Encouraging a stroke patient to quit smoking
    D. Refusing to provide an unproven treatment
    E. Explaining potential side effects to a patient

30. A 73-year-old female with recent myocardial infarction presents with progressive weakness in her arms and legs. She finds it difficult to brush her hair because her arms become fatigued, and she has tea-colored urine. Her examination shows mild proximal weakness in the deltoids and hip flexors bilaterally. Creatine kinase is 7500 U/L (normal is <250 U/L). Which of the following is the most likely diagnosis?

    A. Statin myopathy
    B. Myasthenia gravis
    C. Immune-mediated necrotizing myopathy
    D. Amyotrophic lateral sclerosis
    E. Myotonic dystrophy type 1

31. A healthy 12-year-old Japanese girl develops new left-sided weakness upon awakening. She is found by her mother, who quickly calls 911. In the emergency department, her examination demonstrates a dense left hemiparesis, along with difficulty seeing out of her left visual field. A magnetic resonance image reveals a stroke, prompting an evaluation for the underlying etiology. The digital subtraction angiogram is shown. Which of the following is true regarding this condition?

    A. Adults experience hemorrhage most often and children experience ischemic events.
    B. It is most common in Caucasians.
    C. There is increased risk in trisomy 13.
    D. Treatment options are supportive only.
    E. The main pathology lies within the posterior circulation vessels.

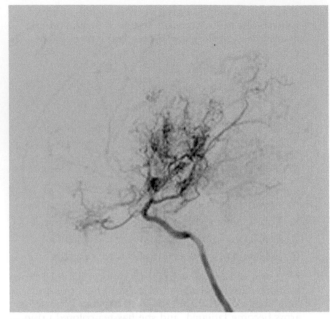

Figure for Question 6.31.

32. An 82-year-old female presents with an 8-month history of progressive memory loss. She has been living independently, but her family is concerned that she can no longer manage this because she forgot to pay several bills and even had her electricity disconnected. She repeats the same stories and asks the same questions to her family. Blood work is normal, including a complete blood count, metabolic panel, liver enzymes, thyroid-stimulating hormone, vitamin B12, and rapid plasma reagin. Her neurological examination is normal, other than scoring a 22/30 on the mini mental state examination. Which of the following is *not* true of Alzheimer disease?

    A. The disease is caused by a buildup of beta amyloid in the brain.

    B. Mutations in presenilin 1 and presenilin 2 lead to the disease.

    C. Biopsy findings include neuritic plaques, neurofibrillary tangles, and amyloid deposition.

    D. Rivastigmine is considered a first-line treatment.

    E. Fluorodeoxyglucose–positron emission tomography (FDG-PET) demonstrates hypometabolism of the occipital lobes.

33. A new blood test for diagnosing multiple sclerosis is used in a clinical trial. The following results are obtained and shown in the table. Which of the following is the positive predictive value of this test?

    A. 90%

    B. 83%

    C. 64%

    D. 50%

    E. 20%

TABLE FOR QUESTION 6.33

	Has multiple sclerosis	No multiple sclerosis
Positive result	50	50
Negative result	10	90

34. Which of the following is an antimuscarinic medication used for detrusor overactivity?

    A. Oxybutynin

    B. Botulinum toxin

    C. Terazosin

    D. Tamsulosin

    E. Vasopressin

35. Which of the following ions directly results in release of acetylcholine from the presynaptic terminal?

    A. Sodium

    B. Potassium

    C. Chloride

    D. Calcium

    E. Magnesium

36. Which of the following is not considered a treatment for complex regional pain syndrome (CRPS)?

    A. Early mobilization of the extremity

    B. Physical therapy

    C. Antiepileptics

    D. Tricyclic antidepressants

    E. Casting

37. For which of the following tumors should an individual with multiple endocrine neoplasia type 1 (MEN1) be monitored?

    A. Glioblastoma

    B. Primary central nervous system (CNS) lymphoma

    C. Hypothalamic hamartoma

    D. Pituitary adenoma

    E. Retinoblastoma

38. A 44-year-old business executive complains of increasing number of headaches. These are pressurelike pain in a band around his head. Whereas they were initially about once per week, their frequency has increased to at least once per day. There is no associated nausea, photophobia, or phonophobia. For the last 3 months, he has required up to four doses of acetaminophen and ibuprofen per day, with less pain relief over time. He reports high levels of work-related stress in recent years and less opportunity for sleep. His neurological and ophthalmological examinations are normal. Which of the following is the most appropriate first step in the care of this patient?

    A. Cranial magnetic resonance imaging (MRI)

    B. Reduce analgesic use

    C. Reduce workload

    D. Initiate riboflavin

    E. Switch to tramadol for abortive therapy

39. A 15-year-old male presents to your outpatient office with complaints of episodic weakness. Several times a week, he will have episodes of generalized weakness lasting approximately 15 minutes. During these episodes, he retains awareness and can breathe, but he seems to be otherwise paralyzed. Weakness can be triggered during rest after exercise or by eating bananas, tomatoes, or baked potatoes. His neurological examination reveals normal strength, sensation, and reflexes. Grip myotonia is present. Which of the following is the most likely diagnosis?

    A. Myotonia congenita

    B. Hypokalemic periodic paralysis

C. Paramyotonia congenita

D. Hyperkalemic periodic paralysis

E. McArdle disease

40. A 60-year-old man with history of atrial fibrillation on warfarin presents with 2 hours of progressive left upper extremity weakness and headache. In this time, his symptoms have progressively worsened, now leaving him with decreased vision in his left visual field and somnolence. On arrival to the emergency department, computed tomography (CT) scan shows a large lobar hemorrhage with some right-to-left midline shift. His international normalized ratio (INR) is 4.5 and blood pressure 172/93 mm Hg. Which of the following is the next best step in this patient's management?

   A. Nicardipine drip for blood pressure

   B. Reverse anticoagulation

   C. Intravenous (IV) tissue plasminogen activator (tPA) for stroke

   D. Intubate for airway protection

   E. Begin levetiracetam for seizure prophylaxis

41. Which of the following is an X-linked disorder?

   A. Niemann-Pick disease

   B. Leigh disease

   C. Neurofibromatosis 1

   D. Fabry disease

   E. Metachromatic leukodystrophy

42. Which of the following has not been a recent Joint Commission on Accreditation of Health Care Organization (JACHO) Patient Safety Goal?

   A. Correct patient identification

   B. Correct surgical site

   C. Safe medication administration

   D. Adequate hospital police force

   E. Safe use of medical alarms

43. The figure demonstrates which of the following developmental abnormalities?

   A. Agenesis of corpus callosum

   B. Schizencephaly

   C. Holoprosencephaly

   D. Lissencephaly

   E. Polymicrogyria

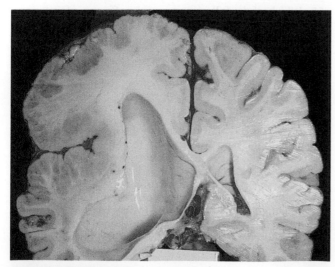

Figure for Question 6.43.

44. A 34-year old woman presents with over 1 year of increasing headaches, followed by increasingly irregular menstrual periods and lactation despite her nulliparous status. Her physical and neurological examinations are normal. Magnetic resonance imaging demonstrates a 6-mm nonenhancing lesion amid the normal structures of the sella, without associated mass effect. Based on her most likely diagnosis, which of the following is the best first-line treatment consideration?

   A. Dopamine agonist

   B. Chemotherapy

   C. Stereotactic radiosurgery

   D. Whole-brain radiation

   E. Dopamine antagonist

45. Which of the following conditions would not be expected to cause positive sharp waves and fibrillation potentials on electromyography (EMG)?

   A. Diabetic polyneuropathy

   B. Myasthenia gravis

   C. Inclusion body myositis

   D. Amyotrophic lateral sclerosis

   E. Carpal tunnel syndrome

46. The primary goal of azathioprine therapy is which of the following?

   A. Removal of B-cells from circulating blood

   B. Removal of T-cells from circulating blood

   C. Removal of immunoglobulins from circulating blood

   D. Removal of all lymphocytes from circulating blood

   E. Inhibition of leukocytes from crossing from peripheral blood to the brain

47. A 75-year-old man with untreated hypertension and diabetes presents to the hospital with sudden retroorbital pain and difficulty opening his right eye. On examination, he has severe ptosis on the right. When you open his lid, his pupils are equal and reactive but there is dysconjugate gaze at rest, with inability to adduct the right eye. Which of the following is the most likely localization for the lesion?

   A. Microvasculature within the oculomotor nerve

   B. Sympathetic chain within carotid sheath

   C. Posterior communicating artery

   D. Oculomotor nucleus within the midbrain

   E. Cavernous sinus

48. A 33-year-old woman is noted to have erratic behavior for the last 2 weeks. She believes the president of the United States can hear her thoughts and that she can control his thoughts. Many times, she is seen responding to voices despite there not being anyone in the same room. After this period of 2 weeks, she no longer responds to internal stimuli but has had poor sleep, has decreased energy, cries all the time, and has no appetite. Which of the following is the most likely diagnosis?

   A. Schizophrenia

   B. Delusional disorder

   C. Schizoaffective disorder

   D. Depression

   E. Schizophreniform disorder

49. A 35-year-old male presents for an evaluation of tremor and rigidity over the last 2 years. On examination the patient has a bilateral resting tremor in both hands and dysmetria on finger-to-nose testing. He is bradykinetic with a festinating gait. A computed tomography (CT) scan of his head is shown here. Which of the following is the most likely diagnosis?

    A. Fahr disease

    B. Idiopathic Parkinson disease

    C. Hemorrhagic stroke

    D. Pantothenate kinase–associated neurodegeneration

    E. Huntington disease

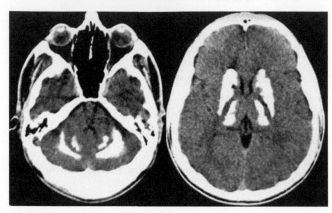

Figure for Question 6.49.

50. Which of the following connects the flow of cerebrospinal fluid (CSF) from the lateral ventricles to the third ventricle?

    A. Foramen of Luschka

    B. Foramen of Monro

    C. Cerebral aqueduct

    D. Fourth ventricle

    E. Foramen of Magendie

51. An 8-month-old infant is admitted for intermittent episodes of generalized stiffening and posturing, which are occasionally associated with apnea and staring. These episodes most commonly present 15–30 minutes after feedings. Which of the following is the most likely diagnosis?

    A. Benign paroxysmal torticollis in infancy

    B. Sandifer syndrome

    C. Spasmus nutans

    D. Breath-holding spell

    E. Seizure disorder

52. A 32-year-old woman presents to the emergency room with chest pain. This has been occurring over the last 3 months each time she steps into an elevator at her place of business. In addition to chest pain, she has diaphoresis, shortness of breath, and nausea. Each time this occurs, she is brought to the emergency room with several negative cardiac workups, including negative troponins, electrocardiogram, transthoracic echocardiogram, and stress test. Now, she avoids work altogether for fear of having another episode while traveling to her office via the elevator. What is the most likely diagnosis?

    A. Generalized anxiety disorder

    B. Panic disorder with agoraphobia

    C. Panic disorder without agoraphobia

    D. Obsessive-compulsive disorder

    E. Posttraumatic stress disorder

53. Which of the following is the correct name for the axonal component indicated by the arrow?

    A. Axon

    B. Soma

    C. Terminal button

    D. Axon hillock

    E. Dendrite

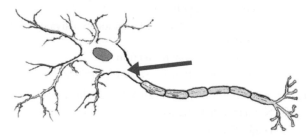

Figure for Question 6.53.

54. A mother brings her 3-month-old boy into the pediatrician's office for a general check-up. She mentions that others have told her that her child's head size appears abnormal. His head circumference is 41 cm, and the remainder of his neurological examination is normal. Which of the following is the best response to the mother?

    A. This is the expected head circumference for a 3-month-old, and he is normal.

    B. His head circumference is enlarged, and he needs a magnetic resonance image (MRI) to further characterize his brain.

    C. His head circumference is less than the expected measurement and could be part of a neurological syndrome.

    D. We can order an MRI because you are concerned about his head size and development.

    E. Because his head is enlarged, I'll need to measure both parents' head circumference.

55. Which of the following transmits afferent information in the muscle stretch reflex?

    A. Gamma motor neuron

    B. Alpha motor neuron

    C. Intrafusal muscle fiber

    D. Extrafusal muscle fiber

    E. Substantia gelatinosa

56. A 29-year-old man presents to the hospital with abdominal pain and is found to have appendicitis. He is admitted to the hospital and scheduled for emergency surgery. Two days after surgery he suffers a generalized tonic-clonic seizure. Neurology is consulted and performs an electroencephalogram (EEG) and magnetic resonance imaging (MRI), both of which are normal. There are no signs of infection, but he is diaphoretic, tremulous, tachycardic, and hypertensive.

He also appears to have visual hallucinations at night. Which of the following is most likely?

A. Postoperative delirium likely due to pain medications

B. Perforated appendix with septic shock

C. Status epilepticus

D. Alcohol withdrawal seizure followed by delirium tremens

E. Cocaine intoxication

57. In the transverse section of the brainstem shown here, the arrow is pointing to which structure?

A. Red nucleus

B. Substantia nigra

C. Nucleus cuneatus

D. Nucleus gracilis

E. Inferior colliculus

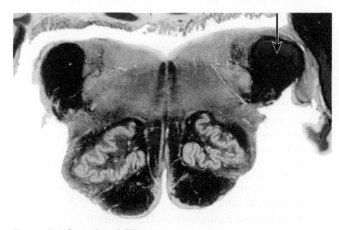

Figure for Question 6.57.

58. A 1-week-old boy remains in the hospital since birth for progressive neurological deterioration. He is now intubated due to coma, poor feeding, and recurrent vomiting. Sepsis has been ruled out. Laboratory analysis reveals decreased serum bicarbonate and hypoglycemia. An organic aciduria is suspected, and urine gas chromatography/mass spectrometry confirms this. Which of the following is *not* true of the organic acidurias?

A. Glutaric acidemia type 1 produces encephalopathy followed by rapid-onset dystonia or chorea with collections of fluid over frontal lobes and subdural hematomas.

B. Propionic acidemia presents with severe metabolic acidosis in the setting of neonatal encephalopathy, as well as blood cell dyscrasias such as thrombocytopenia and neutropenia.

C. Methylmalonic acidemia presents with ketosis, acidosis, and neutropenia but has no hepatomegaly.

D. Respiratory chain deficiencies lead to secondary mitochondrial damage, which leads to further organ damage.

E. Protein restriction is often one treatment modality for organic acidemias.

59. A 21-year-old male presents to the emergency department with generalized weakness. This started 1 hour earlier while the patient was at a seafood restaurant. His friends describe an initial state of euphoria before he began complaining of paresthesias around his lips. He vomited and had difficulty standing. On examination he has bilateral ptosis, bifacial weakness, diffuse extremity weakness, and loss of reflexes. Which of the following is the most likely cause of his symptoms?

A. Ciguatoxin

B. Tetrodotoxin

C. Botulinum toxin

D. Shiga toxin

E. Curare

60. An 18-year-old male presented to the office with progressive weakness over the last 2 years. Initially his left leg went numb for several months. Next he developed a right foot drop. In the last few weeks he has had several falls and noticed decreased grip strength. His neurological examination is remarkable for bilateral lower extremity spasticity, bilateral Babinski signs, brisk reflexes in his arm and legs, and weakness in both his arms and legs without any cranial nerve abnormalities. His magnetic resonance image (MRI) is shown. Which of the following is the most likely diagnosis?

A. Arteriovenous malformation

B. Neuromyelitis optica (NMO)

C. Syrinx

D. Multiple sclerosis

E. Ependymoma

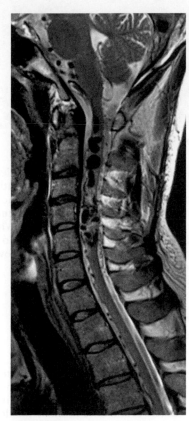

Figure for Question 6.60.

61. A 3-year-old boy presents to the office for evaluation of weakness. Although he developed normally early on, more recently he has become clumsy with falls. On examination, he has diffuse weakness of his lower extremities and enlarged calves. When asked to stand from the floor, he uses his arms to push off his knees to become upright. All of the following are true of this disorder *except?*

    A. X-linked recessive inheritance
    B. Fibrosis of the left ventricle
    C. Muscle biopsy is needed for diagnosis
    D. Creatine kinase is typically above 10,000 mU/mL
    E. Prednisone slows the rate of progression

62. A 45-year-old alcoholic presents with acute confusion. His magnetic resonance imaging (MRI) is shown here. Which of the following is the most likely diagnosis?

    A. Wernicke-Korsakoff syndrome
    B. Multiple sclerosis
    C. Stroke
    D. Marchiafava-Bignami disease
    E. Cerebral autosomal-dominant arteriopathy with subcortical infarcts and leukoencephalopathy (CADASIL)

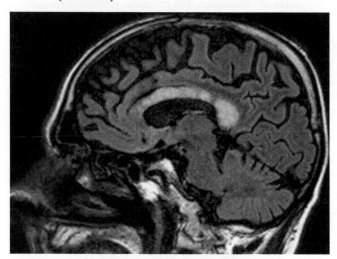

Figure for Question 6.62.

63. A 61-year-old woman with poorly controlled diabetes mellitus type 2 presents to the hospital with acute, severe pain in the midback and urinary incontinence. On examination, she is noted to have a tender, erythematous lesion at the area of pain. While awaiting further diagnostic evaluation, she begins to complain of weakness in her legs. Which of the following is her most likely diagnosis?

    A. Guillain-Barré syndrome
    B. Viral transverse myelitis
    C. Anterior spinal artery stroke
    D. Epidural abscess
    E. Metastatic disease

64. An 82-year-old female presents for evaluation of new-onset headaches and confusion. In the last several months, her family has noticed a decline in her memory but she is still able to make medical decisions for herself. A magnetic resonance image of her brain demonstrates a glioblastoma, suggesting a very poor prognosis. Her family requests keeping the diagnosis from her because it will only upset her. Which of the following is the most appropriate response?

    A. Withhold the diagnosis from the patient.
    B. Ask the patient how much she wants to know before disclosure.
    C. Transfer care to another physician.
    D. Refer the patient to hospice care.
    E. Discharge the patient from the clinic.

65. A 16-year-old young man presents with bilateral lower extremity weakness and spasticity, as well as urinary urgency. The symptoms began about 1 year ago, but have been fairly static for at least 6 months. He has difficulty running without falling, but otherwise his coordination in his arms is fine. He is performing well in school. His paternal grandmother used crutches for most of her life for unknown reasons. Which of the following is the most likely cause of the patient's symptoms?

    A. Tethered cord
    B. Hereditary spastic paraplegia (HSP)
    C. Spinocerebellar ataxia (SCA)
    D. Metachromatic leukodystrophy
    E. Dopa-responsive dystonia

66. An 83-year-old male with a history of atrial fibrillation presents to the emergency room unresponsive after a fall. His computed tomography (CT) scan is shown here. On examination he is somnolent, following no commands. He has a left third nerve palsy with a dilated pupil. Which of the following is the best therapeutic intervention?

    A. Administer intravenous (IV) mannitol
    B. Administer IV 3% NaCl
    C. Switch to aspirin from warfarin
    D. Emergent decompression
    E. Supportive measures alone

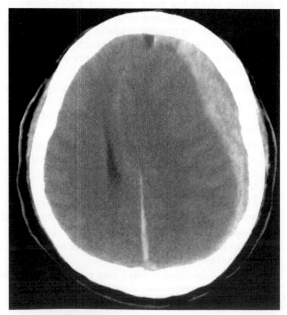

Figure for Question 6.66.

67. A 4-year-old boy with no prior health or developmental concerns is brought to the clinic because of behavioral and developmental concerns. His mother states that he has a hard time speaking to his peers and never seems to look at her in the eyes when she is speaking to him. Unlike his brother and sister, he prefers to be alone and plays with books in his room, frequently turning pages over and over again. She also mentions that anytime they deviate from a plan, such as where to go for dinner, the patient will get angry, almost uncontrollably. What is the most likely diagnosis?

    A. Avoidant personality disorder

    B. Autism

    C. Cerebral palsy

    D. Depression

    E. Absence seizure

68. A 30-year-old female who is 36 weeks pregnant presents to the emergency department with new onset of seizures. Two days before this she complained of a severe headache associated with nausea and vomiting. The headache persisted until today when she developed some blurring of vision. One hour before presentation she had a generalized seizure lasting 5 minutes followed by a second seizure lasting 3 minutes. Her neurological examination demonstrates a somnolent female with no focal findings. Magnetic resonance imaging of the brain performed in the emergency room was unremarkable. Complete blood count and comprehensive metabolic panel were normal. Urinalysis shows no signs of infection, but protein was elevated. Which of the following is the definitive treatment of her condition?

    A. Intravenous (IV) phenytoin load of 20 mg/kg

    B. IV valproic acid load of 20 mg/kg

    C. 2 grams of IV magnesium

    D. Emergency cesarean section

    E. 2 mg of IV lorazepam

69. An injury to the prefrontal cortex would be most likely to affect which type of memory?

    A. Working memory

    B. Episodic memory

    C. Semantic memory

    D. Procedural memory

    E. Declarative memory

70. An eccentric 50-year-old man presents to the neurology clinic with bilateral wrist drop, but no sensory loss. His wife also notes that he's been more confused and forgetful in recent weeks. Other than anemia with an unusual-appearing blood smear, his routine blood work is unremarkable. He notes that he has recently enjoyed a painting class in the style of pointillism. Which of the following is likely to be present in excess and causative of his neurological symptoms?

    A. Arsenic

    B. Lead

    C. Mercury

    D. Zinc

    E. Chromium

71. A 66-year-old female presents for evaluation of memory loss. Her past medical history includes migraine headaches with associated left arm and facial numbness, as well as a small left frontal lobar hemorrhagic stroke from which she recovered well. Her family reports that she's had recent short-term memory loss, word-finding difficulty, and slow mental processing. Her magnetic resonance image (MRI) is shown here. Which of the following is the most likely diagnosis?

    A. Vascular dementia

    B. Alzheimer disease

    C. Cerebral autosomal-dominant arteriopathy with subcortical infarcts and leukoencephalopathy (CADASIL)

    D. Cerebral amyloid angiopathy

    E. Dementia with Lewy bodies

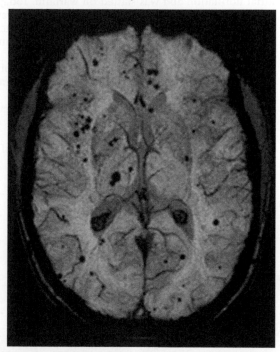

Figure for Question 6.71.

72. A 33-year-old man presents to the emergency room with severe lancinating pain in the left ear and posterior jaw triggered by yawning. He is also scared to eat because chewing can trigger the intense pain. The duration of pain lasts only for seconds. When he does not have the sharp pain, there is a dull ache near the angle of his mandible. His neurological examination is normal, and there is no abnormality seen on otoscopic examination. Temporomandibular joint imaging and magnetic resonance imaging of his cranial nerves are normal. Which of the following is true regarding his condition?

    A. All causes are idiopathic in nature and are usually treated with gabapentin.

    B. Ossification of the stylohyoid ligament can lead to this disorder.

    C. Treatment of choice includes avoidance of triggers.

    D. Attacks usually do not awaken patients from sleep.

    E. Pain is centered around the mandible and usually does not affect the pharynx.

73. A 24-year-old male being treated for tuberculosis presents to the emergency department with painful loss of vision in both eyes. His neurological examination is normal except for finger count acuity in both eyes and loss of red-green differentiation in both eyes. Magnetic resonance imaging of his brain with and without contrast is normal. Which of the following is the most likely cause of his symptoms?

    A. Isoniazid

    B. Rifampin

    C. Streptomycin

    D. Pyrazinamide

    E. Ethambutol

74. A 75-year-old male presents to the emergency department with leg weakness. He was discharged from the hospital 4 weeks ago after his first occurrence of atrial fibrillation and was started on warfarin. Today he fell when trying to get out of bed. Afterward, he was able to walk to the bathroom but could not initiate urination. As the morning progressed his legs became weaker to the point that he could not walk. His neurological examination demonstrates paralysis of his lower extremities with normal arm strength. His cranial nerve examination was normal. He has decreased sensation in his lower extremities with a sensory level from the midabdomen down. A bladder scan demonstrated 800 mL retained in his bladder. His magnetic resonance image is shown here. Which of the following is the most likely diagnosis?

    A. Transverse myelitis

    B. Syringomyelia

    C. Epidural hematoma

    D. Arteriovenous malformation

    E. Spinal stenosis

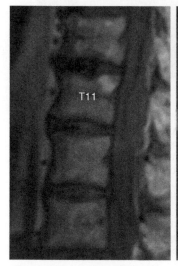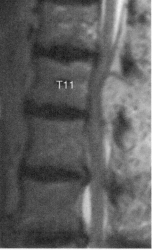

Figure for Question 6.74.

75. A 19-year-old soldier is propelled from a standing position as a result of a nearby explosion. He lands forcefully with a large boulder in the region of his low back. He is found by the unit medic. Examination reveals normal cognitive status, as well as normal arm strength and reflexes. However, he has flaccid, asymmetric weakness in his legs (right is weaker than left), which is worse distally. Similarly, there is patchy numbness in the legs to pin prick and vibration without laterality, although peroneal sensation is intact. His reflexes are asymmetrically decreased with flexor plantar responses. He has urinary incontinence while being examined. Based on the most likely localization, and assuming no orthopedic or penetrating injury, which of the following is probably true regarding this patient?

    A. Bifrontal contusion will improve with time.

    B. Thoracic anterior cord syndrome will lead to spastic paraparesis.

    C. Conus medullaris syndrome is not changed by timing of surgery.

    D. Cauda equina syndrome outcome is not changed by timing of surgery.

    E. Peripheral nerve crush injury leads to both demyelination and axonal loss.

76. After moving furniture, a 69-year-old woman felt sudden pain in her low back and a shooting sensation down to her great toe. Given the most likely injured nerve root, which of the following nerves are likely to be affected?

    A. Femoral nerve

    B. Obturator nerve

    C. Lateral femoral cutaneous nerve

    D. Deep peroneal nerve

    E. Lateral plantar nerve

77. Which of the following is true regarding selective serotonin reuptake inhibitors (SSRIs)?

    A. They increase serotonin by activating serotonin receptors.

    B. The effect of SSRIs typically takes several days to weeks to become apparent.

    C. Erectile dysfunction is not a common side effect in men.

    D. These cannot worsen bipolar disorder.

    E. Sedation is not very likely with SSRIs.

78. A 43-year-old man with a history of complicated migraines and transient ischemic attack (TIA) presents with right upper extremity weakness and slurred speech. His examination shows delayed cognitive processing, right pronator drift, dysarthria, and a slight right facial droop. After his last TIA, his cardiac workup, including transthoracic echocardiogram (TTE), was negative, as was his vessel imaging. He also mentions that his mother had a history of stroke, dementia, and migraines. His magnetic resonance image (MRI) is shown. Given his history, what is the next best diagnostic study to obtain a diagnosis?

    A. No further testing required

    B. Computed tomography (CT) of chest/abdomen/pelvis

    C. Factor V Leiden testing

    D. Brain biopsy

    E. *NOTCH3* mutation testing

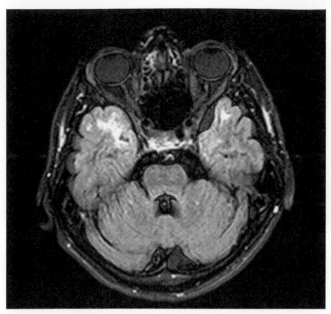

Figure for Question 6.78.

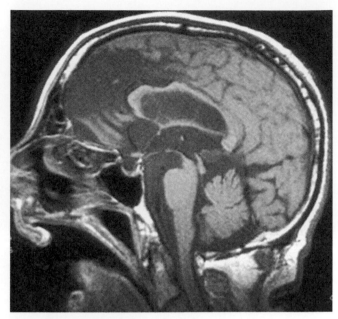

Figure for Question 6.80.

79. A lesion in the subthalamic nucleus is most likely to cause which of the following?

    A. Hemiballismus

    B. Parkinsonism

    C. Essential tremor

    D. Pain syndrome

    E. Vertical gaze palsy

80. A 70-year-old man presents with a 1-year history of frequent falls, most of which have resulted in injuries. Although he denies tremor, he does endorse more shuffling in his gait, hypophonia, and diplopia with difficulty walking down stairs. His wife reports that he frequently chokes while eating. On examination he has a slightly hyperextended neck with slowing of vertical saccades, limited vertical gaze, and lack of convergence. Vertical gaze limitation is overcome by the oculocephalic maneuver. There is contraction of the frontalis with some difficulty opening his eyes. Rigidity is more prominent in the axial musculature than in the upper extremities. There is pivoting of his gait when turning, followed by retropulsion. The patient's magnetic resonance image is shown. Which of the following is the most likely diagnosis in this patient?

    A. Multiple system atrophy (MSA)

    B. Normal pressure hydrocephalus

    C. Progressive supranuclear palsy (PSP)

    D. Idiopathic Parkinson disease

    E. Corticobasal ganglionic degeneration

81. A 15-year-old boy joins his football team at the urging of his parents. He quickly excels at the sport, but his grades fall from As to Cs. His teachers complain about his irritability and "quick temper" in class. When asked, the boy's football coach seconds the concern of irritability, and also notes that the boy has developed muscle hypertrophy and worsening acne. Which of the following is most likely the reason for his personality change?

    A. Methamphetamines

    B. Depression

    C. Misuse of exogenous steroids

    D. Physical abuse

    E. Stress from parental pressure

82. When performing cold water calorics on an awake individual with intact vestibular function, other than causing severe nausea, which of the following is true?

    A. Head should deviate away from the stimulated ear

    B. Fast phase of nystagmus should be upward

    C. No nystagmus should occur

    D. Fast phase of nystagmus should be toward the stimulated ear

    E. Fast phase of nystagmus should be away from the stimulated ear

83. A 78-year-old female presents to clinic for evaluation of progressive memory loss. Six months ago she had a small right parietal stroke. Immediately after the stroke, she had short-term memory deficits, which have persisted. Then, 3 months ago she developed a new slowing of her cognitive processing. Two weeks ago, her family noticed that she no longer knew how to use her kitchen appliances. A magnetic resonance imaging (MRI) showed subcortical white matter disease but no acute strokes and no evidence of prior hemorrhages. Which of the following is the most likely diagnosis?

    A. Alzheimer disease

    B. Cerebral amyloid angiopathy

    C. Vascular dementia

    D. Frontotemporal dementia

    E. Cerebral autosomal-dominant arteriopathy with subcortical infarcts and leukoencephalopathy (CADASIL)

84. In comparison to rapid eye movement (REM) sleep, all of the following physiological changes occur during non-REM (NREM) sleep *except*?

    A. Decrease in sympathetic activation

    B. Bradycardia

    C. Decreased blood pressure

    D. Decreased cerebral blood flow

    E. Decrease in parasympathetic activation

85. A 42-year-old man presents to the emergency room with recurrent episodes of excruciating, searing pain on the right side of his face. Brushing his teeth and walking into the wind seem to trigger the pain. He has upwards of 10 episodes per day, although each lasts only seconds. Which of the following would be unlikely as an underlying cause of this symptom?

    A. Trigeminal nerve compression by enlarged blood vessel

    B. Multiple sclerosis

    C. Paraneoplastic syndrome

    D. History of facial trauma

    E. Cerebellopontine angle tumor

86. After leaving the cochlear nucleus, which structure do auditory signals pass next?

    A. Lateral lemniscus

    B. Inferior colliculus

    C. Superior olivary complex

    D. Medial geniculate body

    E. Superior colliculus

87. Which of the following reflexes does *not* involve the trigeminal nerve?

    A. Corneal reflex

    B. Jaw jerk reflex

    C. Lacrimal reflex

    D. Oculocardiac reflex

    E. Gag reflex

88. During a microvascular decompression for trigeminal neuralgia, brainstem auditory evoked potentials are monitored. Which of the following is the most likely reason for loss of wave I during the procedure?

    A. Lateral pontine infarct

    B. Midbrain infarct

    C. Stretch injury to vestibular nerve

    D. Displaced acoustic stimulator

    E. Normal variant

89. At what age should a child be able to smile spontaneously, copy facial expressions, babble, reach for a toy with one hand, and push up to elbows when lying on the stomach?

    A. 2 months

    B. 4 months

    C. 6 months

    D. 9 months

    E. 1 year

90. A 17-year-old male recently passed away from refractory seizures. Three years ago he developed quick jerking movements of his arms. These brief movements caused him to drop items or throw things across the room. He developed frequent generalized tonic-clonic seizures. He went from being a straight A student to barely passing. His seizures became so frequent he died from status epilepticus. A periodic acid–Schiff–stained slide from brain autopsy is shown here. Which of the following is the most likely diagnosis?

    A. Myoclonic epilepsy with ragged red fibers

    B. Juvenile myoclonic epilepsy

    C. Medial temporal sclerosis

    D. Lafora body disease

    E. Creutzfeldt-Jakob disease (CJD)

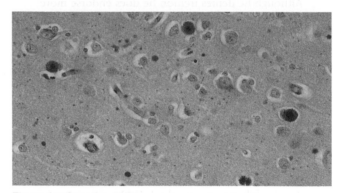

Figure for Question 6.90.

91. Which is the best test for determining one's intelligence quotient?

    A. Wechsler Intelligence Scale

    B. California Verbal Learning Test

    C. Boston Naming Test

    D. Trail-Making Test

    E. Wisconsin Card Sorting Test

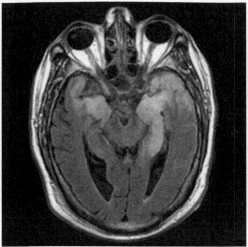
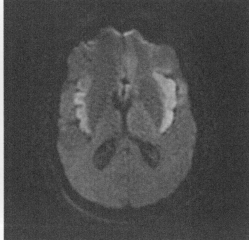

Figure for Question 6.92.

92. A 27-year-old man is brought to the hospital with 2 days of fever, malaise, confusion, and hallucinations. This morning he had his first generalized tonic-clonic seizure. On examination, outside of confusion and poor memory, he demonstrates normal strength, sensation, and reflexes. Spinal fluid reveals normal glucose, slightly elevated red blood cells (RBCs), and markedly elevated protein with a lymphocyte-predominant pleocytosis. Cytology is pending. A magnetic resonance image (MRI) is obtained in the emergency room and fluid attenuated inversion recovery and diffusion weighted imaging sequences are shown here. Based on this, computed tomographies of the chest, abdomen, and pelvis are performed and reveal no obvious abnormalities. Which of the following is the next best course of action?

    A. Initiate antipsychotic therapy

    B. Initiate intravenous corticosteroids

    C. MRI of the spine with and without contrast

    D. Initiate intravenous acyclovir therapy

    E. Perform testicular ultrasound

93. A 3-year-old boy is evaluated for loss of milestones. He is generally docile and sleeps soundly (albeit sonorously) through the night. On examination, he is a very calm young man, less than 2nd percentile for height, and in the 80th percentile for weight. He has hepatosplenomegaly, coarse facies, corneal clouding, macroglossia, and decreased hearing bilaterally. A female cousin had similar symptoms. His image is shown here. Which of the following is the deficient enzyme?

    A. Ornithine transcarbamoylase

    B. Alpha-L iduronidase

    C. Iduronate-2-sulfatase

    D. Heparan sulfamidase

    E. Fumarase

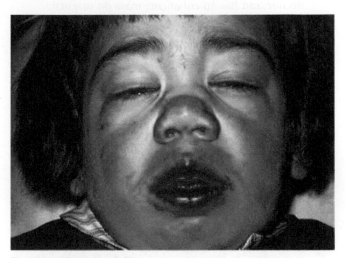

Figure for Question 6.93.

94. An 18-month-old boy presents to the neurology clinic for gait difficulty. He did not start attempting to walk until he was 15 months old. He continues to have frequent falls, and tends to walk on his toes. His mother also notes that he bounces when he walks. His history is notable for a full-term birth, but he had a nuchal cord and low Apgar scores. His examination is notable for spasticity in the bilateral lower extremities, as well as ankle clonus bilaterally. In addition, he has weakness in his hip flexors and knee flexors bilaterally. Which of the following is true regarding his most likely condition?

    A. Magnetic resonance images (MRIs) are often normal.

    B. His neurological deficits will likely progress with age.

    C. There are no cognitive or developmental delays seen in this condition generally.

    D. Regression in motor skills is a common manifestation of this condition.

    E. Seizures are often associated with this condition.

95. A 16-year-old male is an exceptional football player and is taken off the field during the first quarter of the state championship with a concern for a concussion. As the sideline physician, you determine that the patient likely suffered a mild concussion without loss of consciousness. The patient's coach says the team will lose without putting him back in the game. The patient is eager to return to the field. Which of the following is the most appropriate action?

    A. Allow the patient to return to the game.
    B. Hold the patient out until halftime and then allow return to play.
    C. Withhold the patient from the game.
    D. Allow return to play as long as he is not given the ball.
    E. Immediately transfer the patient to the emergency room.

96. A 54-year-old immunosuppressed man was in the hospital 1 week ago for an elective ventriculoperitoneal shunt placement for idiopathic intracranial hypertension. He returns now with severe neurological decline and has an enhancing mass on magnetic resonance imaging (MRI). He undergoes removal of the enhancing mass, the pathology from which is demonstrated here. Which of the following is the most likely cause of his acute decline?

    A. Toxic/metabolic encephalopathy
    B. Bacterial abscess
    C. Residual surgical debris
    D. Shunt malfunction
    E. Fungal infection

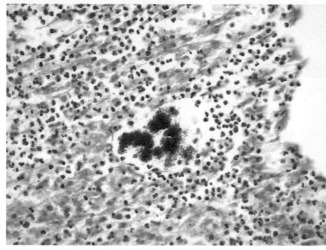

Figure for Question 6.96.

97. A 1-month-old presents to the hospital with lethargy and is found to have *Escherichia coli* septicemia. History provided by his mother includes poor growth since birth and a diagnosis of cataracts. He appears jaundiced and is noted to have hepatomegaly. Laboratory examination reveals liver dysfunction and hypoglycemia. Which of the following is true regarding this condition?

    A. The mainstay of care is to discontinue ingestion of fructose-containing formulas.
    B. This condition often remains occult on the newborn screen.
    C. Once diagnosed, the neurological deficits will progress despite restriction of the initial substrate.
    D. It results from a deficiency in glutaryl-CoA dehydrogenase.
    E. It results from a deficiency in galactose-1-phosphate uridyltransferase (GALT) deficiency.

98. A comatose patient who suffered a traumatic car accident has midposition pupils that do not respond to light. What is the most likely localization of the causative injury for his pupillary abnormality, as well as his coma?

    A. Bilateral pons
    B. Cerebrum
    C. Bilateral diencephalon
    D. Bilateral midbrain tegmentum
    E. Bilateral oculomotor nuclei

99. A 22-year-old female with a history of chronic headaches and substance abuse presents to the emergency department for evaluation. In the last few hours she has had lacrimation, rhinorrhea, nausea, abdominal cramps, and diarrhea. She is noted to be restless and irritable. Her neurological examination is normal except for dilated pupils. She believes this reaction is from her medications. Which of the following is the most likely cause?

    A. Amitriptyline
    B. Oxycodone withdrawal
    C. Topiramate
    D. Alcohol withdrawal
    E. Propranolol withdrawal

100. Which of the following immunotherapies acts through a purine analog metabolite?

    A. Azathioprine
    B. Cyclophosphamide
    C. Cyclosporine
    D. Rituximab
    E. Methotrexate

Questions 101-105: Match the gene to its associated channelopathy.

101. *SCN4A*

102. *CLCN1*

103. *CACNA1A*

104. *GLRA1*

105. *KCNA1*

    A. Hereditary hyperekplexia
    B. Familial hemiplegic migraine
    C. Episodic ataxia type 1
    D. Hypokalemic periodic paralysis
    E. Myotonia congenita

ANSWERS

1. C. Myotonic dystrophy is a disorder marked by myotonia (grip myotonia and percussion myotonia), prominent facial weakness, frontal balding, and distal weakness. This disorder can cause cataracts, sleep apnea, diabetes, and cardiac arrhythmias, which are a significant cause of mortality in these patients. The EMG shows myopathic units along with diffuse myotonia, which is spontaneous activity with a waxing and waning quality. This is an autosomal-dominant disorder with anticipation due to a CTG repeat. The responsible gene is the *DMPK* gene on chromosome 19. *SOD1* mutations are associated with hereditary amyotrophic lateral sclerosis (*see* Bradley's NiCP, 7th edn, Ch. 110, pp. 1915–1956).

2. A. Myelin basic protein (MBP) has long been considered the primary candidate for an autoimmune cause of multiple sclerosis. Whereas normal individuals have MBP-targeting T-cells in peripheral blood, this population may be increased in patients with active disease. Further, the primary animal model for studying multiple sclerosis, EAE, is created with autoimmunity toward MBP. The other proteins may also contribute to multiple sclerosis autoimmunity, but to a lesser extent. Proteolipid protein accounts for 50% of central nervous system myelin protein, whereas myelin-associated glycoprotein, myelin oligodendrocyte glycoprotein, and cyclic nucleotide phosphodiesterase account for a small percent of myelin proteins (*see* Bradley's NiCP, 7th edn, Ch. 51, pp. 676–695).

3. D. Whereas birth order has not been associated with risk for MS, all of the other factors have been considered potential links for disease development. Smoking has been shown to increase the risk of MS in multiple case control studies. Vitamin D deficiency, as well as the related factor of latitude of residence (and sun exposure), have been associated with MS risk in several studies. Evidence of prior infections, especially with Epstein-Barr virus, has been associated with MS risk. Immune system genetics, including certain classes of major histocompatibility proteins and human leukocyte antigen (HLA), such as HLA class I A3 and B7, have also been associated with MS risk (*see* Bradley's NiCP, 7th edn, Ch. 51, pp. 676–695).

4. D. In normal adults, the average CSF volume is between 125 and 150 mL (*see* Bradley's NiCP, 7th edn, Ch. 88, pp. 1261–1278).

5. B. The key point in this question is to realize that the patient's neurological condition has continued to worsen, which would go against the typical course of cerebral palsy. The next key point is to recognize the description of diurnal variation (symptoms worsen as the day goes on with relief after sleep). Her symptoms in the arms and legs describe dystonia. Given these facts, a dopa-responsive dystonia (DYT-5) is the most likely diagnosis. This often presents with gait dysfunction in childhood with diurnal variation, parkinsonism, and extrapyramidal dysfunction such as hyperreflexia and increased tone. This condition is often misdiagnosed as cerebral palsy, but does not remain static. DYT-5 is exquisitely sensitive to levodopa. The diagnosis can be confirmed by sending for cerebrospinal fluid neurotransmitters (GTP cyclohydrolase 1 deficiency or tyrosine hydroxylase deficiency). Although a trial of physical therapy may be useful, a treatment should first be offered in this case. A referral to a genetic

counselor could be considered given that GTP cyclohydrolase 1 deficiency is autosomal dominant and tyrosine hydroxylase deficiency is autosomal recessive, but treatment should not be withheld. Wilson disease, an autosomal-recessive defect in copper metabolism that can present with dystonia, parkinsonism, psychiatric symptoms, and liver failure, typically does not have a diurnal variation as in this case. It is treated with chelation therapy (penicillamine or triethylenetetramine dihydrochloride; *see* Bradley's NiCP, 7th edn, Ch. 23, pp. 223–249).

6. B. Peroneal (fibular) compression at the fibular head is a relatively common disorder in pregnancy. It occurs as a consequence of compression of the peroneal (fibular) nerve from positioning during delivery, particularly with prolonged labor and epidural anesthesia. Prognosis is usually favorable without specific treatments. Normal recruitment in the tibialis posterior, gluteus medius, and short head of the biceps femoris in combination with reduced recruitment in the tibialis anterior and peroneus longus localizes the lesion to the fibular head rather than to the lumbar plexus or to a specific nerve root. Nerve conduction studies would show a conduction block of the peroneal (fibular) nerve around the fibular head. Fibrillations and positive sharp waves would not be seen until 7–14 days after the initial injury. Retroperitoneal hematomas can lead to lumbosacral plexopathy or femoral neuropathy. Epidural hematomas and ischemic strokes should be considerations in the postpartum period, but EMG findings of reduced recruitment localize the lesion to the peripheral nervous system (*see* Bradley's NiCP, 7th edn, Chs. 112, pp. 1791–1865 and 107, pp. 1973–1991).

7. E. The image demonstrates a classic oligodendroglioma with round nuclei and perinuclear halos, causing a "fried egg" appearance. Meningioma histology is notable for meningothelial whirls and psammoma bodies. Pilocytic astrocytoma is a grade I astrocytoma with no mitoses, but with Rosenthal fibers, which are a marker of chronic inflammation and gliosis. CNS lymphoma is a lymphoproliferative disease, most commonly with large CD20+ B-cells intracerebrally. Schwannomas are notable for arising from the nerve sheath eccentrically in an encapsulated mass and compressing the underlying nerve, as opposed to neurofibromas, which also arise from the nerve sheath, but are unencapsulated and more of a tortuous plexus of Schwann cells and axons (*see* Bradley's NiCP, 7th edn, Ch. 72, pp. 1026–1044). Figure from Daroff RB, Jankovic J, Mazziotta JC, Pomeroy SL 2016 *Bradley's Neurology in Clinical Practice*, 7th edn, Elsevier, with permission.

8. C. Hemoglobinopathies are an important consideration for pediatric strokes. The prior admission for finger pain was likely a sickling-related dactylitis. Whereas sickle cell disease, the most common hemoglobinopathy, is autosomal recessive, his family history does not necessarily rule this out. Although cardiac structural irregularities may cause strokes, they do not cause dactylitis. *NOTCH3* mutations are associated with cerebral autosomal-dominant arteriopathy with subcortical infarcts and leukoencephalopathy (CADASIL). This disease, as the name indicates, does cause strokes but is not present in our current case due to the autosomal-dominant nature and the unlikelihood of associated dactylitis. Lipid screening

would identify evidence of a familial dyslipidemia, which increases stroke risk, although that is not the most likely answer in this case. Although mitochondrial disorders, such as mitochondrial encephalomyopathy with lactic acidosis and strokes, are associated with strokes, generally patients are also of short stature with associated weakness, seizures, or vomiting. Because this syndrome is mitochondrial, his mother would be likely to have shown symptoms thereof (*see* Bradley's NiCP, 7th edn, Ch. 68, pp. 996–1006).

9. D. The following muscles are predominantly innervated by the C7 root: triceps, pronator teres, anconeus, extensor carpi radialis, and flexor carpi radialis.

10. E. Hypervitaminosis A, along with the use of tetracyclines or hormonal contraceptives, are several of the known causes of increased intracranial pressure. Discontinuing the offending agent should result in resolution of the symptoms. Topiramate, acetazolamide, and weight loss are common treatments for idiopathic intracranial hypertension. Although snoring may indicate sleep apnea, and sleep apnea is a risk factor for idiopathic intracranial hypertension, snoring alone is not a risk for increased intracranial pressure (*see* Bradley's NiCP, 7th edn, Ch. 103, pp. 1686–1719).

11. C. The patient's physical examination demonstrates chronic progressive weakness of eye motility that does not follow a specific anatomical or cranial nerve pattern, which is typical of an external ophthalmoplegia. This, in combination with hearing loss and pigmentary retinopathy, suggests a mitochondrial disorder, with Kearns-Sayre syndrome as the most likely cause. Oculopharyngeal muscular dystrophy (OPMD) can cause similar eye movement abnormalities, but typically other signs are present, such as ptosis, dysarthria, or dysphagia. Notably, OPMD is not a mitochondrial disorder and is not associated with hearing loss or pigmentary retinopathy. Myasthenia gravis and the Miller Fischer variant of Guillain-Barré syndrome can cause similar eye movement abnormalities, but hearing loss and retinopathy are not present. MELAS is a mitochondrial disorder associated with muscle weakness, lactic acidosis, headaches, and stroke-like episodes involving hemiparesis or vision loss. Eye motility disorders, retinopathy, and hearing loss are uncommon with MELAS (*see* Bradley's NiCP, 7th edn, Ch. 93, pp. 1349–1364).

12. D. Rett syndrome is a genetic pervasive developmental disorder caused by a mutation in the *MECP2* gene on the X chromosome. Patients with Rett syndrome often have abnormally small hands and feet, as well as microcephaly. The majority of patients never walk or talk. Hand-wringing stereotypes are commonly seen in this disorder. It is notable that the majority of cases of Rett syndrome are sporadic rather than inherited from either parent. *FMR1* mutations are associated with fragile X syndrome (*see* Bradley's NiCP, 7th edn, Chs. 50, pp. 648–675 and 90, pp. 1301–1323).

13. C. When membrane potential reaches 55 mV, voltage-gated sodium channels open, causing rapid influx of sodium ions into the cell, which causes depolarization. As further depolarization occurs, more sodium channels open, accelerating depolarization quickly. Once membrane potential reaches approximately +60 mV the sodium channels close quickly and K$^+$

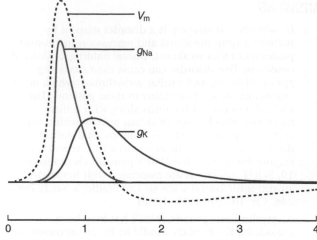

Figure for Answer 6.13 When the resting membrane voltage (V_m) is depolarized to threshold, voltage-gated sodium channels are opened, increasing Na$^+$ conductance (g_{Na}), resulting in an influx of sodium and further depolarization. The action potential, however, is short lived, due to the inactivation of the sodium channels within 1–2 ms and an increase in K$^+$ conductance (g_K). These changes, along with the Na$^+$/K$^+$ pump, allow the axon to reestablish the resting membrane potential (*see* Bradley's NiCP, 7th edn, Ch. 34–35, pp. 349–391). *(Action potential, from Preston DC, Shapiro BE 2013* Electromyography and Neuromuscular Disorders, *3rd edn, Elsevier, with permission.)*

channels open. The removal of K$^+$ from the cell and discontinuation of Na$^+$ intake causes repolarization. The K channels are slow in closing, which causes the overshoot hyperpolarization and refractory period. The Na-K ATPase pump helps return the cell to the starting resting concentrations.

14. E. The patient presents with signs and symptoms concerning for meningitis or encephalitis with a lumbar puncture consistent with viral meningitis or encephalitis. The EEG demonstrates bitemporal periodic lateralized epileptiform discharges, with a predominance over the right side, which is common in herpes encephalitis due to the predilection for the temporal lobes. Tuberculous meningitis and strep pneumonia do not have typical EEG findings. Subacute sclerosing panencephalitis (SSPE) demonstrates synchronous 2- to 3-second bursts of high-amplitude slow waves associated with myoclonic jerks occurring every 5–10 seconds. The EEG in Creutzfeldt-Jakob disease demonstrates 1- to 2-Hz triphasic periodic sharp wave complexes with a low voltage and slow background (*see* Bradley's NiCP, 7th edn, Ch. 78, pp. 1121–1146). Figure from Daroff RB, Jankovic J, Mazziotta JC, Pomeroy SL 2016 *Bradley's Neurology in Clinical Practice*, 7th edn, Elsevier, with permission.

15. A. This EEG demonstrates periodic bursts of high-amplitude slow wave complexes, which are typical of subacute sclerosing panencephalitis (SSPE), a severe consequence of measles infection. Absence epilepsy is characterized by a generalized 3-Hz spike and wave discharges. Hepatic encephalopathy and other metabolic encephalopathies can show a slow background with triphasic waves. Herpes encephalitis will show bitemporal periodic lateralized epileptiform discharges (PLEDs). Benign epilepsy with centrotemporal spikes shows exactly what the name

says—centrotemporal spikes during sleep, which can be bilateral, be independent, and have a horizontal dipole (*see* Bradley's NiCP, 7th edn, Ch. 34, pp. 348–365). Figure from Buchanan R, Bonthius DJ 2012 Measles virus and associated central nervous system sequelae. *Seminars in Pediatric Neurology* 19(3): pp. 107–114, with permission.

16. B. Schizoid personality disorder is a disorder marked by emotional detachment from society and even family. These patients tend to hold jobs in which there is little human interaction. There is no discomfort or fear of a relationship as is present with avoidant personality disorder, and there is no paranoia as is present with paranoid personality disorder. This is differentiated from schizophrenia by the lack of hallucinations and lack of disorganized thought processes. Patients with autism may prefer solitude because of their impaired social skills, but those with schizoid personality disorder are able to interact normally.

17. A. NCL is a group of autosomal-*recessive* disorders characterized by myoclonic epilepsy, blindness, and psychomotor retardation. Extrapyramidal symptoms may also occur. Several gene mutations lead to various forms of this disorder. The most well-known form is the juvenile form (Batten disease), which is characterized by visual loss, seizures, myoclonus, and psychomotor retardation beginning between the ages of 4 and 10 years old. Commonly, "fingerprint bodies," or granular osmophilic deposits, are seen on electron microscopy. Magnetic resonance imaging shows only cerebral atrophy, whereas cerebellar atrophy occurs later in the course of the disease. EEG generally shows a disorganized background with spike and slow wave complexes. Both enzyme levels and genetic sequencing can be tested to help facilitate the diagnosis of NCL. The treatment is supportive, mostly consisting of epilepsy management (*see* Bradley's NiCP, 7th edn, Ch. 91, pp. 1324–1341).

18. E. The vein of Labbé is a superficial cerebral vein that anastomoses the middle cerebral vein to the transverse sinus. The vein of Trolard anastomoses the middle

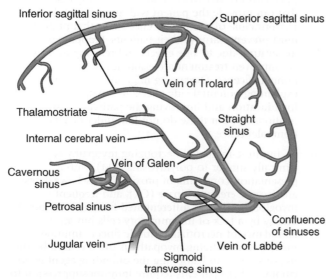

Figure for Answer 6.18 *(from Lemkuil BP, Drummond JC, Patel PM 2013 Central nervous system physiology: cerebrovascular. In: Hemmings HC, Egan TD (eds.) Pharmacology and Physiology for Anesthesia, pp. 123–136, Elsevier, with permission.)*

cerebral vein with the superior sagittal sinus. The figure demonstrates the major venous anatomy of the brain.

19. C. Given the history of alcoholism and ascites, paired with encephalopathy and asterixis, the most likely cause of his trouble is hepatic encephalopathy. Hyperparathyroidism may lead to hypercalcemia. When severe, hypercalcemia can cause depression, encephalopathy, or even coma, among other medical complications. There is no indication in the current patient of hyperparathyroidism. Intoxication is a possibility in a patient with history of alcoholism, although his problem is progressive over several days. Further, fever and abdominal pain are not generally associated with intoxication. Although uremic encephalopathy may also cause depressed levels of consciousness and asterixis, this patient would be at higher risk of hepatic trouble with his new ascites. Myxedema, related to chronic hypothyroidism, may cause depressed level of consciousness, but generally in the setting of progressive weight gain, fatigue, peripheral edema, and constipation (*see* Bradley's NiCP, 7th edn, Ch. 58, pp. 814–834).

20. D. In cirrhotic patients, spontaneous bacterial peritonitis is a common precipitant of hepatic encephalopathy. It is important to note that the ammonia level needn't be extremely high in hepatic encephalopathy if the case is otherwise consistent. Fever of unknown origin may cause an encephalopathy in an otherwise susceptible patient, although an abdominal source seems more likely given the scenario. Alcohol withdrawal would more likely cause tachycardia, agitation, and hallucinations. Excessive dietary protein may lead to an elevated ammonia level and encephalopathy in a severely cirrhotic patient, although it wouldn't account for abdominal pain and fever. Tylenol overdose may cause an acute liver failure with encephalopathy, although this isn't the most likely choice given the patient's history.

21. C. The most likely answer of the given choices is an ependymoma. The clinical picture demonstrates a young patient with acute onset of cervical dystonia. Imaging demonstrates a lesion in the cervical cord that is intramedullary, expansive, edematous, and avidly takes up contrast, which are all typical of ependymomas (and other tumors like lymphoma). Genetic torsion dystonia (DYT1) presents similarly but with normal imaging. MS presents with lesions within the spinal cord; however, these are not typically expansive lesions with as much edema as is present in the images presented, and MS would be quite rare in a patient of this age. Meningiomas are extramedullary tumors that avidly enhance with contrast with a dural tail. Spinal cord infarct causes severe weakness with loss of pain and temperature sensation while preserving vibration and proprioception (*see* Bradley's NiCP, 7th edn, Ch. 75, pp. 1065–1083). Figures from van den Hauwe L, van Goethem JW, Balériaux D, De Schepper AM 2015 *Grainger & Allison's Diagnostic Radiology*, Elsevier, with permission.

22. B. Penicillin G is the treatment of choice in cases of neurosyphilis, which is more common in patients with a history of HIV. This disease is marked by chronic meningitis, multiple cranial neuropathies, embolic infarcts, and multiple intracranial aneurysms. Cerebrospinal fluid (CSF) testing is usually nonspecific

with an elevated white cell count (mononuclear pleocytosis), protein, and mildly low glucose. Venereal disease research laboratory (VDRL) testing of the CSF can help make the diagnosis. Amphotericin B is used in the treatment of fungal meningitis, including cryptococcal meningitis, which is a common infection in immunocompromised and acquired immunodeficiency disease (AIDS) patients. This commonly presents with worsening headaches, bilateral papilledema, and greatly elevated opening pressures in patients with HIV. Vancomycin is frequently used in empiric treatment of presumed bacterial meningitis, but this will not treat neurosyphilis. Acyclovir is used in the treatment of herpes encephalitis, which can present in a similar fashion but would not be associated with multiple aneurysms. Highly active antiretroviral therapy is important for all HIV patients to protect against opportunistic infections and should be started, but this will not treat neurosyphilis (*see* Bradley's NiCP, 7th edn, Ch. 79, pp. 1147–1158).

23. B. Dexamethasone is often used in cases of primary or secondary CNS tumors for several reasons, including its low mineralocorticoid activity (less sodium absorption and potassium excretion), longer half-life than prednisone, and its lower tendency to induce psychosis. The main reason to institute dexamethasone in cancer patients is to reduce the *vasogenic* edema surrounding primary and secondary CNS tumors, as well as to provide pleotropic antiinflammatory effects. Cytotoxic edema is often found in strokes as well some abscesses, and does not generally improve with steroids. Knowing the physiological dose of dexamethasone is helpful for neurologists in order to understand dosing when beginning or weaning dexamethasone.

24. A. All of the following are known risk factors for OSA: male gender, increasing age, menopause, body mass index >25, male neck circumference >17 inches, female neck circumference >16 inches, alcohol, smoking, nasal allergies, craniofacial abnormalities, and race (Hispanics, African Americans, and Pacific Islanders). Hypertension is not a risk factor for OSA, but it can be a consequence of untreated OSA (*see* Bradley's NiCP, 7th edn, Ch. 102, pp. 1615–1685).

25. A. An illusion is a misinterpretation of true sensory input, most commonly by mistaking obscure visual input for something unrelated. This is in contrast to a hallucination, which is a sensory experience without a true stimulus (e.g. seeing something that does not exist). Although patients with dementia and delirium may be at increased risk of visual hallucinations, there is insufficient evidence in the stem to make such a diagnosis. Delusions are fixed false beliefs, maintained even when confronted with reality.

26. D. Surgery for temporal lobe epilepsy can be an effective treatment to provide seizure freedom. The best candidates include patients with abnormalities seen on MRI, especially mesial temporal sclerosis. Surgical outcome is best when it can be localized only to one side, so unilateral ictal or interictal discharges are a positive predictor. PET scans are typically performed in the evaluation for surgery, and interictal hypometabolism suggests an area of dysfunction. If this correlates with EEG abnormalities, this is also another good prognostic sign. Normal postoperative EEGs don't predict success; however, abnormal postoperative EEGs

suggest a higher chance of seizure recurrence. A history of head trauma as the cause of refractory seizures is an unfavorable predictor of surgical success (*see* Bradley's NiCP, 7th edn, Ch. 101, pp. 1563–1614).

27. D. The image is a hematoxylin and eosin stain showing neurofibrillary tangles composed of tau within neocortical neurons, which appear as pale basophilic fibrillary cytoplasmic inclusions. Also present in Alzheimer disease are beta-amyloid plaques. Pick disease would have pick bodies, which are intracytoplasmic eosinophilic inclusions made of tau. Creutzfeldt-Jakob disease would be associated with microvacuolar degeneration and occasional prion protein deposition or kuru plaques. Parkinson disease is classically associated with Lewy bodies, which are alpha-synuclein inclusions, as well as loss of dopaminergic neurons in the substantia nigra. Huntington disease is marked by neuronal loss, but little other histological change specific to the disease (*see* Bradley's NiCP, 7th edn, Ch. 95, pp. 1380–1421). Figure from Ma JM 2010 Biopsy pathology of neurodegenerative disorders in adults. In: *Practical Surgical Neuropathology: A Diagnostic Approach*, Churchill Livingstone, pp. 551–572, with permission.

28. C. Labyrinthitis is generally thought to result from a viral infection of the vestibulocochlear nerve. It is distinguished from vestibular neuritis, whose etiology is likely the same, by the presence of hearing loss in addition to vertigo. Vestibular schwannoma may cause similar symptoms, but not generally so abruptly. A stroke involving the labyrinthine artery territory may cause vertigo and hearing loss, but this would be less likely than labyrinthitis in the wake of fevers. Finally, aneurysmal rupture generally leads to subarachnoid hemorrhage, which should present with headache before other neurological deficits (*see* Bradley's NiCP, 7th edn, Ch. 46, pp. 583–604).

29. C. The principle of beneficence demands that physicians perform actions that benefit the patient's well-being. This can be giving medications or performing procedures that improve health, or other interventions, like discussions on smoking cessation, that can provide the patient with great health benefits. The principle of nonmaleficence states that physicians must prevent harm to their patients. Stopping a medication due to side effects and refusing to provide an unproven treatment are examples of nonmaleficence. Discussing migraine causes or explaining potential side effects to a patient are good for education and improving the patient–physician relationship, but these do not fall under beneficence or nonmaleficence.

30. C. Immune-mediated necrotizing myopathy is clinically similar to polymyositis (PM), with a presentation consisting of proximal muscle weakness, an elevated creatine kinase (CK), and frequent myoglobinuria. It is differentiated from PM on muscle biopsy by a lack of inflammatory cells but an abundance of necrotizing muscle fibers. Immune-mediated necrotizing myopathy is often caused by the use of statins, and stopping the offending agent is not curative. These patients require immunosuppression to halt the disease. Statin myopathy is less aggressive and typically causes mild weakness, minimally elevated CKs (<1000 U/L), and improves with discontinuation of the offending agent. Statin myopathies are more likely to

occur with the concurrent use of fibrates, niacin, erythromycin, and cyclosporine. Myasthenia gravis can cause proximal muscle weakness, but it is not associated with CK elevations. Amyotrophic lateral sclerosis can also cause proximal weakness, but CK elevations are usually <1000 U/L. Myotonic dystrophy is an autosomal-dominant condition caused by CTG trinucleotide repeats on chromosome 19 in the *DMPK* gene. This disorder is marked by bifacial weakness, grip weakness, and percussion myotonia, but CKs are not usually elevated to 7500 U/L and myoglobinuria does not occur (*see* Bradley's NiCP, 7th edn, Ch. 101, pp. 1563–1614).

31. A. The digital subtraction angiogram shown depicts a large number of collateral vessels consistent with moyamoya disease. This is a vasculopathy that results from distal stenosis and intimal thickening of the internal carotid arteries. The name comes from the appearance of the collateral vessels that look like a "puff of smoke" which is *moyamoya* in Japanese. Although it can occur in any ethnicity, it is more common in those of Asian descent. Moyamoya syndrome occurs in those with risk factors including sickle cell disease, neurofibromatosis type 1, radiation to the brain, and Down syndrome (trisomy 21). There is no documented increased risk of moyamoya syndrome with trisomy 13, however. Moyamoya disease may also occur in those without known risk factors. Typically, children have ischemic events, whereas adults have hemorrhagic events due to rupture of fragile collateral vessels. There is no standardized treatment, but most are treated with antiplatelet agents. Others go on to have surgical revascularization with external carotid artery (usually the superficial temporal artery) directly or indirectly anastomosed to the distal brain tissue, bypassing the stenotic regions of the internal carotid artery (*see* Bradley's NiCP, 7th edn, Ch. 65, pp. 920–967). Figure from Smith ER, Scott RM 2010 Moyamoya: epidemiology, presentation, and diagnosis. *Neurosurgery Clinics of North America* 21(3): 543–551, with permission.

32. E. Alzheimer disease is a neurodegenerative condition caused by a buildup of amyloid protein in the brain, resulting in pathological findings of neuritic plaques and neurofibrillary tangles. Typical patterns of memory loss include episodic memory loss, anomic aphasia, and visuospatial impairment while procedural memory and working memory remain relatively intact early in the disease. Genetic predispositions to Alzheimer disease involve mutations in the amyloid precursor protein and presenilin 1 and presenilin 2 genes. Although no clinical test can confirm Alzheimer disease, imaging can provide clues to the diagnosis. Magnetic resonance imaging may show marked atrophy of the temporoparietal region in the setting of global atrophy. FDG-PET scans show hypometabolism of the temporoparietal region in Alzheimer disease whereas occipital hypometabolism is seen in dementia with Lewy bodies (*see* Bradley's NiCP, 7th edn, Ch. 95, pp. 1380–1421).

33. D. The positive predictive value is calculated by dividing the true positives by the true positives plus the false positives: 50/(50 + 50) = 0.50. Specificity is a measure of the true negatives divided by the true negatives plus the false positives. A test with a high specificity helps rule in a disorder if the test is positive. In this example there are 90 true negatives and 50 false positives, so 90/(90 + 50) = 0.64. High sensitivity helps

rule out a disorder if the result is negative. Sensitivity is calculated by dividing the true positives by the true positives plus the false negatives (83%). The negative predictive value is calculated by dividing the true negative by the true negative rate plus the false negative rate (90%). The following chart shows the equations used in these calculations.

TABLE FOR ANSWER 6.33

	Disease is present	Disease is not present
Positive result	True positive (TP)	False positive (FP)
Negative result	False negative (FN)	True negative (TN)

Specificity = TN/(FP + TN)
Sensitivity = TP/(TP + FN)
Positive predictive value = TP/(FP + TP)
Negative predictive value = TN/(FN + TN)

34. A. Each of the listed drugs is used, in some capacity, for the treatment of bladder dysfunction. Oxybutynin is an antimuscarinic medication that reduces detrusor overactivity, and may be helpful in neurogenic bladder from suprapontine and cord lesions. Botulinum toxin prohibits local release of acetylcholine, and may be injected into the walls of the bladder to reduce overactivity. Terazosin and tamsulosin are alpha-antagonists that relax the internal urethral sphincter and allow urinary flow. Although these may be used for the treatment of neurogenic bladder, their effect is likely greatest in the setting of bladder outflow obstruction (e.g. prostate hyperplasia). Vasopressin (DDAVP) is a naturally produced hormone that may be taken synthetically to reduce urinary production. This is most commonly used to prevent nocturnal incontinence in the setting of neurogenic bladder dysfunction (*see* Bradley's NiCP, 7th edn, Ch. 47, pp. 605–621).

35. D. Voltage-gated calcium channels open when the synaptic terminal is depolarized, leading to an influx of calcium into the presynaptic terminal. Calcium activates soluble NSF attachment protein receptor proteins (SNARE) to dock to the presynaptic terminal membrane and results in release of acetylcholine into the synapse. Sodium, potassium, and chloride are involved in axonal propagation of action potentials, but it is calcium that directly leads to the release of neurotransmitters. Magnesium at higher concentrations inhibits release of acetylcholine from the presynaptic terminal (*see* Bradley's NiCP, 7th edn, Ch. 109, pp. 1896–1914).

36. E. CRPS is a complex disorder that is accompanied by vasomotor dysregulation, skin color changes, and pain out of proportion to the severity of the inciting event (if such an event is identified). Many risk factors have been associated with CRPS, including postsurgical pain, strokes, fractures, and casting. Early postoperative mobilization may reduce the incidence of CRPS, and physical and occupational therapies accelerate CRPS recovery. There is also growing evidence that vitamin C supplementation may reduce postoperative CRPS incidence. There are several pharmacological approaches to the treatment of CRPS, including topical anesthetics, bisphosphonates, glucocorticoids, antiepileptics, tricyclic antidepressants, and clonidine. Additionally, there are invasive therapeutic strategies such as tender point injections, nerve or spinal cord stimulators, or regional sympathetic nerve blocks. The

goal of any symptomatic therapy is to allow patients to participate in rehabilitation and restore strength and movement in the affected limb (*see* Bradley's NiCP, 7th edn, Ch. 54, pp. 720–741).

37. D. MEN1 is associated with tumors of the anterior pituitary, parathyroid, and pancreatic islet cells. MEN2 is associated with tumors of the thyroid, adrenal gland (pheochromocytoma), and parathyroid. Syndromes associated with glioblastoma include neurofibromatosis type 1 and Turcot syndrome, which is also associated with medulloblastoma, multiple colonic polyps, and colon cancer. There are no known syndromes with increased risk of primary CNS lymphoma. There are no known syndromes with increased risk of hypothalamic hamartoma. Retinoblastoma risk is increased with genetic *Rb* mutation, but is not associated with MEN1 (*see* Bradley's NiCP, 7th edn, Ch. 71, pp. 1018–1025).

38. B. Medication overuse headache is a common secondary headache type in the setting of an underlying primary headache disorder. It is associated with frequent use of analgesics or opioids. The most important first step in the treatment of medication overuse headache is reduction of the offending agent(s). Further, it is prudent to avoid the addition of other agents that may exacerbate the symptoms, such as tramadol. Such a reduction may be accomplished in either isolation or with the initiation of an appropriate preventive therapy for the suspected underlying headache disorder. Although riboflavin has shown efficacy in the prevention of migraine headaches, this patient likely has underlying tension headaches, for which riboflavin is not commonly used. Reducing the patient's workload may improve his stress levels and/or tension headaches, but is a difficult therapy to initiate in isolation. MRI is an important diagnostic tool in cases suspicious of an intracranial lesion. However, this patient's history and examination are not worrisome for an intracranial lesion, and so MRI could be avoided unless standard therapies are not effective or his symptoms change (*see* Bradley's NiCP, 7th edn, Ch. 103, pp. 1686–1719).

39. D. This patient has *hyper*kalemic periodic paralysis. This disorder typically presents in the first or second decade with frequent and brief attacks of weakness. The attacks usually last <1 hour and happen multiple times a week. Some describe paresthesias before the attacks. Later in life they can develop a progressive proximal myopathy. The episodes are triggered during rest after exercise and by eating foods high in potassium such as bananas, tomatoes, potatoes, raisins, and nuts. *Hypo*kalemic periodic paralysis starts at a later age than hyperkalemic paralysis. It is triggered by large carbohydrate loads or rest after exercise. The attacks usually happen a couple of times a month and last longer than the hyperkalemic attacks. Myotonia congenita and paramyotonia congenita involve myotonia that is either warm or cold induced without episodes of weakness like hypokalemic periodic paralysis and hyperkalemic periodic paralysis. McArdle disease is not associated with myotonia and causes pain with intense muscle contractions after a few minutes of exercise. It also demonstrates the "second-wind" phenomenon which occurs if the person lowers exercise intensity for a few minutes; he or she can then resume a higher level of activity without cramps or pain (*see* Bradley's NiCP, 7th edn, Ch. 99, pp. 1519–1537).

40. D. In intracerebral hemorrhages (ICHs), the first considerations are the ABCs (airway, breathing, circulation). Given this patient's progressing somnolence, he should be intubated for airway protection. His blood pressure is also high and should be slowly lowered, keeping in mind that overly decreasing the blood pressure may drop cerebral perfusion pressure. Most providers will aim to reduce blood pressure to <140 mm Hg. It is also important to reverse the INR in this patient, given the propensity to progress. The most commonly used agents are vitamin K 10 mg IV in addition to fresh frozen plasma (FFP; usually 4–6 units). Prothrombin complex concentrate is becoming more widely used, given that is has less infusion volume and faster onset than FFP, but it has limited availability. Glucose should be controlled, as well as temperature. Typically, surgical clot evacuation of supratentorial ICH is not performed unless clots are within 1 cm of the surface. However, for infratentorial hemorrhages, posterior fossa decompression should be performed if the hemorrhage is >3 cm and there is impending compression. If intracranial pressure (ICP) begins to rise, then ICP monitoring devices should be placed, and the patient should be managed accordingly. Although lobar hemorrhages do increase the risk of seizures (especially if cortical), there is no indication to begin anticonvulsants prophylactically. IV tPA is not indicated in this case despite the good time frame, given the contraindications of hemorrhage and INR >1.6 (*see* Bradley's NiCP, 7th edn, Ch. 66, pp. 968–980).

41. D. Fabry disease is an X-linked lipid storage disorder. Metachromatic leukodystrophy and Niemann-Pick disease are both autosomal-recessive enzyme deficiencies. Leigh disease is a mitochondrial disorder, and neurofibromatosis 1 is an autosomal-dominant disorder (*see* Bradley's NiCP, 7th edn, Chs. 50, pp. 648–675 and 107, pp. 1791–1866).

42. D. Although maintaining an adequate security organization may be important for campus security and, occasionally, for individual patient security, this is not a specific goal of JACHO. Aside from the items listed here, other recent and important JACHO patient safety goals include improving staff communication, preventing iatrogenic infections, and identifying individual patient risks.

43. E. The image demonstrates focal polymicrogyria with localized loss of white matter and associated hydrocephalus. The corpus callosum is present in this image. Schizencephaly is an abnormal cleft in the brain lined with cortex. Holoprosencephaly is impaired hemispheric differentiation. Lissencephaly is an abnormally smooth brain due to a migrational abnormality (*see* Bradley's NiCP, 7th edn, Ch. 89, pp. 1279–1300). Figure from Finkbeiner WE, Ursell PC, Davis RL, Connolly AJ 2009 *Atlas of Autopsy Pathology*, 2nd edn, Elsevier, with permission.

44. A. The woman most likely is suffering from a prolactin-secreting pituitary adenoma. Pituitary adenomas are the third most common primary intracranial tumor, and prolactin is the most commonly secreted hormone among these. A tumor <1 cm in size is classified as a microadenoma, and may be treated with dopamine agonist therapy as the first-line choice (such as bromocriptine or cabergoline), which provides negative feedback on prolactin

production. Giving a dopamine antagonist, on the other hand, may increase prolactin levels even further. Chemotherapy is not generally used for these tumors. Stereotactic radiosurgery may also be used for pituitary adenomas, although it is often reserved for recurrent tumors after surgical resection due to associated risk of radiation exposure to the normal surrounding pituitary, as well as the optic pathways. Whole-brain radiation is rarely used for a single mass lesion, and would cause excessive toxicity without clear benefit in this case (*see* Bradley's NiCP, 7th edn, Ch. 74, pp. 1049–1064).

45. B. Abnormal spontaneous activity on EMG (fibrillations and positive sharp waves) comes from irritability of the muscle membrane from denervation. The connection between the muscle and the nerve can be damaged either by axon loss, as is the case in neuropathies such as diabetes, amyotrophic lateral sclerosis (ALS), or carpal tunnel syndrome. The connection can also be lost in cases of myopathy, such as inclusion body myositis, where inflammation in the muscles disconnects the motor neuron from the muscle membrane. In myasthenia gravis the neuromuscular junction malfunctions, but the nerve and muscle are in contact so no abnormal spontaneous activity should be seen (*see* Bradley's NiCP, 7th edn, Ch. 35, pp. 366–390).

46. D. Azathioprine, a purine antimetabolite, removes both B- and T-cells from circulation and may be used for various autoimmune diseases (e.g. myasthenia gravis) or for immunosuppression following organ transplantation. Other drugs that remove both B- and T-lymphocytes from circulation include alemtuzumab, an anti-CD52 antibody, or fingolimod, which sequesters lymphocytes in the lymph system and out of the circulating blood. Tacrolimus and cyclosporine are two examples of drugs that primarily deplete T-cells. Rituximab is an anti-CD20 monoclonal antibody that specifically depletes B-cells. Immunoglobulins may be removed from the circulating blood either with intravenous immunoglobulins or with plasma exchange. Inhibition of leukocytes from crossing the blood-brain barrier is the mechanism of action for natalizumab, an anti–cell adhesion molecule α4 antibody that is also approved for relapsing multiple sclerosis (*see* Bradley's NiCP, 7th edn, Ch. 109, pp. 1896–1914).

47. A. A pupil-sparing third nerve palsy that is otherwise complete is most commonly associated with microvascular infarcts within the third nerve. These tend to relate to hypertension and diabetes. Improvement comes gradually over 4–6 weeks, with the main intervention being risk factor modification. A lesion in the sympathetic chain would cause Horner syndrome, including ptosis (usually mild, affecting Müller muscle only), miosis, and anhidrosis on the ipsilateral face. Posterior communicating artery aneurysms may cause compressive third nerve palsies, but generally include mydriasis due to the exterior representation of parasympathetic fibers on the oculomotor nerve. The oculomotor nucleus may be affected by mass lesions in the region or with uncal herniation, but generally causes a complete third nerve palsy, including pupillary involvement. Cavernous sinus localization would generally cause a complete third nerve palsy, including pupillary involvement. Further, lesions in the cavernous sinus would generally cause additional cranial neuropathies (including trochlear, ophthalmic, maxillary, or abducens), given

the density of structures within this small space (*see* Bradley's NiCP, 7th edn, Chs. 18, pp. 179–189 and 104, pp. 1720–1735).

48. C. Schizoaffective disorder is characterized by at least 2 weeks of psychosis (delusions in this case) without prominent mood symptoms, followed by a clear onset of mood symptoms (depression in this case). The mood symptoms can alternatively be mania or mixed episodes. Schizoaffective disorder is distinguished from schizophrenia, delusional disorder, and schizophreniform disorder, both by the duration of psychosis and by the prominence of mood dysfunction. Further, this is distinguished from a depressive episode by the presence of psychosis.

49. A. Fahr disease is a disorder marked by idiopathic calcification of the basal ganglia and cerebellum leading to a parkinsonlike disorder. Idiopathic Parkinson disease has no typical CT scan findings. The hyperdense lesions on the scan are the same density as the skull, indicating mineralization rather than hemorrhage (which is usually a lower density than bone). Pantothenate kinase–associated neurodegeneration results in excessive iron deposition in the globus pallidus, seen best on magnetic resonance imaging susceptibility weighted imaging as the "eye of the tiger sign." Huntington disease is associated with caudate atrophy, but does not show excessive mineralization (*see* Bradley's NiCP, 7th edn, Ch. 96, pp. 1422–1460). Figure from Alemdar M, Selek A, İşeri P, Efendi H, Komsuoğlu SS 2008 Fahr's disease presenting with paroxysmal nonkinesigenic dyskinesia: a case report. *Parkinsonism and Related Disorders* 14(1): 69–71.

50. B. After CSF production by the choroid plexus in the lateral ventricles, the flow thereafter is lateral ventricle → foramen of Monro → third ventricle → cerebral aqueduct → fourth ventricle → foramina of Luschka (lateral) and Magendie (medial) → cisterna magna → cerebral sinuses → arachnoid granulations for reabsorption. The figure demonstrates the ventricular anatomy and CSF flow.

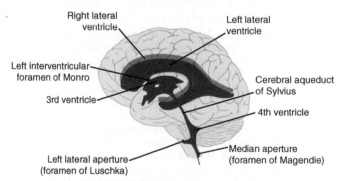

Figure for Answer 6.50 (*from O'Meara WP, Borkar SA, Stambuk HE, Lymberis SC 2007 Leptomeningeal metastasis.* Current Problems in Cancer *31(6): 372–424, with permission.*)

51. B. The patient has Sandifer syndrome, which is characterized by intermittent paroxysmal spells of generalized stiffening and posturing (especially with neck extension) in infants due to gastroesophageal reflux. Occasionally, these spells can be associated with apnea, staring, or extraneous movements of the extremities. They generally occur within 30 minutes of

eating. Given the history of provoking spells by eating, seizure disorder is less likely. Workup for Sandifer syndrome includes an evaluation for gastroesophageal reflux with a pH probe and treatment with an H2 blocker such as ranitidine. Benign paroxysmal torticollis involves paroxysmal episodes of cervical dystonia that begin and end suddenly, with no alteration of mental status and no provocation by feeding. Spasmus nutans consists of nystagmus, head nodding, and head tilt that fluctuate during the course of the day but with retained consciousness. Breath-holding spells may look similar to Sandifer syndrome and can have similar posturing, but are usually preceded by cyanosis and apnea and are associated with intense emotions such as crying or fear.

52. B. In this case the patient has recurring episodes of panic attacks, defined by the discrete episodes of symptoms that include intense fear with palpitations, diaphoresis, shortness of breath, sensation of choking, chest pain, nausea, dizziness, or fear of dying. Each episode usually lasts 5–30 minutes and typically leads to frequent emergency room visits, prompting large, medically negative workups. Recurring panic attacks with the concern for having more attacks fits with a diagnosis of panic disorder. Agoraphobia is anxiety in settings in which escape may be difficult or help is unavailable, such as in this case. Treatment usually includes benzodiazepines or beta-blockers. There is no history of excessive worrying or recurring compulsions that would suggest either generalized anxiety disorder or obsessive-compulsive disorder. In addition, there is no mention of prior exposure to a catastrophic or traumatic event that would predispose to hyperarousal or flashbacks, making posttraumatic stress disorder unlikely.

53. D. The arrow indicates the axon hillock, which is at the junction of the cell body (soma) and the axon. The dendrites are the branched processes off of the soma of the neuron that receive input from surrounding cells. The terminal buttons create the synapses at the end of the axonal processes. Figure from De Nicola AF, et al. 2009 Progesterone neuroprotection in traumatic CNS injury and motoneuron degeneration. *Frontiers in Neuroendocrinology* 30(2): 173–187, with permission.

54. A. A normal size head circumference of a full-term newborn is approximately 35 cm. For the first 3 months of life, the head will increase in size by 2 cm/month for the first 6 months, followed by approximately 1 cm/month until the first year. This makes a head circumference of about 41 cm a target size in a normal full-term 3-month-old. Macrocephaly is defined as a head circumference greater than at least two standard deviations above the mean, whereas microcephaly is defined as at least two standard deviations below the mean. The provider should be concerned when a child has abnormal development, an abnormal neurological examination, or is crossing lines on a growth chart. If any of these is present, further evaluation to characterize the macro/microcephaly should prompt neuroimaging and consideration for further serological tests if other physical features are present (abnormal facies, short stature, heart murmurs, etc.) Many conditions are associated with macrocephaly, including obstructive hydrocephalus, nonobstructive hydrocephalus, pseudotumor cerebri, and fragile X syndrome, to name a few. Benign familial megalencephaly is one potential cause of macrocephaly in a normally developed child who has parents with macrocephaly. Microcephaly is associated with mental retardation and a number of both acquired and genetic conditions, including but not limited to in-utero alcohol exposure, TORCH infections, and multiple chromosomal abnormalities.

55. C. Intrafusal muscle fibers contain muscle spindles, which determine how quickly a muscle is changing in length. This is the afferent portion of the muscle stretch reflex. When the spindle detects a change in muscle length, signals are sent through the sensory nerve back to the cord through the dorsal horn. Without synapsing in the dorsal portion of the cord, these neurons synapse directly on alpha motor neurons in the anterior horn, which are the efferent part of the reflex. Gamma motor neurons help provide innervation to the intrafusal muscle spindles. Alpha motor neurons innervate the extrafusal muscle spindles and result in muscle movements. The substantia gelatinosa is in the dorsal horn of the spinal cord and acts as a relay for sensory signals to be routed to the cerebellum and thalamus (*see* Bradley's NiCP, 7th edn, Ch. 110, pp. 1915–1955).

56. D. The patient in the clinical scenario is most likely in alcohol withdrawal. Minor symptoms begin within 6–36 hours from the last drink, and can sometimes include tremors, diaphoresis, nausea, diarrhea, agitation, and headache. Alcohol withdrawal seizures occur mostly in the first 12–48 hours from the last drink, and are usually generalized in nature. These often respond to benzodiazepines, because they work on the same receptor that alcohol effects (gamma aminobutyric acid A). Also around 12–48 hours, patients can have visual (and auditory) hallucinations. Delirium tremens occurs at 2–5 days and can cause agitation, encephalopathy, autonomic instability, and arrhythmias. Beta-blockers, calcium channel blockers, benzodiazepines, and antipsychotics are the mainstay of treatment. Admission to the hospital is a common time for alcohol withdrawal, emphasizing the importance of an accurate social history. Given this patient's seizure, postoperative delirium is less likely. Septic shock is also less likely, given a lack of hypotension. Status epilepticus would be unlikely with a history of waxing and waning mental status, single seizure, and normal EEG. Finally, although cocaine intoxication can also cause autonomic dysfunction, one would expect to see changes on the MRI, such as cocaine-induced hypertensive hemorrhage or posterior reversible encephalopathy syndrome, to explain his seizure.

57. D. The nucleus gracilis contains the second-order neurons of the medial lemniscus system, including vibratory and proprioceptive sensory input from the legs. The nucleus cuneatus is just medial to the nucleus gracilis in the medulla and carries the vibration and proprioception input from the arms. The red nucleus is farther rostral in the midbrain and is involved in motor coordination. The substantia nigra is posterior to the red nucleus, in the cerebral peduncle, and is also important in motor function. The inferior colliculus is in the anterior midbrain and is important in auditory function. Figure from Nolte J 2013 *Human Brain in Photographs and Diagrams*, Elsevier, with permission.

58. C. Methylmalonic acidemia and propionic acidemia are both autosomal-dominant diseases and present with severe metabolic acidosis, ketosis, and blood cell

dyscrasias. However, methylmalonic acidemia is associated with hepatomegaly and requires vitamin B12 as a cofactor due to a deficiency in methylmalonyl-CoA mutase. The deficient enzyme in propionic acidemia is propionyl-CoA carboxylase. Glutaric acidemia type 1 is an autosomal-recessive deficiency in glutaryl-CoA dehydrogenase deficiency, ultimately leading to decreased gamma aminobutyric acid and progressive extrapyramidal syndromes. This is sometimes confused with nonaccidental trauma due to bifrontal fluid collections and subdural hemorrhages. Any of the organic acidurias may lead to mitochondrial damage due to accumulation of disease-specific substrates. Treatment for all organic acidurias includes a low-protein diet to reduce accumulation of amino acid–related substrates (*see* Bradley's NiCP, 7th edn, Ch. 85, pp. 1226–1236).

59. B. Tetrodotoxin is a voltage-gated sodium channel blocker that affects nerves, skeletal muscles, and cardiac muscle. This toxin comes from newts, shellfish (particularly in Japan), and pufferfish. Mild intoxication causes a state of euphoria along with paresthesias around the lips, which is the intended effect when eating pufferfish. However, an overdose results in nausea, vomiting, diffuse weakness, and even death from respiratory failure or cardiac arrhythmias within 30 minutes of ingestion. Ciguatoxin is also a voltage-gated sodium channel blocker that binds to presynaptic sodium channels in the nodes of Ranvier, stopping action potentials. This toxin is acquired through ingestion of infected shellfish. Clinically this can cause nausea, vomiting, myalgias, and predominant sensory paresthesias and pain. There can be paradoxical temperature sensation where hot is felt as cold and cold as hot. Ciguatoxin-associated illness is usually short lived and recovery is in a few days. Botulinum toxin blocks the release of acetylcholine from the presynaptic terminal, leading to diffuse weakness. This should not cause paresthesias or euphoria, as seen in our patient. Shiga toxin comes from an infection with shigella, leading to profound diarrhea and potentially hemolytic uremic syndrome. However, there are no neuromuscular effects of shiga toxin. Curare is a nicotinic acetylcholine receptor blocker that can result in profound weakness and respiratory depression without sensory abnormalities (*see* Bradley's NiCP, 7th edn, Ch. 86, pp. 1237–1253).

60. A. The patient presents with a stepwise progression of neurological deficits that localize to the cervical spinal cord. The MRI image is a T2 image showing multilobulated lesions of mixed intensity within and around the cord from C2–C5. This represents engorged blood vessels and hemorrhage, which cause myelopathy through both ischemia and venous congestion (leading to cord edema or impingement). Multiple sclerosis can present with a cervical myelopathy and stepwise neurological deficits; however, the MRI in MS shows T2 hyperintense lesions within the cord. NMO is also a consideration, but the MRI in NMO shows a longitudinally extensive transverse myelitis. A syrinx appears as a hyperintense lesion of the same intensity as cerebrospinal fluid on T2 imaging in the central portion of the cord. These can be quite large and extend down the entire length of the spinal cord. A spinal ependymoma would present on MRI as a hyperintense lesion within the cord that enhances with contrast (*see* Bradley's

7th edn, Ch. 69, pp. 1007–1014). Figure from Fatterpekar G 2012 *The Teaching Files: Brain and Spine*, Saunders, with permission.

61. C. Duchenne muscular dystrophy (DMD) is an X-linked recessive disorder causing an absence of dystrophin in muscle fibers, typically presenting in boys between the ages of 2 to 3 years. Initially patients with DMD have normal development but display progressive loss of muscular strength and coordination. Common signs on examination include pseudohypertrophy of the calves and Gower's sign (using hands to help rise from the floor). In addition to skeletal muscle abnormalities, cardiac conduction abnormalities and left ventricular fibrosis are often seen. Creatine kinase levels are usually quite elevated, often above 10,000 mU/mL. Prednisone at a dose of 0.75 mg/kg has been shown to slow the progression of the disease for up to 3 years. Genetic testing has replaced muscle biopsy for diagnosis in most cases (*see* Bradley's NiCP, 7th edn, Ch. 110, pp. 1915–1955).

62. D. Marchiafava-Bignami is a rare disorder seen in alcoholics involving injury to the corpus callosum, which is presumed to be from a nutritional deficiency. Marchiafava-Bignami results in a syndrome that includes coma, seizures, subacute chronic memory loss, and ataxia. The MRI shows T2/FLAIR (fluid attenuated inversion recovery) hyperintensities in corpus callosum in the acute setting, and atrophy of the corpus callosum in the chronic setting. Wernicke-Korsakoff is a more common condition found in alcoholics, but causes MRI abnormalities in the bilateral mammillary bodies, periaqueductal gray matter, and bilateral medial thalami. Strokes and multiple sclerosis can cause lesions in the corpus callosum, but the history of alcoholism points toward Marchiafava-Bignami. CADASIL is a genetic arteriopathy that causes subcortical strokes, and the MRI typically demonstrates T2/FLAIR hyperintensities in the anterotemporal lobes (*see* Bradley's NiCP, 7th edn, Ch. 87, pp. 1254–1260). Figure from Remollo S, Puig J, Aguirregomozcorta M, Gich J, Blasco G, Serena J 2010 Value of diffusion-tensor imaging and fiber tractography in the diagnosis and follow-up of Marchiafava-Bignami disease. *European Journal of Radiology Extra* 73(2): e41–e43, with permission.

63. D. An epidural abscess is the most likely diagnosis based on the patient's poorly controlled diabetes (a particular susceptibility to epidural abscesses) and cutaneous evidence of an abscess on examination. The patient should have emergent spine magnetic resonance imaging, with and without contrast, followed by broad antibiotic coverage to cover at least staphylococcal and streptococcal species. Further, most patients will require emergent surgery for debridement in order to prevent spinal compression and infarction. Although anterior spinal artery stroke, viral transverse myelitis, and metastatic disease may present with similar symptoms, none should have an overlying skin abscess. Guillain-Barré syndrome may cause intense neuropathic pain and rapidly progressive weakness, but the skin infection at the site of her pain should point towards an epidural abscess as the cause (*see* Bradley's NiCP, 7th edn, Ch. 79, pp. 1147–1158).

64. B. Honest communication with patients is important for the patient–physician relationship. The ethical response to this situation is to ask the patient how

much she would like to know and then inform her in a manner she can understand. This may need to be done over the course of a few visits rather than just one visit. Withholding information from patients without their consent is unethical. Transferring to another physician to avoid a difficult conversation with a patient or the family is unethical. Discharging the patient from the clinic because you disagree with the family is also unethical. A referral to hospice may be in order, but only after there has been a discussion of the diagnosis.

65. B. HSP encompasses a group of hereditary disorders that cause bilateral lower extremity spasticity and weakness with urinary bladder dysfunction. A number of genes are associated with HSP, which may lead to disease transmission through autosomal-dominant, autosomal-recessive, X-linked, or mitochondrial inheritance. Tethered cord may lead to lower extremity weakness and bladder dysfunction, but would likely worsen as the child grows, and is not usually inherited. SCAs are another group of disorders, including Machado-Joseph disease (SCA-3), that cause ataxia of the limbs, trunk, eyes, and speech, as well as peripheral neuropathy. These may be either autosomal dominant or autosomal recessive, depending on the specific disease. SCA is less likely for the patient noted here due to the lack of ataxia. Metachromatic leukodystrophy is caused by arylsulfatase A deficiency and is associated with weakness, hypotonia, clumsiness, slurred speech, incontinence, and behavioral changes. This disease is transmitted in an autosomal-recessive manner. Dopa-responsive dystonia is an autosomal-dominant condition of childhood-onset dystonia with dramatic and sustained response to low-dose levodopa. This usually begins with foot dystonia, gait disturbance, and diurnal exacerbation that is often confused initially for cerebral palsy. Unless treated, it will often progress to parkinsonism and generalized dystonia (*see* Bradley's NiCP, 7th edn, Ch. 98, pp. 1484–1518).

66. D. The patient presents with an acute subdural hematoma as shown on the CT scan. With his history of atrial fibrillation, it is reasonable to assume he has likely been anticoagulated. Although reversal of anticoagulation is important, because of his poor neurological status and unresponsiveness, the first measure should be evacuation and drainage of the hematoma before herniation and death occur. Mannitol and 3% NaCl can be used to reduce cerebral edema, although this patient's symptoms are not from edema, but rather a space-occupying hematoma. Supportive measures alone are not indicated because death could occur without immediate decompression (*see* Bradley's NiCP, 7th edn, Ch. 39, pp. 411–459 and Ch. 55, pp. 742–758). Figure from Naidich TP, Castillo M, Cha S, Smirniotopoulos JG (eds.) 2013 *Imaging of the Brain* (Expert Radiology Series), Saunders, with permission.

67. B. The diagnosis of autism involves impairment of communication and social skills, and may involve motor stereotypies, including repetitive actions with mechanical devices such as wheels and other motorized parts. Other mannerisms include frequent rocking back and forth. There is also a lack of flexibility in day-to-day activities where structure is often important. As part of the communication deficit, patients with autism do not seek out social interactions and frequently have language dysfunction, including

echolalia (repeating others' phrases), palilalia (repeating the patient's own phrases), and/or aprosody (absence of normal variation in speed, tone, and emphasis of speech). Autism is distinguished from Asperger's syndrome, which is a milder phenotype on the spectrum, by patients often having normal language development and intelligence quotient (IQ), but there is some difficulty with social interactions. Personality disorders are typically not diagnosed in this age group. There is no indication of birth trauma in this patient to indicate cerebral palsy, which would be a static neurological condition. Depression should be considered in any child or adult who prefers seclusion and has dysfunction in social interactions, but would not be characterized by language dysfunction or motor stereotypies. Finally, there is no indication of frequent staring or automatisms that would make seizures likely.

68. D. This patient presents with eclampsia. This condition presents with elevated blood pressures, proteinuria, headaches, visual disturbances, and seizures. Seizures are necessary for the conversion from preeclampsia to eclampsia. Although magnesium can be a temporizing measure, the definitive treatment of eclampsia is delivery of the baby. Phenytoin, valproic acid, and lorazepam can be helpful to acutely stop seizures. However, they are not considered the definitive treatment of eclampsia (*see* Bradley's NiCP, Ch. 112, pp. 1973–1991).

69. A. The prefrontal cortex is most involved in working memory, which is information kept in conscious awareness without active memorization, such as hearing a telephone number and then immediately dialing it. Episodic memory is also referred to as *short-term memory* and *declarative memory*. This is housed in the mesial temporal lobes, requiring an intact hippocampus for both storage and retrieval. Episodic memory involves the ability to recall specific details or words after several minutes or even hours. Semantic memory is also known as *long-term memory* and is housed in the lateral temporal lobe and broader cortical areas, but it does not require the use of the hippocampus for retrieval. Procedural memory lies in the cerebellum and basal ganglia. This type of memory involves learned motor skills such as using tools, complex learned movements like throwing a ball, or even driving (*see* Bradley's NiCP, 7th edn, Ch. 7, pp. 57–65).

70. B. Lead poisoning is associated with motor neuropathy, sideroblastic anemia, encephalopathy, constipation, and nephropathy. The patient probably had lead exposure through paint ingestion in his art class (similar to Vincent Van Gogh). Arsenic poisoning causes more of a sensory neuropathy with paresthesias. Later, patients may complain of muscle cramping. Further, patients may have pigmentary changes, as well as hyperkeratosis of the palms and soles. Mercury poisoning may cause neuropsychiatric symptoms, as well as renal and pulmonary disease. Neuropathy is not generally problematic, however. Zinc toxicity is not directly problematic. However, too much zinc causes decreased copper absorption, which may cause myelopathy or myeloneuropathy. There are no neurological symptoms associated with excessive chromium (*see* Bradley's NiCP, 7th edn, Ch. 86, pp. 1237–1253).

71. D. The MRI shows a susceptibility weighted sequence demonstrating small multifocal areas of hypointensity

consistent with multiple microhemorrhages, which is the hallmark image of cerebral amyloid angiopathy. This condition is marked by microhemorrhages, lobar hemorrhages, migraines with strokelike symptoms, seizures, and a dementia consisting of slow processing and short-term memory loss. Vascular dementia results from multiple ischemic, not hemorrhagic, injuries. This can result in a stepwise deterioration in memory and cognitive function with periods of relative stability. Magnetic resonance imaging for vascular dementia would show diffuse white-matter hyperintensities on T2/FLAIR (fluid attenuated inversion recovery) imaging. Alzheimer disease has no specific MRI correlate, although diffuse atrophy or even focal atrophy of the temporoparietal junction can be seen. Cerebral autosomal-dominant arteriopathy with subcortical infarcts and leukoencephalopathy is caused by a mutation in the *NOTCH3* gene, which leads to multifocal infarcts, migraine headaches, and dementia. On MRI, CADASIL typically is associated with T2/FLAIR hyperintense lesions in the anterotemporal poles. Dementia with Lewy bodies, like Alzheimer disease, does not have any specific MRI findings (*see* Bradley's NiCP, 7th edn, Ch. 39, pp. 411–458). Figure from Gray ZA, Greenberg SM, Press DZ 2014 rTMS for treatment of depression in a patient with cerebral amyloid angiopathy: a case report on safety and efficacy. *Brain Stimulation* 7(3): 495–497, with permission.

72. B. The patient has glossopharyngeal neuralgia. This is a condition characterized by recurring paroxysmal attacks lasting from a few seconds to 2 minutes and is severe in intensity, usually with pain located in the posterior tongue, tonsillar fossa, pharynx, beneath the angle of the lower jaw, or in the ear. It can be idiopathic or secondary to demyelinating lesions, cerebellopontine angle tumors, peritonsillar abscess, carotid aneurysm, or Eagle syndrome, which is characterized by lateral compression of the glossopharyngeal nerve by a calcified stylohyoid ligament. This condition is often triggered by swallowing, coughing, talking, or yawning. The treatment of choice is largely the same as it is for trigeminal neuralgia and includes gabapentin, carbamazepine, oxcarbazepine, or baclofen (*see* Bradley's NiCP, 7th edn, Ch. 103, pp. 1686–1719).

73. E. Ethambutol is a common agent used in multi-drug treatment of tuberculosis. Serious side effects of ethambutol include peripheral neuropathy and retrobulbar optic neuritis. Isoniazid is one of the common agents used to treat tuberculosis in combination with rifampin and ethambutol. The main neurological side effect of isoniazid is peripheral neuropathy caused by pyridoxine deficiency. Isoniazid causes increased excretion of pyridoxine, so supplementation is recommended. Rifampin does not have any significant neurological side effects, but it is a liver enzyme inducer, so it could increase metabolism of seizure medications. Pyrazinamide is a nicotinamide analog that has no significant neurological side effects. Streptomycin is an aminoglycoside that can cause tinnitus, decreased hearing, and ataxia (*see* Bradley's NiCP, 7th edn, Ch. 79, pp. 1147–1158).

74. C. This patient presents with an acute-onset myelopathy in the setting of recent anticoagulation, which should be concerning for an epidural hematoma. The imaging demonstrates a large extradural mass posterior to the spinal cord, which is isointense on T1 and hyperintense on T2 imaging, which is most consistent with an epidural hematoma. This emergent condition must be recognized and acted upon immediately in order to reduce the risk of prolonged neurological deficits. Transverse myelitis presents as a T2 hyperintense lesion within the spinal cord. Syringomyelia presents as a T2 hyperintense lesion in the central portion of the spinal cord with similar signal characteristics to cerebrospinal fluid. A spinal arteriovenous malformation usually demonstrates enlarged hypointense blood vessels along with spinal cord hyperintense hemorrhagic lesions. This patient does have a bulging disc below the level of the epidural hematoma, but the epidural is the most significant lesion (*see* Bradley's NiCP, 7th edn, Ch. 69, pp. 1007–1014). Figure from Aoki Y, Yamagata M, Shimizu K, et al. 2012 An unusually rapid spontaneous recovery in a patient with spinal epidural hematoma. *The Journal of Emergency Medicine* 43(2): e75–e79, with permission.

75. D. The patient's asymmetric weakness, sensory loss, hyporeflexia, and flaccid bladder are classic for cauda equina syndrome. This may result from trauma to the lumbar spine below the level of the conus medullaris. There is no definitive evidence that performance of surgery changes outcomes of cauda equina syndrome, or that early versus late surgery has different outcomes. Because nerve roots and peripheral nerves are more resilient than the cord, cauda equina syndrome is more likely to improve with time than would a myelopathy. A bifrontal localization could include paraparesis, but the greater weakness distally is unlikely given the deep location of the feet on the homunculus. Bladder dysfunction may present from frontal injury, but tends to be quite deep, pericallosal white matter localization. Further, sensory loss would be a parietal location. Anterior cord syndrome affects the corticospinal and spinothalamic tracts, thus disrupting movement in an upper motor neuron pattern, as well as pin prick sensation. However, the dorsal columns (and therefore vibration) remain intact. Conus medullaris syndrome generally causes a mixed picture of upper- and lower-motor neuron weakness, absent leg reflexes, and saddle anesthesia. Peripheral nerve crush injury causes motor and sensory loss only in the region provided by the affected nerve. The patient's presentation does not localize to any of these other listed sites, although each of their listed outcomes would be true (*see* Bradley's NiCP, 7th edn, Ch. 63, pp. 881–902).

76. D. The L5 nerve root is among the most commonly affected by disc herniation and usually causes pain in the L5 dermatome (including the great toe). Among the nerves listed, the deep peroneal nerve (innervating the tibialis anterior, extensor digitorum longus, extensor hallucis longus, and extensor digitorum brevis) is the only one that derives input from the L5 root by way of the sciatic nerve. The femoral nerve receives input from L1–L4 and innervates the iliopsoas and quadriceps femoris. The obturator nerve receives input from the L2–L4 roots and innervates the adductor muscles, including the external obturator, pectineus, adductor longus, adductor brevis, adductor magnus, and gracilis. The lateral femoral cutaneous nerve is derived from L2 and L3 and only has sensory function over the lateral thigh. The lateral plantar nerve is derived from S1 and S2, and innervates the small/intrinsic muscles of the feet. The figure depicts the

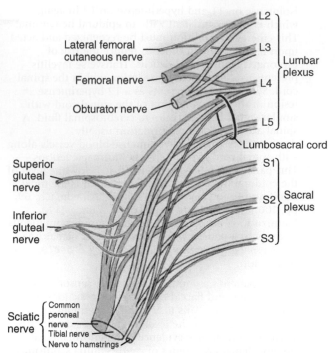

Lateral femoral cutaneous nerve
Femoral nerve
Obturator nerve
L2
L3
L4
L5
Lumbar plexus
Lumbosacral cord
Superior gluteal nerve
Inferior gluteal nerve
S1
S2
S3
Sacral plexus
Sciatic nerve
Common peroneal nerve
Tibial nerve
Nerve to hamstrings

Figure for Answer 6.76 *(from Canale ST, Beaty JH 2008 Campbell's Operative Orthopaedics, 11th edn, Mosby, with permission.)*

regional anatomy. Contribution of L1 not shown (*see* Bradley's NiCP, 7th edn, Ch. 106, pp. 1766–1791).

77. B. Selective serotonin reuptake inhibitors are medications that work by inhibiting the serotonin transporter, allowing for more serotonin to be available in the postsynaptic region. This class of medication tends to be excellent for treating a variety of conditions and symptoms, including depression, anxiety, eating disorders, obsessive-compulsive disorders, functional or psychogenic disorders, pain, posttraumatic stress disorder, and even premature ejaculation. Common side effects include nausea (likely from 5HT3 receptor action), sexual dysfunction (including erectile dysfunction in men), increased suicidality (especially in undiagnosed bipolar disorder), and sedation. A few notable points regarding SSRIs: (1) fluvoxamine and paroxetine are the most sedating of the SSRIs; (2) fluoxetine and sertraline are the most activating SSRIs; (3) citalopram and sertraline have the fewest drug–drug interactions; (4) fluoxetine has the longest half-life and is good for those who miss doses; (5) escitalopram and sertraline appear to be the best-tolerated SSRIs in terms of fewer side effects.

78. E. This patient has a family history of migraines, dementia, and stroke, along with a personal history of recurring vascular events and complicated migraines. This history in the setting of an MRI that shows confluent subcortical white matter changes affecting the anterior temporal lobes, points toward cerebral autosomal dominant arteriopathy with subcortical infarcts and leukoencephalopathy. This is caused by a mutation in the *NOTCH3* gene on chromosome 19, typically diagnosed with a skin biopsy or genetic testing of the blood. Often, the leukoencephalopathy spares the U-fibers on MRI. It would be incorrect to do no further testing because a young person who has

recurring vascular events should be evaluated for secondary stroke prevention. A CT of the chest/abdomen/pelvis could be used to evaluate for an occult malignancy, which would make someone more prone to strokes. However, given this MRI and family history, choice E is better. A brain biopsy could be performed if primary central nervous system vasculitis is suspected, although headaches are generally more indolent and family history absent in this condition. Although factor V Leiden testing could be useful with recurring infarcts, the imaging finding and family history make *NOTCH3* mutation more likely (*see* Bradley's NiCP, 7th edn, Ch. 65, pp. 920–968). Figure from Dericioglu N, Vural A, Agayeva N, et al. 2013 Cerebral autosomal dominant arteriopathy with subcortical infarcts and leukoencephalopathy (CADASIL) in two siblings with neuropsychiatric symptoms. *Psychosomatics* 54(6): 594–598, with permission.

79. A. Hemiballismus is classically associated with a lesion of the subthalamic nucleus. Parkinsonism can be related to depletion of dopamine from the substantia nigra. Treatment may include medications to increase dopamine in the brain, or with deep brain stimulation to the globus pallidus interna or the ventral intermedius nuclei. Essential tremor is a hereditary condition rather than a consequence of a specific lesion, although deep brain stimulation to the ventral intermedius nucleus may treat the condition. Lesions to the thalamus may cause a pain syndrome such as Dejerine-Roussy syndrome; this is not the case with hypothalamic lesions. Weakness may arise from injury to various locations, especially involving the corticospinal tract (*see* Bradley's NiCP, 7th edn, Ch. 96, pp. 1422–1460).

80. C. PSP is a tauopathy that is characterized by severe postural instability early in the course, frequent falls, impairment of vertical gaze, and symmetrical parkinsonism that is typically unresponsive to levodopa. PSP can be associated with retrocollis of the neck, apraxia of eyelid opening, pseudobulbar affect (emotional incontinence), and frontal lobe dysfunction associated with perseveration (as seen with the applause sign). Imaging typically shows atrophy of the midbrain in the sagittal section (hummingbird sign). PSP is distinguished from idiopathic Parkinson disease by early postural instability. In the current case, there is no evidence of autonomic dysfunction that would point toward MSA. Normal pressure hydrocephalus is usually characterized by apraxia of gait rather than vertical eye movement abnormalities as seen in this patient. Cortical basal ganglionic degeneration does share some overlap with PSP, but is typically associated with unilateral dystonic posturing, alien hand syndrome, myoclonus, and cortical abnormalities such as agraphesthesia or hemispheric atrophy (*see* Bradley's NiCP, 7th edn, Ch. 96, pp. 1422–1460). Figure from Berlot R, Kojović M 2015 Palatal tremor in progressive supranuclear palsy: a case report. *Parkinsonism and Related Disorders* 3(21): 335–336, with permission.

81. C. The sudden change in the boy's personality and physical appearance should prompt suspicion of illicit drug use. Both recreational drugs (i.e. marijuana, heroin, methamphetamines, cocaine) and performance-enhancing drugs (anabolic steroids, testosterone, growth hormone) can be found in schools. The patient's mood changes, acne, and muscle

hypertrophy suggest anabolic steroids as the most likely source of his changes. Other potential side effects of anabolic steroids in men include gynecomastia, alopecia, and testicular atrophy. Women taking anabolic steroids may experience a deeper voice, clitoral hypertrophy, hirsutism, and amenorrhea. Both men and women may have aggressive behavior, liver damage, severe acne, and hypertension. The other choices are common considerations for personality changes in teenagers, but would not account for all of the changes noted in the question.

82. E. Introduction of cold water into the external auditory canal creates a temperature gradient with the endolymph, mostly within the semicircular canal, which is closest to the middle ear. This gradient moves and hyperpolarizes the hair cells and activates the vestibulooccular reflex. With normally functioning vestibular and cortical input, a normal reflex can be remembered by the mnemonic COWS (cold-opposite; warm-same). This means that the fast phase of nystagmus normally goes away from cold stimulation or toward warm stimulation. In a comatose patient, the eyes tend to deviate toward a cold stimulus or away from a warm stimulus, with no nystagmus (*see* Bradley's NiCP, 7th edn, Ch. 46, pp. 583–604).

83. C. Vascular dementia is a non-neurodegenerative dementia in which there is a stepwise progression of cognitive deficits not necessarily related to specific ischemic insults, but related to the cumulative burden of ischemic disease. This can occur with cortical strokes, subcortical white matter disease, hypoperfusion, or arteriopathies. Subcortical patterns of ischemic disease are the most common and clinically present with motor and sensory deficits, extrapyramidal symptoms, pseudobulbar palsy, depression, urinary incontinence, and slow mental processing. Alzheimer disease leads to progressive, not stepwise, deficits in memory, language, visuospatial defects, and executive function. Cerebral amyloid angiopathy can cause dementia but most often presents

with a lobar intracerebral hemorrhage and evidence of multifocal hemorrhages. Frontotemporal dementia has varied presentations, but most often presents with behavioral disturbances and poor executive function in the sixth or seventh decade of life. CADASIL can also cause a vascular dementia, but this typically presents in the young with migraines, strokes, seizures, and an MRI pattern showing anterior temporal lobe white matter disease (*see* Bradley's NiCP, 7th edn, Ch. 95, pp. 1380–1421).

84. A. During NREM and REM sleep a variety of physiological changes can be seen. The differences between them include the following: NREM has increased sympathetic activity, whereas REM has a decrease; REM has a lack of thermoregulation, and NREM involves bradycardia, whereas REM can involve tachyarrhythmia as well as bradycardia; REM involves increased cerebral blood flow; and REM involves penile or clitoral tumescence. The following table shows all the physiological changes that occur during wakefulness, NREM, and REM (*see* Bradley's NiCP, 7th edn, Ch. 102, pp. 1615–1685).

85. C. The patient is suffering from trigeminal neuralgia (also known as *tic douloureux*). Magnetic resonance imaging is indicated after diagnosis of this condition to identify any reversible or potentially dangerous cause. Many cases of trigeminal neuralgia are believed to result from vascular compression of the trigeminal nerve, and microvascular decompression is performed as a therapy in these cases. Multiple sclerosis is another cause of trigeminal neuralgia, with local demyelination of the trigeminal nerve leading to aberrant activation and pain. Facial trauma similarly may result in axonal loss along the trigeminal nerve and lead to this syndrome. Tumors in the cerebellopontine angle, such as schwannomas or others, may cause local compression of the trigeminal nerve. Paraneoplastic disorders are highly unlikely to cause trigeminal neuralgia, with only two case reports to date (*see* Bradley's NiCP, 7th edn, Ch. 103, pp. 1686–1719).

TABLE FOR ANSWER 6.84 Physiological changes during wakefulness, NREM sleep, and REM sleep

Physiology	Wakefulness	NREM sleep	REM sleep
Parasympathetic activity	++	+++	++++
Sympathetic activity or variable (++)	++	+	Decreases
Heart rate	Normal sinus rhythm	Bradycardia	Brady/tachyarrhythmia
Blood pressure	Normal	Decreases	Variable
Cardiac output	Normal	Decreases	Decreases further
Peripheral vascular resistance	Normal	Normal or decreases slightly	Decreases further
Respiratory rate	Normal	Decreases	Variable; apneas may occur
Alveolar ventilation	Normal	Decreases	Decreases further
Upper airway muscle tone	++	+	Decreases or absent
Upper airway resistance	++	+++	++++
Hypoxic and hypercapnic ventilatory responses	Normal	Decreases	Decreases further
Cerebral blood flow	++	+	+++
Thermoregulation	++	+	–
Gastric acid secretion	Normal	Variable	Variable
Gastric motility	Normal	Decreases	Decreases
Swallowing	Normal	Decreases	Decreases
Salivary flow	Normal	Decreases	Decreases
Migrating motor complex (a special type of intestinal motor activity)	Normal	Slow velocity	Slow velocity
Penile or clitoral tumescence	Normal	Normal	Increases markedly

+, mild; ++, moderate; +++, marked; ++++, very marked; –, absent; *NREM*, non–rapid eye movement; *REM*, rapid eye movement.
From Daroff RB, Jankovic J, Mazziotta JC, Pomeroy SL 2016 Bradley's Neurology in Clinical Practice, *7th edn, Elsevier, with permission.*

86. C. The pathway of auditory signals from the cochlea to the final destination in the temporal lobe is as follows: cochlea, vestibular nerve, cochlear nucleus, superior olivary nucleus, inferior colliculus, medial geniculate nucleus of the thalamus, and radiations to the temporal lobe. The superior colliculus is involved in the visual pathway, not the auditory pathway (*see* Bradley's NiCP, 7th edn, Ch. 34, pp. 349–365).

87. E. The gag reflex involves the glossopharyngeal nerve for the afferent component and the vagus nerve for efferent. The corneal reflex is a consensual disynaptic reflex involving V1. The jaw jerk reflex is a monosynaptic myotatic reflex involving V3. The lacrimal reflex involves both V1 and the facial nerve. The oculocardiac reflex involves V1 and the vagus nerve (*see* Bradley's NiCP, 7th edn, Ch. 104, pp. 1720–1735).

88. D. Wave I of the brainstem auditory evoked potential is primarily generated by the cochlea. This wave should be present in all patients, unless they have ear canal blockage or damage to their middle or inner ear. Frequently during surgery the acoustic stimulators in the ear may be displaced with patient repositioning, causing a normal study to appear abnormal. In prolonged surgeries, anesthesia may also reduce this waveform. If there were a clinically significant event, such as an injury to the cochlear nerve or brainstem, wave I would be present, but there would be loss of all waves afterward, prolongation of the wave I–III latency, or prolongation of the wave III–V latency (*see* Bradley's NiCP, 7th edn, Ch. 34, pp. 348–365 and Ch. 38, pp. 407–410).

89. B. At 4 months, children should smile spontaneously; copy facial expressions; babble; cry in different ways to express hunger, pain, and tiredness; reach for a toy with one hand; use hands together; and watch faces closely. They should be able to hold the head upright unsupported, bring the hands to the mouth, shake toys, and push up to the elbows when lying on the stomach. At 2 months, children may coo or make gurgling sounds, may smile, pay attention to faces, and can hold the head up when on the tummy. They may not be able to support the head independently and will not follow objects at a distance. At 6 months, children will recognize familiar faces, respond to others' emotions, string vowels together when babbling, respond to their name, pass objects from hand to hand, and sit without support. At 9 months, children show fear of strangers, understand "no," copy sounds, point, play peek-a-boo, use pincer grasp, crawl, and pull to stand. At 1 year, a child will be nervous when away from parents or around strangers, play games like "peek-a-boo," use simple gestures to communicate, have very few words, can rise to a sitting position without help, and may stand alone or even walk (*see* Bradley's NiCP, 7th edn, Ch. 8, pp. 66–72).

90. D. This patient had Lafora body disease. This presents with a progressive myoclonic epilepsy with early dementia and refractory seizures. This comes from a mutation in laforin. Patients die within a few years of the onset of this disorder. The pathology slide shows intensely staining central bodies with a spiculated outline and surrounding zone of less intensely stained material (Lafora bodies). Juvenile myoclonic epilepsy does not cause dementia as was seen in this case. Myoclonic epilepsy with ragged red fibers has myoclonus, ataxia, generalized seizures, and a myopathy with predominant ragged red fibers. Mesial temporal sclerosis is not associated with myoclonus. CJD can present with myoclonus and frequent seizures in the setting of dementia. However, this biopsy does not show spongiform changes (*see* Bradley's NiCP, 7th edn, Ch. 101, pp. 1563–1614). Figure from Ellison D, Love S, Chimelli L, et al. 2013 *Neuropathology*, 3rd edn, Elsevier, with permission.

91. A. The Wechsler Intelligence Scale is the most commonly used test to determine one's intelligence quotient. The California Verbal Learning Test is a memory test. The Boston Naming Test is a test of language. The Trail-Making Test and the Wisconsin Card Sorting Test examine executive function.

92. D. The patient is most likely presenting with a viral encephalitis, such as herpes zoster, which has a particular predilection for mesial temporal lobe and insular involvement. Evidence pointing toward this diagnosis includes preceding malaise and fever, as well as lymphocytic pleocytosis and elevated protein and RBCs, but normal glucose in the cerebrospinal fluid. The scans of the abdomen and pelvis in the emergency room were red herrings, looking for systemic malignancy in case this was limbic encephalitis. Intravenous antiviral therapy is the best course of action for this patient. Antipsychotic therapy may be necessary in the course of his treatment if he demonstrates psychosis, but does not treat the underlying infection. Intravenous steroids also will not treat the underlying infection. MRI of the spine would be useful if staging a central nervous system (CNS) cancer, or if there were evidence of myelopathy to suggest multifocal CNS infection. Finally, testicular ultrasound would be important if paraneoplastic limbic encephalitis were at the top of the differential diagnosis (*see* Bradley's NiCP, 7th edn, Ch. 78, pp. 1121–1146). Figure from Rath TJ, Hughes M, Arabi M, Shah GV 2012 Imaging of cerebritis, encephalitis, and brain abscess. *Neuroimaging Clinics of North America* 22(4): 585–607, with permission.

93. B. The child described in the question has Hurler syndrome, also known as *mucopolysaccharidosis type 1* (MPS I), which is an autosomal-recessive disease causing a deficiency in alpha-L iduronidase and resultant accumulation of glycosaminoglycans. This disease may be treated with bone marrow transplantation or with enzyme replacement. Ornithine transcarbamoylase (OTC) deficiency is an X-linked recessive disease and the most common deficiency in the urea cycle. Symptoms usually begin in the first few days of life, and include progressive irritability, lethargy, and metabolic encephalopathy from hyperammonemia. Therapy for OTC deficiency includes low-protein diet, nitrogen-scavenging agents like sodium benzoate, and supplementation of arginine. Iduronate sulfatase deficiency is seen in the X-linked recessive Hunter syndrome, which leads to an accumulation of heparin sulfate and dermatan sulfate. Although Hunter syndrome is clinically similar to Hurler syndrome, two key differences include the pattern of inheritance and the presence of corneal clouding in Hurler syndrome. Heparan sulfamidase deficiency is the cause of autosomal-recessive Sanfilippo syndrome (MPS III). Children with Sanfilippo syndrome generally have coarse facial features and developmental delay, but with marked behavioral disturbance, including aggressive behavior,

destructiveness, and hyperactivity. Additionally, Sanfilippo syndrome commonly presents with severe sleep disturbance, which is a significant challenge for parents, given their children's aggressive behavior, even at night. Fumarase deficiency, an autosomal-recessive disorder of the Krebs cycle, is generally apparent during pregnancy with polyhydramnios, and then in the newborn period with poor feeding and hypotonia and radiographic findings of lissencephaly and pachygyria. Then, infants develop encephalopathy without reaching developmental milestones, blindness due to optic atrophy, and seizures (*see* Bradley's NiCP, 7th edn, Ch. 91, pp. 1324–1341). Figure from Nannini V 2014 Metabolic and autoimmune syndromes. *Atlas of the Oral and Maxillofacial Surgery Clinics of North America* 22(2): 123–134, with permission.

94. E. The case describes an 18-month-old with history of full-term birth but an eventful delivery with poor Apgar scores due to a nuchal cord. The patient now presents with delayed motor milestones, including delayed ambulation, and spastic paraparesis. These symptoms are most consistent with a diagnosis of cerebral palsy (CP), spastic diplegia. The etiology of his CP was likely hypoxic-ischemic injury from his nuchal chord, which would generally be seen as encephalomalacia on an MRI of the brain. CP is a static neurological deficit, with neither regression nor progression over time. Patients with CP may present with abnormal muscle tone (initially hypotonia followed by spasticity), early hand preference before 1 year of age, asymmetric crawling, failure to thrive, or abnormal gait. Seizures and cognitive delay, especially mental retardation, are also common. CP is generally classified by the involved limbs and muscle tone, including spastic diplegia, spastic hemiplegia, spastic quadriplegia, choreoathetoid CP, mixed CP, and hypotonic truncal or extremity CP. Treatment is supportive and often includes physical and occupational therapy, cognitive therapy, muscle relaxants, botulinum toxin injections for the motor symptoms, and antiepileptics for seizures (*see* Bradley's NiCP, 7th edn, Ch. 90, pp. 1301–1323).

95. C. Physicians serving at sporting events have an ethical obligation to protect the patient's health despite pleas from coaches, parents, and patients. With regard to this patient, most would recommend the patient refraining from physical activity for the rest of the day, or possibly the next week, to prevent a devastating second injury. Any return to activity, even noncontact play without rest, could place the patient at risk of a second injury. There is nothing in the question to suggest the patient needs to be transferred to the emergency department.

96. B. Bacterial abscess is the most likely scenario based on his immunosuppressed state and the enhancing mass on MRI. The photomicrograph demonstrates inflammatory infiltrate with a colony of gram-positive cocci. Encephalopathy is not associated with focal abnormalities in the brain. Although surgical debris may cause similar problems, it does not account for the bacteria shown on the photomicrograph. Shunt malformation would not cause a focal lesion in the brain. Fungal infection is also a possibility, but not compatible with the photomicrograph (*see* Bradley's NiCP, 7th edn, Ch. 79, pp. 1147–1158). Figure from Camelo-Piragua S, Hedley-White ET 2010 Infections of the Nervous System. In: Kradkin RL (ed.) *Diagnostic Pathology of Infectious Disease*, pp. 483–518, Elsevier, with permission.

97. E. The constellation of hypoglycemia, hepatomegaly, jaundice, cataracts, and *E. coli* septicemia are classic for a diagnosis of galactosemia. This is one of the most common disorders of carbohydrate metabolism. It is an autosomal-recessive deficiency of GALT function, which leads to an elevation of galactose. Other clinical manifestations not included in the question include poor feeding, diarrhea, and vomiting, which are often prominent in children with galactosemia. The diagnosis is usually made on a newborn screen, but may also be made by identification of hypoglycemia and galactosuria. Removal of lactose and galactose from the diet leads to resolution of clinical features and can potentially prevent neurological deficits (*see* Bradley's NiCP, 7th edn, Ch. 91, pp. 1324–1341).

98. D. Pupillary light response may help localize a coma-inducing lesion. Midbrain tegmental injury is associated with fixed midposition pupils. Pontine lesions are associated with fixed pinpoint pupils. Global cerebral injury, as in diffuse anoxic injury or toxic/metabolic injury, tends to cause small but reactive pupils. Diencephalic injury similarly leads to small but reactive pupils. Injury to the oculomotor nuclei, especially in the case of uncal herniation and compression, causes a fixed and dilated ipsilateral pupil (*see* Bradley's NiCP, 7th edn, Ch. 5, pp. 34–50).

99. B. Opioid withdrawal presents with lacrimation, rhinorrhea, nausea, abdominal cramps, diarrhea, and irritability. Opioid withdrawal is not life threatening, but is very uncomfortable. Opioid use causes pinpoint pupils, whereas withdrawal causes dilated pupils. Amitriptyline use has several side effects, including depression; QT prolongation; and anticholinergic effects like dry eyes, dry mouth, and constipation, but does not generally affect pupils. Topiramate can cause metabolic acidosis or nephrolithiasis, but has no effect on pupils. Alcohol withdrawal involves tachycardia, tremor, hypertension, encephalopathy, autonomic dysfunction, and potentially seizures. Propranolol withdrawal could cause rebound tachycardia and hypertension (*see* Bradley's NiCP, 7th edn, Ch. 87, pp. 1254–1260).

100. A. Azathioprine is a prodrug for mercaptopurine, a purine analog that inhibits DNA synthesis. This most strongly affects lymphocytes, given their rapid division. Cyclophosphamide is a nitrogen mustard alkylating agent that leads to DNA crosslinking and disruption of cellular replication. It also strongly inhibits lymphocytes. Cyclosporine specifically depletes T-cells by interfering with their production of interleukins and downstream activation. Rituximab is a monoclonal antibody against CD20 that specifically depletes B-cells. Methotrexate is thought to work by two mechanisms: in autoimmune disorders, it inhibits purine metabolism and T-cell activation, and in cancers (e.g. primary central nervous system lymphoma), it competitively inhibits dihydrofolate reductase (*see* Bradley's NiCP, 7th edn, Ch. 109, pp. 1896–1914).

101. D. Hypokalemic periodic paralysis.

102. E. Myotonia congenita.

103. B. Familial hemiplegic migraine.

104. A. Hereditary hyperekplexia.

105. C. Episodic ataxia type 1.

Index

Page numbers followed by "*f*" indicate figures, and "*t*" indicate tables.